T0144608

Translating Biomaterials for Bone Graft

Bench-top to Clinical Applications

Edited by
Joo L. Ong • Teja Guda

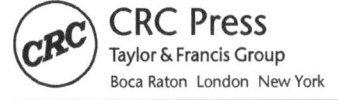

CRC Press
Taylor & Francis Group
Boca Raton London New York

CRC Press is an imprint of the
Taylor & Francis Group, an **informa** business

CRC Press
Taylor & Francis Group
6000 Broken Sound Parkway NW, Suite 300
Boca Raton, FL 33487-2742

First issued in paperback 2020

© 2017 by Taylor & Francis Group, LLC
CRC Press is an imprint of Taylor & Francis Group, an Informa business

No claim to original U.S. Government works

ISBN-13: 978-1-4665-9862-1 (hbk)
ISBN-13: 978-0-367-65824-3 (pbk)

Visit the Taylor & Francis Web site at
http://www.taylorandfrancis.com

and the CRC Press Web site at
http://www.crcpress.com

Contents

Part IV   Clinical Considerations

Part V   Translational Pathways for Bone Graft Development

Preface

Bone grafts meet the continually increasing therapeutic demand to heal large and small defects in bone tissue and restore patients to a better quality-of-life. This edited book is designed to present the current translational research in the field of bone tissue engineering, from bench top designs to clinical applications. All stages of the therapy development pipeline ranging from materials, drugs, and biologic delivery used for bone graft applications to preclinical and clinical considerations as well as the current translational pathways for bone graft development are discussed. The chapters are written by basic materials scientists, clinicians, and researchers and consultants in the medical device industry in order to provide a holistic understanding of the field. As such, this book is intended for use as a reference of the state-of-the-art in current technologies and/or clinical practices related to bone therapy and should be of interest to clinicians, scientists, and students interested in the current research and/or practices in the field of bone regeneration and restoration.

The book delves into the ongoing transition within the field of bone tissue engineering, beginning with the development of various classes of novel biomaterials and transitioning to more mature combinatorial therapies in the later chapters. These include not only synthetic grafts, but also the controlled release of drugs and growth factors or the incorporation of biologics and stem cells, all targeted at accelerating healing. The long-term patency of tissue engineered graft substitutes is highly dependent not only on the ability to integrate with native bone, but also on the infiltration of host vasculature. The specific needs for bone graft functionality vary based not only on whether the deficit sites are located in the extremities, the spine, or the craniofacial skeleton, but also on the nature of the defect's etiology: whether it originated due to tissue trauma, congenital defects, or as a result of cancerous resection. The incorporation of antibiotics is often required to avoid further complications of infection that would result in graft failure. Specific targeted applications require equally specialized preclinical models for effective evaluation of both native biology as well as functional restoration. Finally, the book discusses the regulatory approval pathways for bone graft development and translation into clinical use, which involves consideration of the class of devices: whether they are similar to existing solutions, involve minimal manipulation of donor tissue, or are completely novel materials, drugs, and biologics. These considerations drive the ability to successfully transition the latest generations of bone graft materials into clinics.

Joo L. Ong, Ph.D.

Teja Guda, Ph.D.

About the Editors

Joo L. Ong is the Associate Dean for Administration for the College of Engineering at the University of Texas at San Antonio (UTSA). He is also the USAA Foundation Distinguished Professor of Biomedical Engineering at UTSA. His research focuses on modification and characterization of biomaterial surfaces of dental and orthopedic implants, use of ceramic and composite scaffolds for bone regeneration, and protein–biomaterials and bone–biomaterials interactions. He is a Fellow of the American Institute for Medical and Biological Engineering.

Teja Guda is an Assistant Professor of Biomedical Engineering at the University of Texas at San Antonio (UTSA). He is also Assistant Director of the Center for Innovation, Technology and Entrepreneurship at UTSA. His research focuses on the development of biomaterials for musculoskeletal tissue engineering, the biomechanical stimulation and characterization of orthopedic tissues, and the nondestructive characterization of porous material architectures.

Contributors

L. Actis
Department of Biomedical
  Engineering
University of Texas at San Antonio
San Antonio, Texas

Kazuhisa Bessho
Department of Oral and
  Maxillofacial Surgery
Graduate School of Medicine
Kyoto University
Kyoto, Japan

Joel D. Bumgardner
Department of Biomedical
  Engineering
University of Memphis
Memphis, Tennessee

David L. Carnes, Jr.
Department of Periodontics
University of Texas Health Science
  Center at San Antonio
San Antonio, Texas

Laura Gaviria
Department of Biomedical
  Engineering
University of Texas at San Antonio
San Antonio, Texas

Teja Guda
Department of Biomedical
  Engineering
University of Texas at San Antonio
San Antonio, Texas

Scott A. Guelcher
Department of Chemical and
  Biomolecular Engineering

Vanderbilt University
Nashville, Tennessee

Warren O. Haggard
Department of Biomedical
  Engineering
University of Memphis
Memphis, Tennessee

Su-Gwan Kim
Department of Oral and
  Maxillofacial Surgery
School of Dentistry
Chosun University
Gwangju, South Korea

Jennifer S. McDaniel
Extremity Trauma and Regenerative
  Medicine Task Area
U.S. Army Institute of Surgical
  Research
Fort Sam Houston
San Antonio, Texas

Antonios G. Mikos
Department of Bioengineering
Rice University
Houston, Texas

Sergio A. Montelongo
Department of Biomedical
  Engineering
University of Texas at San Antonio
San Antonio, Texas

Shantikumar V. Nair
Amrita Centre for Nanosciences
Amrita Institute of Medical Sciences
  and Research Centre

Amrita Vishwa Vidyapeetham
  University
Kochi, India

Ji-Su Oh
Department of Oral and
  Maxillofacial Surgery
School of Dentistry
Chosun University
Gwangju, South Korea

Joo Ong
Department of Biomedical
  Engineering
University of Texas at San Antonio
San Antonio, Texas

Joshua A. Parry
Department of Orthopedic Surgery
  and Biomedical Engineering
Mayo Clinic
Rochester, Minnesota

Joseph J. Pearson
Department of Biomedical
  Engineering
University of Texas at San Antonio
San Antonio, Texas

Marcello Pilia
Extremity Trauma and Regenerative
  Medicine Task Area
U.S. Army Institute of Surgical
  Research
Fort Sam Houston
San Antonio, Texas

James W. Poser
JW Poser & Associates L.L.C.
San Antonio, Texas

Christopher R. Rathbone
Extremity Trauma and Regenerative
  Medicine Task Area
U.S. Army Institute of Surgical
  Research

Fort Sam Houston
San Antonio, Texas

Binulal N. Sathy
Amrita Centre for Nanosciences
Amrita Institute of Medical Sciences
  and Research Centre
Amrita Vishwa Vidyapeetham
  University
Kochi, India

Sarita R. Shah
Department of Bioengineering
Rice University
Houston, Texas

Junya Sonobe
Department of Oral and
  Maxillofacial Surgery
Graduate School of Medicine
Kyoto University
Kyoto, Japan

Larry D. Swain
Department of Biomedical
  Engineering
University of Texas at San Antonio
San Antonio, Texas

Patsy J. Trisler
Trisler Consulting
Chevy Chase, Maryland

Carlos M. Wells
Department of Biomedical
  Engineering
University of Memphis
Memphis, Tennessee

Michael J. Yaszemski
Department of Orthopedic Surgery
  and Biomedical Engineering
Mayo Clinic
Rochester, Minnesota

Part I

Introduction

1

Bone Grafting Evolution

Laura Gaviria, L. Actis, Teja Guda, and Joo Ong

CONTENTS

1.1 Introduction and Clinical Need

Bone is a dynamic and highly vascularized tissue that provides structural support to the body by carrying major biomechanical loads and playing many roles which are essential for the body. The skeleton protects internal organs, supports muscular contraction to create motion, and acts as a stored mineral reservoir that is capable of rapid mobilization on metabolic demand.[1,2] Therefore, it is reasonable to conclude that major alterations in bone's structure dramatically affect a patient's health and quality of life.[1]

All these functions have made bone the ultimate smart composite material, by which most of its outstanding properties are related to its dual composition: a mineralized inorganic component and a non-mineralized or organic component. The mineral component comprises about 65–70% of the bone matrix and is primarily made up of biological apatites. Representing the non-mineralized or organic component is mainly type I collagen. Several different types of proteins such as glycoproteins, proteoglycans and sialo-proteins are also present in the non-mineralized component.[1–3] This composite structure of tough and flexible collagen fibers reinforced by biological apatite is integral to achieve the characteristic compressive strength and high fracture toughness of bone.[2]

In general, bone has a unique regenerative capacity to heal and remodel following trauma or disease without any surgical intervention and without leaving a scar, which is especially true in younger people.[1–4] However, in the case of extensive tissue damage (caused by a high-energy traumatic event, large bone resection for pathologies such as tumor or infection, or severe nonunion fractures), bone defects are unable to heal without intervention.[2–5] Furthermore, musculoskeletal disorders and diseases are the second greatest cause of disability globally[6] and are the leading cause of disability in people older than 50 years of age in the United States. The number of patients with chronic musculoskeletal diseases are 60% greater than that of the number of patients with chronic circulatory diseases and more than twice that of number of patients with all chronic respiratory diseases. Unfortunately, the cost for treating musculoskeletal diseases are also associated with many direct and indirect expenditures, and these expenditures are predicted to continue growing in the next 25 years as the worldwide population rapidly ages.[1,7] In 2006 alone, the sum of the direct and indirect expenditures related to musculoskeletal diseases was estimated to be about 7.4% of the US gross domestic product.[7–9]

With this motivation, many bone regeneration strategies have been investigated in order to improve the patient's quality of life and to minimize the medical and socioeconomic challenges associated with bone damage.[2,3,8] Significant bone defects require the use of bone grafts in order to fuse joints, prevent movement in the spine and extremities, repair bone in delayed unions or nonunions, repair fractures with significant bone loss, and repair bone voids caused by surgery, traumatic disease or infection.[5,10]

1.2 Past and Present of Bone Grafting in Orthopedic Surgery

Orthopedic techniques and bone grafting have been practiced for thousands of years.[11] Some first evidence on the use of bone graft substitutes has been found in prehistoric skulls with metal plates and coconut shells in the sites of cranial defects.[12] In fact, some of them have shown evidence of xenografts with regrowth around the grafted bone.[11]

The Egyptians were also advanced in dental and bone surgery; mummies from 656–525 BC showed evidence of orthopedic operations and prostheses that were inserted while the patients were still alive. Further analysis indicated that the prostheses and artificial limbs were made out of iron, resins and wood. Although simple in design, these solutions were efficacious and allowed the patients to live for many years after the operation. Similarly, Aztec skulls with metal plates have been found, as well as ancient documents that described the treatment of bone fractures by realigning and splinting, in addition to placing of wooden prostheses in the case of failure. Later, during 300–200 BC, ancient Greeks from the Alexandrian school studied surgery extensively and performed difficult operations such as limbs amputation and tumor resection.[11]

Modern attempts of bone grafting started in 1668 when Job van Meekeren, a Dutch surgeon, documented the filling of a bony defect in a soldier's cranium with a piece of skull from a dog. The surgery was successful, but the patient was excommunicated by his church because of the use of xenotransplant.[11,13,14] In order to be allowed back to his church, the patient requested that the bone graft be removed 2 years after implantation. Later, in 1820, Philips von Walter, a German surgeon, performed the first autologous graft by replacing a fragment of the cranium after trepanation.[11] Other examples of autografts documented in the late 1800s include the use of tibial periosteal flaps by Dr. Seydel to close a cranial defect and the use of a fibular graft by Dr. Bergmann to close a tibial defect.[12]

One of the most important contributions during the nineteenth century was made in 1861 by Leopold Ollier, a French surgeon, who studied the phenomenon of bone regeneration and described the term "bone graft" for the first time. Most importantly, Ollier postulated his theories on the possibility to regenerate bone by inducing cartilage to ossify.[11,15] By that time, most popular grafts were of autologous origin, and non-autologous grafts were not taken into consideration until 1880 when William Macewen, a Scottish surgeon, implanted a tibial allograft from one child to another.[11] In February 1891, Dr. A.M. Phelps of New York reported the successful insertion of a piece of bone from a dog into the tibial defect of a boy.[11,12,15]

Between 1912 and 1940, an Italian surgeon by the name of Vittorio Putti did research in all the major orthopedic problems and introduced new methods and surgical instruments for the improvement of graft integration.[11,16] With more than 1600 autograft procedures documented by the early 1920s, modern tools of internal and external fixation were not yet available then and the role of vascularization in the repair process was still not clear, adding to the number of limitations and failures.[11,12] Between 1915 and 1932, Fred Houdlett Albee, an American surgeon, introduced a series of rules and principles for using bone grafts and published articles describing the 810 successful operations performed on nonunions of the limbs using autografts. By 1942, many autologous and homologous transplants had been already performed, and the fundamental concepts about immune response and storage of bone material were already known.[11] These new concepts established the beginning of a new era in bone grafting.

1.3 Recent Progress in Bone Grafting

1.3.1 Autologous Bone Grafts

Harvested from the patient itself, autografts has been established as the gold standard for bone grafting for many decades, offering structural support with no potential for disease transmissions or immunogenic responses.[17] The most common harvesting sites for autogenous cancellous bone grafts are the iliac crest, the humeral greater tubercule and the greater trochanter of femur. For cortical bone autografts, harvesting sites are the fibula, rib, distal ulna and iliac wing.[15,18]

Autografts have shown good results in bone formation, mainly because the presence of osteoblasts provides direct osteogenesis, the availability of bone matrix allows for osteoconduction, and the presence of osteoinductive growth factors improves healing and regeneration.[1,15,18] Nonetheless, their structures can be altered during the transportation process, and cells inside the autografts will not survive more than 2 hours.[19] Additionally, an additional surgical site is required to harvest the limited graft material.[1,10,12,17] Other complications for the patient include donor site morbidity as a result of blood loss, hematoma and arterial injury, nerve injury and numbness, hernia formation, fracture and pelvic instability, cosmetic defects, chronic pain and infection.[10,12,18,20]

1.3.2 Allogenic Bone Grafts

Allografts come mainly from two different sources of bone: (1) bone from living donors, and (2) multi-organ donors.[19] Prior to the 1980s, allografts were the second most important alternative for bone repair and were primarily used as substitutes for autografts in large defect sites. Yet by 2006, at least one-third of all bone grafts used in North America were allografts,[12,13,19,21] accounting for about 300,000 implanted grafts worldwide every year.[19]

Allografts have become very popular due to their osteoconductive properties and their availability in various shapes and sizes without sacrificing host structures or leading to donor-site morbidity.[17] Unfortunately, the major concern with allografts is that they carry the risk for disease transmission and immune rejection.[1,15,19] It is also known that some tissue processing techniques that seek to eliminate the risk of disease transmission can alter the graft's biomechanical and biochemical properties.[10,13,17]

1.3.3 Allograft-Based Alternatives

With the motivation to replace autografts and allografts, other allograft- and cell-based solutions for bone repair have been investigated. Demineralized bone matrix (DBM) is an allograft-based alternative consisting of cortical bone that has been demineralized via acid extraction, leaving behind collagenous and non-collagenous proteins and a low concentration of growth factors.[10] Since its antigenic surface is destroyed during demineralization, DBM does not evoke any appreciable local foreign-body immunogenic reactions.[19] DBM became very popular in the first decade of the twenty-first century because of its osteoinductive properties. However, its ability to produce bone can be affected by the processing, storage and sterilization methods used, and these methods can vary from product to product.[10,21]

Another allograft-based alternative is the use of bone marrow aspirate, which can either be used alone or in conjunction with other graft substitutes. Bone marrow aspirate represents a good source of osteogenic precursor cells with the potential to differentiate into osteoblasts capable of producing new bone tissue. However, besides being a very invasive procedure, the major drawback of this technique is that it might be difficult to obtain enough bone marrow with a sufficient number of osteoprogenitor cells necessary for bone healing.[10,22]

The use of platelet-rich plasma (PRP) is another allograft-based alternative. The PRP is derived from the patient's own plasma and has been mechanically treated to increase the concentration of platelets compared to whole blood. The higher concentration of platelets provides a locally increased concentration of growth factors and cytokines that are contained within the platelets themselves. Examples of commonly used growth factors are nerve growth factor, platelet-derived growth factor, epidermal growth factor, fibroblast growth factor-2, vascular endothelial growth factor and transforming growth factor-β. These growth factors have been found to stimulate the proliferation of osteoblast progenitors, increase type I collagen synthesis, and enhance angiogenesis as well as vascularization.[10,23,24] Many studies have supported the use of PRP for regenerative treatments, especially as pre- and post-operative support for augmentation of bone grafts. However, current literature on the use of PRP is inconclusive regarding standardization of study protocols, processing techniques and outcome measures.[23,25–27]

1.3.4 Synthetic Materials

To replace autogenous and allogenic bone grafts, several synthetic materials have been utilized, especially in the last 2 decades, either as bone graft substitutes or internal fixation devices.[2,12] More recently, between 2004 and 2010, the use of bone substitutes became more popular as the use of allografts diminished substantially and the efforts towards the development of graft alternatives increased.[21] Subsequent sections below discuss the different groups of synthetic biomaterials that can be used as bone graft substitutes.

1.3.4.1 Ceramics

Ceramics, especially bioactive ceramics, have been widely used in the biomedical engineering and bone substitution/regeneration field because of their similarity in composition to the mineral phase of bone.[2,10] These ceramics allow osteoblast cells to attach, proliferate and differentiate. Not surprisingly, the major attraction towards these ceramics is their possession of osteoconductive and/or osteoinductive properties.[28] These materials can be designed with specific resorption rates and can be tailored to deliver ions capable of activating signaling pathways involved in cell differentiation and osteogenesis.[2,10,28] Among the many bioactive ceramics, tricalcium phosphate (TCP), hydroxyapatite (HA), calcium sulfates, bioactive glasses and their combinations are the ceramics of clinical interest.[2,12] These ceramics are available in granular, bulk, or paste forms and are present as a porous or solid material.[1,10,29,30] However, due to their brittle nature, bioactive ceramics possess low mechanical stability and thus cannot be used for load-bearing, large bone defect applications.[1,2,31,32] Furthermore, due to the osteoclastic activity of bone, the dissolution rates of bioactive ceramics can be hard to predict and control. The inability to control degradation is problematic since the mechanical stability of the ceramic construct or scaffold could be compromised if it degrades too rapidly. A rapid degradation of the calcium phosphate scaffold or construct could also induce a dramatic increase in the concentration of extracellular calcium and phosphate ions which may be cytotoxic.[1,29,30,33]

In addition to the granular or powder form, bioactive ceramics can also be fabricated as injectables. For example, calcium phosphate cements (CPCs) are an interesting evolution of calcium phosphates ceramics that have been fabricated as injectable cements. These injectable cements are formed when a dry calcium phosphate powder reacts with a liquid component (i.e., an inorganic or organic acid, or sodium phosphate solutions) under physiologic pH and temperatures. The major attractiveness of these pastes or cements is their versatility in terms of degradation and manageability.[34,35] In the clinics, CPCs allow the surgeon to easily fill irregular defects and shape the material during surgery in order to achieve reasonable aesthetic contours. Recently, these injectable cements have also been used as drug delivery systems.[36] Nonetheless, CPCs have the potential risk of paste extruding into the surrounding tissues. Additionally, the CPCs also have many problems associated with the rate of degradation and mechanical stability.[10,29,30,33]

1.3.4.2 Polymers

Representing different physical, mechanical and chemical properties, there are many polymers that are potential candidates for bone graft substitutes. These polymers can be loosely divided into natural polymers and synthetic polymers. Synthetic polymers can be further divided into degradable and nondegradable polymers.[12]

Natural polymers, such as collagen and hyaluronic acid, are interesting candidates for tissue engineering since they provide innate biological informational guidance to cells favoring cell attachment and promoting chemotactic responses. In addition to low cost, natural polymers are biodegradable and possess high renewability potential. However, concerns with the use of natural polymers include immunogenicity, potential risk of disease transmission, sourcing and poor handling, and weak mechanical properties. To overcome these drawbacks, resorbable synthetic polymers with predictable and reproducible properties were developed.[37]

Unlike natural polymers, not all synthetic polymers are degradable. Examples of degradable synthetic polymers include polylactic acid (PLA), polyglycolic acid (PGA), copolymers of PLA and PGA (PLGA) and polycaprolactone. These degradable synthetic polymers offer a versatile alternative since they are biocompatible, and properties such as rate of degradation, pore size, porosity, interconnectivity and hydrophobicity/hydrophilicity can be tailored depending on their applications. In addition, their ability for cell attachment and morphology can be easily manipulated through surface modifications.[30,33,38] Other synthetic polymers such as polyethylene glycol or alginate-based materials are also popular for use as biomaterials since they can often be delivered in a minimally invasive manner and gel in situ (e.g., photocrosslinked or ionically) to provide a three-dimensional cellular microenvironment with high water content.[2,31] Despite their advantageous properties, these polymers do not possess osteogenic, osteoconductive or osteoinductive properties, do not offer mechanical stability, and can cause inflammatory reactions due to their degradation by-products.[30,33]

1.3.4.3 Composite Materials

Composite materials are materials consisting of two or more different components at a micro or macro size range having a distinct interface separating them. The advantage of using composite materials is their ability to combine the best properties of both components in terms of biomechanical properties, biological properties and degradation profiles. At present, composites used in bone repairs use particle- or fiber-reinforced combinations of metals and ceramics or ceramics and polymers. The inspiration for the development of composite materials is bone itself, which is a natural composite.[2,12,39,40]

1.4 Clinical Need for Engineered Bone

There are three primary reasons to develop bone tissue engineering alternatives. First, although bone has an inherent ability to regenerate, there is a need of bone grafts in cases such as excessive bone loss. Second, there is a need for better materials that can be used in the reconstruction of large bony defects.[1–3,31,41] Although autologous bone graft is known to be the "gold standard" for bone repair,[31,43] it cannot be used in cases that involve large bone loss or large bone defects due to the limited graft materials that can be harvested. Like autologous bone grafts, there are a limited number of donors for allogenic bone grafts and thus they can not satisfy the clinical demand[31,44] for graft materials. Additionally, allogeneic bone grafts carry the potential risks of pathogen transmission and immune rejection. A final reason for developing bone tissue engineering alternatives is the need to cover the growing demand for bone graft materials. Additionally, the drive to develop synthetic bone grafts is not only to fill gaps in demand, but also to improve functionality and move toward the development of improved bone graft materials.[3] Of the 3 million musculoskeletal procedures performed annually in the United States, it has been estimated that about half of them require the use of bone graft in order to achieve union. Worldwide, approximately 2.2 million bone graft procedures are performed each year to repair bone defects, and these procedures equate to a yearly estimated cost of $2.5 billion.[40,42] The demand for bone graft materials is predicted to continue growing on a global basis, along with the shortage in the availability of musculoskeletal donor tissues traditionally used in bone reconstructions. It is no surprise that researchers and biomaterials companies are getting more and more interested in the market for bone graft substitutes, which is growing at a rapid rate.[1,13,15,17,31]

A major research focus has been integrating bone graft materials with biomolecules, cells and/or antibiotics in order to promote and enhance functional tissue regeneration.[2,45,46] Over the past few decades, great progress in the development of engineered bone has been achieved. In particular, major efforts have been undertaken in the research of biocompatible and biodegradable scaffolds, cell sources, identification of growth factors to induce endogenous osteogenesis and angiogenesis, and bioreactors to enhance in vitro osteogenic priming. Although numerous preclinical trials have produced optimistic results, the lack of translation for clinical use suggests that significant issues remain and that there is still a real need for developing better solutions for bone grafting.[31,47]

1.5 Overview of Bone Tissue Engineering Field

The term "tissue engineering" was defined in 1993 by Langer and Vacanti as "an interdisciplinary field of research that applies the principles of engineering and the life sciences towards the development of biological substitutes that restore, maintain, or improve tissue function."[48] This approach aims to induce the formation of new functional tissues through the understanding of tissue formation and regeneration by integrating knowledge in physics, chemistry, engineering, materials science, biology and medicine. From the biological perspective, new bone growth requires the availability of cells, extracellular matrix, intercellular communications, cell-matrix interactions and growth factors.[49] However, in bone tissue engineering, these factors alone cannot create new bone. Cells do not grow in a three-dimensional (3D) fashion in vitro, and this thus requires the use of a 3D construct or scaffold to mimic bone structures for new 3D bony tissue formation.[50] Additionally, all of these single-cell components must be well-coordinated spatially and combined in a time-dependent fashion in order to achieve a successful result.[1,31,51] Researchers have given the greatest attention to the synergistic combination of cell therapy and biomaterials to achieve this goal.[2]

1.5.1 Requirements and Properties and Biomaterial Design

The diamond concept, proposed by Giannoudis, describes the following four elements necessary for bone formation: (1) osteoconductive scaffolds, (2) osteogenic cells, (3) growth factors and (4) mechanical stability.[19,52–54] Therefore, modern approaches use these elements as combinatorial therapies for bone repair.[1]

Apart from the mechanical properties, biomaterials used for the fabrication of bone scaffolds should be biocompatible, bioresorbable, osteogenic, osteoconductive, osteoinductive, structurally similar to bone, easy to use and manufacture and cost-effective.[1,10,17,39] Chemical and biomechanical properties, as well as morphology and degradation kinetics, should be also considered in the scaffold design. In terms of macro- and microstructural properties, the scaffold should possess a porous interconnected pore network with surfaces optimized for cellular attachment, migration, proliferation, differentiation and survival as well as to enable the transport of nutrients and metabolic waste.[1] The degree of interconnecting pores and their interconnecting characteristics are crucial to facilitate neovascularization and capillary ingrowth. However, the degree of porosity can influence other properties of the scaffold such as its mechanical stability. As such, the mechanical needs of the particular regenerated tissue must be taken into consideration.[28] Moreover, the initial mechanical strength of the scaffold must be sufficient to account for the loss of mechanical function of the tissue and to allow the implant to survive the mechanical stress of the environment.[1,3,31]

Scaffolds must also have a controllable rate of degradation that is complimentary to cell/tissue growth and maturation.[1,3,31] It is ideal that the degradation by-products be non-cytotoxic, non-hemolytic and non-inflammatory,[42] and that undesirable responses such as irritation, sensitization and fibrous tissue formation be avoided.[51] Recent research focus has also included the development of scaffolds with antibacterial properties and modified surfaces.[1,51]

Finally, biomaterials used in the development of 3D scaffolds must satisfy both commercial requirements and clinical needs. As such, the biomaterials used must be scalable to allow for cost-effective manufacture since low-income and middle-income countries carry 80% of the worldwide disease burden.[51] Additionally, since most biomaterials alone show limitations in terms of biological and biomechanical properties, researchers are currently relying on various composite materials as well as diverse fabrication methods in order to achieve optimized performance in bone tissue engineering applications.[31]

1.5.2 Incorporation of Cells

A fundamental concept in tissue engineering is combining the scaffold with living cells and/or biologically active molecules to form a "tissue-engineered construct" (TEC) that will promote repair and/or tissue regeneration.[1] Although some scaffold materials have been shown to induce bone formation without prior cell implantation, it has been suggested that large bone defects may require the implantation of cells to promote bone healing and regeneration.[1,12]

Because of their non-immunogenicity, the first choice of cells is osteoblasts. Autologous osteoblasts can be isolated from biopsies and then expanded in vitro. Unfortunately, this methodology is very time consuming, given the low number of cells that can be obtained and the relatively low expansion rates. Furthermore, in certain bone-related diseases, osteoblasts may not be an appropriate cell choice for transplantation because of their lower than expected protein expression profile.[1,49] As an alternative to autologous cells, the use of cells obtained from non-human donors (xenogeneic cells) has been proposed.[1] However, the immunogenicity of these cells and the possibility of transmission of infectious agents have made this technique unattractive.[1]

Over the last few decades, stem cells have emerged as one of the key players in tissue engineering, and several studies have been conducted to compare the different cell sources. Adult bone marrow and adipose cells can be easily obtained and they have medium osteogenic and mineral deposition capacity. However, since their proliferation rates are low, these cell lines have been found to have limited efficiency. Cells from the periosteum and cord blood or embryonic and fetal bone marrow stem cells all have higher proliferation rates and osteogenic and mineral deposition capacity. However, some disadvantages of stem cells in general are related to the form, quantity and ease in which they can be obtained.[31]

1.5.3 Growth Factors and Surface Modification

Many inductive molecules and chemoattractants in bone regulate cellular activity by binding to receptors on cell surfaces to stimulate the intracellular environment. These molecules can be delivered locally from scaffolds in order to control production and resorption of bone as well as to produce angiogenesis.[1,12,15,17]

In past years, isolation and synthetic production of growth factors have allowed for the examination of the function of a single factor as well as multiple factors. The promoting signaling molecules can be categorized into the following three groups: (1) pro-inflammatory cytokines, (2) TGF-β superfamily and other growth factors, and (3) angiogenic factors.[55] The ability to isolate and synthesize growth factors from bone has created many possibilities in the bone engineering field.[12,56] Other molecules can also be incorporated into scaffolds in order to generate appropriate osteo-inductive cues for attracting a patient's own stem cells.[2,51] Additionally, topographic cues such as grooves, ridges, wells and other features at the micron scale and, more recently, the nanoscale can influence cell behavior from cell adhesion to modulation of the intracellular signaling pathways that regulate transcriptional activity and gene expression.[57] Modification of biomaterials can take on different levels of complexity, from relatively simple changes in the hydrophilicity of the material to functionalization with charged groups, peptides or proteins. The arginine-glycine-aspartic acid (RGD) tripeptide motif and lysine-arginine-serine-arginine (KRSR) motif are perhaps the most commonly adopted surface modification strategies to enhance functionality. RGD is present on many ECM proteins including collagen type I, fibronectin, vitronectin, bone salio-protein and osteopontin and can have an impact on osteoblast adhesion, migration, gene and protein expression and mineralization. KRSR binds to transmembrane proteoglycans and could improve cell attachment and spreading.[2,57,58]

1.5.4 The Need for Vascularization

Currently, the attention on tissue engineering has gradually shifted to strategies for improving vascular formation. Having a network of blood vessels within a tissue-engineered graft is important for maintaining cellular survival and hence bone repair. However, this strategy still represents a big challenge in tissue engineering with a bright future for clinical applications.[31,59] At present, several strategies for improving vascularization in tissue engineered grafts are under investigation, including the induction of vascularization in vivo through exogenous administration of growth factors (i.e., VEGF),[43,46] the design of interconnected scaffolds to improve vascularization, and pre-vascularization using three-dimensional co-culture systems.[31]

Vascularization of clinically relevant sized tissue engineering constructs remains both a limit in the transfer of tissue engineering from in vitro to in vivo and in the transfer from animal to human systems. In addition, administration of growth factors involved in angiogenesis is still problematic since it is very costly and can have undesirable effects caused by suboptimal release kinetics, supraphysiological concentrations and a short half-life.[2]

1.6 Translational Requirements

Natural and synthetic bone grafts are deemed medical devices. In the United States, the Food and Drug Administration (FDA) is given the mandate to provide a reasonable assurance of the safety and effectiveness of medical devices. Before the Medical Device Amendments of 1976 (MDA), there were no provisions to regulate medical device safety or claims made regarding such devices. Most of the activity of the Food and Drug Administration (FDA) was towards protecting the American people from fraudulent devices. Due to the lack of safety regulations, devices such as defective cardiac pacemakers and intraocular lenses were not uncommon. With the passing of the MDA, the first legislation was passed which addressed the review of medical devices. The MDA provided a definition for the term "device" and established requirements for all devices, referred to as general controls. Furthermore, the FDA was directed to classify medical devices into one of three classes according to risk: Class I, Class II and Class III, which represent low-, moderate-, and high-risk medical devices, respectively. Based on their risk, requirements for market approval of medical devices vary, making it easier for low-risk medical devices to reach the market when compared to high-risk medical devices. Later, with the passing of the Safe Medical Devices Act of 1990 (SMDA), post-market requirements for medical devices were established. However, a product that has been deemed to be a human tissue, such as some bone grafts, can go directly to market providing that it complies with the rules established for tissue banks, which generally includes testing of the tissues for diseases.[60,61]

The process to approve the use and marketing of medical devices in the United States is somewhat different from that in the European Union (EU). The provision of evidence that the medical device works as intended may be sufficient to grant marketing approvals of even high-risk medical devices in the EU, whereas the approvals from the FDA are a lot more stringent. As a result, patients in the EU have access to certain high-risk medical devices sooner than patients in the United States. It must be noted that products marketed under less rigorous regulatory guidelines may have a greater chance of later-identified adverse events.[61,62]

1.7 Concluding Remarks

The bone tissue engineering field has experienced great advances in recent decades, with an expansion in knowledge of bone biology, biomaterials for bone repair and their applications, and diverse strategies for repairing large and small bone defects. Currently, most research efforts are put towards the use of growth factors and the understanding of their interactions with different growth factors, with cells and with intracellular pathways. At the same time, the development of techniques to enhance vascularization and of vascularized grafts are also of great interest since they present many challenges and opportunities for achieving optimal performance, both in vitro and in vivo, as well as in clinics. The motivation for translating bone engineering concepts from bench to bedside is rooted in the limitations in solving the increasing and somewhat difficult issues related to orthopedic and craniofacial reconstructions. In this book written by world renowned scientists, researchers and clinicians, current translational research in the field of bone tissue engineering is discussed.

References

1. Salgado, A.J., Bone Tissue Engineering: State of the art and future trends. *Macromol. Biosci.*, 2004, 4: 743–765.
2. Stevens, M.M., Biomaterials for bone tissue engineering. *Materials Today*, 2008, 11(5): 18–25.
3. Woodruff, M.A., Bone tissue engineering: From bench to bedside. *Materials Today*, 2012, 15(10): 430–435.
4. Jakob, M. Perspective on the evolution of cell-based bone tissue engineering tragegies. *European Surgical Research*, 2012, 49: 1–7.
5. Calori, G.M. The use of bone-graft substitutes in large bone defects: Any specific needs? *Injury*, 2011, 24: S56–S63.
6. Vos T.F. Years lived with disability (YLDs) for 1160 sequelae of 289 diseases and injuries 1990–2010: A systematic analysis for the Global Burden of Disease Study 2010. *Lancet*, 2012, 380: 2163–96.
7. Jacobs J.J. United States Bone and Joint Initiative. Burden of musculoskeletal diseases overview. In *The Burden of Musculoskeletal Diseases in the United States*, AAOS (ed.), 2011, Rosemont, IL: AAOS, pp. 1–20.
8. Katz S.I. United States Bone and Joint Initiative. Preface. In *The Burden of Musculoskeletal Diseases in the United States*, AAOS (ed.), 2011, Rosemont, IL: AAOS, pp. i–x.
9. Lidgren, L. The bone and joint decade and the global economic and healthcare burden of musculoskeletal disease. *Journal of Rheumatology*, 2003, 67: 4–5.
10. Beamen F. Bone graft materials and synthetic substitutes. *Radiol Clin North Am*, 2006 May; 44(3): 451–61.
11. Donati, D. Bone grafting: Historical and conceptual review, starting with an old manuscript by Vittorio Putti. *Acta Orthopaedica*, 2007, 78(1): 19–25.
12. Laurencin, C.T. *Bone Graft Substitutes*. 2003, West Conshohocken, PA: ASTM International, p 315.
13. Jahangir, A.A. Bone-graft substitutes in orthopedic surgery. *AAOS Now*, 2008, 7(10): 5.
14. Williams, A. Bone transplantation. *Orthopedic Blue Journal*, 2004, 27(5): 488–495.
15. Kaveh, K. Bone grafting and bone graft substitutes. *J. Anim. Vet. Adv.*, 2010, 9(6): 1055–1067.

16. Karabuda, C. Historical and clinical evaluation of 3 different grafting materials for sinus lifting procedure based on 8 cases. *Journal of Periodontology*, 2001, 72(10): 1436–1442.
17. Greenwald, A.S. The evolving role of bone-graft substitutes. *J. Bone Joint Surg. Am.*, 2001, 83(2): 98–103
18. Dimitriou, R. Complications following autologous bone graft harvesting from the iliac crest and using the RIA: A systematic review. *Injury, Int. J. Care Injured*, 2011, 42: S3–S15.
19. Zimmermann, G. Allograft bone matirx versus synthetic bone graft subtitutes. *Injury*, 2011, 42: S16–S21.
20. Mendenhall S. Bone grafts and bone substitutes. *Orthopedic Network News*, 1999, 10(4): 10–17.
21. Mendenhall S. 2010 bone grafts and bone substitutes. *Orthopedic Network News*, 2010, 21(4): 16–19.
22. Jager, M. Bridging the gap: Bone marrow aspiration concentrate reduces autologous bone grafting in osseous defects. *Journal of Orthopaedic Research*, 2010, 29(2): 173–180.
23. Saucedo, J.M. Platelet-rich plasma. *Brief CME*, 2012, 37A: 587–589.
24. Kim, Y.H. Enhancement of bone regeneration by dual release of a macrophage recruitment agent and platelet-rich plasma from gelatin hydrogels. *Biomaterials*, 2014, 35: 214–224.
25. Rosalyn T., Nguyen, J.B.-S., McInnis, K. Application of platelet-rich plasma in musculoskeletal and sports medicine: An evidence-based approach. *PM&R*, 2011, 3(3): 226–250.
26. Ujash Sheth, N.S., Klein, G., Fu, F., Einhorn, T.A. et al. Efficacy of autologous platelet-rich plasma use for orthopaedic indications: A meta-analysis. *The Journal of Bone and Joint Surgery*, 2012, 94(4): 298–307.
27. Intini, G. The use of platelet-rich plasma in bone reconstruction therapy. *Biomaterials*, 2009, 30: 4956–4966.
28. Hannink, G. Bioresorbability, porosity and mechanical strength of bone substitutes: What is optimal for bone regeneration? *Injury*, 2011, 42: S22–S25.
29. Goodrich, J. A review of reconstructive materials for use in craniofacial surgery bone fixation materials, bone substitutes, and distracters. *Childs Nerv Syst*, 2012, 28: 1577–1588.
30. Cho, Y.R. Biomaterials in craniofacial reconstruction. *Clin. Plastic Surg.*, 2004, 31: 377–385.
31. Bao, C.L.M. Advances in bone tissue engineering. In *Regenerative Medicine and Tissue Engineering*, J.A. Andrades, (ed.), 2013, Rijeka, Croatia: INTECH. pp. 599–614.
32. Blokhuis, T.J. Bioactive and osteoinductive bone graft substitutes: Definitions, facts and myths. *Injury, Int. J. Care Injured*, 2011, 42: S26–S29.
33. Kretlow, J.D., Young, S.Y., Klouda, L., Wong, M., Mikos, A.G. Injectable biomaterials for regenerating complex craniofacial tissues. *Advanced Materials*, 2009, 21: 3368–3393.
34. Bose, S. Calcium phosphate ceramic systems in growth factor and drug delivery for bone tissue engineering: A review. *Acta Biomaterialia*, 2012, 8: 1401–1421.
35. Kurien, T. Bone graft substitutes currently available in orthopaedic practice: The evidence for their use. *Bone Joint J*, 2013, 95-B(5): 583–597.
36. Bose, S. Calcium phosphate ceramics in drug delivery. *JOM*, 2011, 63(4): 93–98.

37. Puppi, D. Polymeric materials for bone and cartilage repair. *Progress in Polymer Science*, 2010, 35: 403–440.
38. Middleton, J.C. Synthetic biodegradable polymers as orthopedic devices. *Biomaterials*, 2000, 21: 2335–2346.
39. Vagaska, B. Osteogenic cells on bio-inspired materials for bone tissue engineering. *Physiol. Res.*, 2010, 59: 309–322.
40. Kolk, A. Current trends and future perspectives of bone substitute materials—From space holders to innovative biomaterials. *Journal of Cranio-Maxillo-Facial Surgery*, 2012, 40: 706–718.
41. Burg, K. Biomaterial developments for bone tissue engineering. *Biomaterials*, 2000, 21: 2347–2359.
42. Bohner, M. Resorbable biomaterials as bone graft substitutes. *Materials Today*, 2010, 13(1–2): 24–30.
43. Tsigkou, O. Engineered vascularized bone grafts. *PNAS*, 2010, 107(8): 3311–3316.
44. Seong, J.M. Stem cells in bone tissue engineering biomedical research. *Biomedical Materials*, 2010, 5: 1–15.
45. Carulli, C. Tissue engineering applications in the management of bone loss. *Clinical Cases in Mineral and Bone Metabolism*, 2013, 10(1): 22–25.
46. Bose, S. Recent advances in bone tissue engineering scaffolds. *Trends in Biotechnology*, 2012, 30(10): 546–554.
47. Fisher, M. Tissue engineering and regenerative medicine: Recent innovations and the transition to translation. *Tissue Engineering*, 2013, 19(1): 1–13.
48. Neligan, P.C. Tissue engineering. In *Plastic Surgery: Volume One: Principles*, P.C. Neligan, (ed.), 2012, Philadelphia, PA: Elsevier.
49. Janinki, P. What should be the characteristics of the ideal bone graft substitute? Combining scaffolds with growth factors and/or stem cells. *Injury*, 2011, 42: S77–S81.
50. Dvir, T. Nanotechnological strategies for engineering complex tissues. *Nature Nanotechnology*, 2011, 6: 13–22.
51. Bhatia, S.K, (ed.). *Biomaterials for Clinical Applications*. 2010, NY: Springer, p. 295.
52. Giannoudis, P.V. Bone regeneration strategies: Current trends but what the future holds? *Injury*, 2013, 44: S1–S2.
53. Yu, N. Biodegradable poly(a-hydroxy acid) polymer scaffolds for bone tissue engineering. *Journal of Biomedical Materials Research*, 2010, 93B(1): 285–295.
54. Giannoudis, P.V. Fracture healing: The diamond concept. *Injury*, 2007, 38(S4): S3–S6.
55. Calori, G.M. Enhancement of fracture healing with the diamond concept: The role of the biological chamber. *Injury*, 2011, 42: 1191–1193.
56. Nandi, S.K. Orthopaedic applications of bone graft & graft substitutes: A review. *Indian J Med. Res.*, 2010, 132: 15–30.
57. Hayes, J.S. The cell–surface interaction. *Adv Biochem Engin/Biotechnol*, 2011, 126: 1–31.
58. Palchesko, R.N. Optimization of calcium aluminate for use as a bone scaffold material through physical and chemical surface modification (doctoral dissertation). Bayer School of Natural and Environmental Science, 2011, Duquesne University, Pittsburgh, PA. Retrieved from ProQuest Dissertations Publishing, 2011.
59. Liu, Y. Review: Development of clinically relevant scaffolds for vascularised bone tissue engineering. *Biotechnology Advances*, 2013, 31: 688–705.

60. Johnson, J.A. *FDA Regulation of Medical Devices.* 2012, Washington, DC: Congressional Research Service.
61. U.S. Food and Drug Administration. Guidance for Industry and FDA Staff— Class II Special Controls Guidance Document: Dental Bone Grafting Material Device. Draft, 2013, Washington, DC: USFDA, [cited November 26, 2013]. Available from: http://www.fda.gov/MedicalDevices/DeviceRegulationandGuidance /GuidanceDocuments/ucm071842.htm.
62. Kramer, D.B., Xu, S., Kesselheim, A.S. Regulation of medical devices in the United States and European Union. *New England Journal of Medicine*, 2012, 366(9): 848–855.

Part II

Materials for Bone Graft Applications

Part II

2

Designing Scaffolds for Bone Tissue Engineering

Binulal N. Sathy, Sarita R. Shah, Antonios G. Mikos,
and Shantikumar V. Nair

CONTENTS

2.1 Introduction

Tissue engineering has been described as "an interdisciplinary field that applies the principles of engineering and life science towards the development of biological substitutes that restore, maintain, or improve tissue or organ function."[1] The history of this emerging field began in the early 1970s and gained popularity in the 1980s through the experimental initiatives of Langer and Vacanti.[2] In 1993, Langer and Vacanti described the utilization of a branching network of synthetic biocompatible/biodegradable polymers configured as scaffolds seeded with viable cells, a seminal paper that became the foundation for current advances in the field of tissue engineering.[1]

The goal of tissue engineering is to restore the structure and function of damaged tissues by augmenting the body's inherent healing capabilities with bioactive molecules, scaffolds, cells, or a combination of these components[3]. Currently, auto/allografts are the gold standards for tissue replacement.[4-7] Their clinical success is attributed to the unique combination of suitable cells within a native extracellular matrix (ECM), spatial distribution of functional vessels, and availability of bioactive molecules. However, the limited availability of grafts, donor site morbidity, and risk of disease transmission necessitates viable alternatives to meet with the increasing demand for tissue replacements.[8–10] Tissue engineering solutions present a promising alternative to autografts and allografts. Successful solutions rely on mimicry of the structural and functional features of native tissues by using a variety of combinatorial approaches, especially composites of different biomaterials with or without exogenous stem/progenitor cells.[11–13]

2.1.1 Tissue Engineering Scaffolds

Scaffolds form the basis of recent tissue regeneration approaches. The design of appropriate scaffolds for tissue engineering applications relies heavily on advances in the field of biomaterials sciences in order to exploit not only new materials but also new fabrication techniques. Effective scaffolds are three-dimensional structures fabricated from synthetic, natural, or semi-synthetic materials with ECM-mimicking properties.[13–15] They are temporary matrices for cell proliferation, differentiation, ECM deposition, and vascularization, and are expected to degrade in concert with tissue in-growth and maturation[16–17]. Literature indicates that the success of tissue engineering scaffolds depends on the extent of similitude between their structural and functional properties to that of native ECM.[13,14–18] As a result, different materials and engineering strategies have been employed to engineer scaffolds that are biocompatible, bio-functional, and biodegradable.

An ideal scaffold should mimic the structural, functional, and mechanical properties of native ECM. The functions of ECM in native tissues and the general role of scaffolds in engineered tissues have been reviewed elsewhere.[19–22] In tissues, cells reside in a complex three-dimensional network of fibrillar proteins, proteoglycans, and glycosaminoglycans (GAGs) which are collectively termed as the ECM.[23] Proteins such as collagen and elastin fibers are ten to several hundred nanometers in diameter, and the basement membrane, an important type of ECM in human tissues, is a flexible thin mat of 40 to 120 nm thickness composed mainly of type IV collagen and laminin nanofibers embedded in heparin sulphate proteoglycan hydrogels.[11] In addition to the nanofibers, the pores, ridges, and grooves are all at the nanoscale order.[24] ECM also plays a crucial role in cell signaling and maintenance of tissue homeostasis by serving as a reservoir of water, nutrients, cytokines, and growth factors and providing stimuli to cells in the form of integrins and/or mechanosensitive ion channels.[19,25] In addition to providing cells with a tissue-specific architecture and environment to reside, the overall structural design, features, and composition of the matrix contribute to the mechanical properties of the ECM.[25,26] The unique functionality of native ECM is due to the combinatorial effect of its structure, composition and the resident bioactive molecules. Therefore, the challenge for tissue engineers is to develop a scaffold analogue to native ECM that can simulate ECM properties and dimensions. This chapter describes the influence of biomaterial characteristics and scaffold architecture on scaffold properties and cell response.

2.2 Combinatorial Biomaterials in Scaffold Development

Many scaffold fabrication techniques and biomaterials are available for the development of tissue engineering scaffolds, which have been reviewed extensively.[14,27] Biomaterials that lack cytotoxicity and support tissue-specific cell-biomaterial interactions have been generally defined as biocompatible. However, in tissue engineering, biocompatibility indicates that the scaffold material and its degradation products will not elicit toxicity or provoke any rejection, inflammation, or immune response, in addition to the above mentioned features.[28,29] As biocompatibility is an essential feature of tissue engineering scaffolds, there has been increasing interest in the use of biocompatible materials and less toxic fabrication processes and surface modifications.

Biocompatible materials from a variety of sources, such as natural and synthetic polymers, ceramics, and metals, are currently used to fabricate tissue engineering scaffolds. However, these materials by themselves often fail to mimic the complex physicochemical and biological properties of desired tissue types. Therefore, a combinatorial approach using multiple types of biomaterials in a composite is an attractive alternative for developing scaffolds with properties that will suit the demands of the target tissue.

2.2.1 Physicochemical Properties

Scaffolds are designed to fulfill the essential physicochemical requirements, such as hydrophilicity, degradability, and mechanical strength, for a specific tissue engineering application. Recent research in the field aims to improve the tunability of these properties by creating hybrid or composite scaffolds.[30,31] The final composite properties are usually different from those of the individual base materials.

Hydrophilicity of the scaffolding material is a crucial parameter that determines its wetability, which in turn is a major factor that influences important biological outcomes such as cell adhesion and proliferation.[32] Incorporation of proteins such as collagen and gelatin into hydrophobic matrices are understood to facilitate improvements in hydrophilicity of composite scaffolds. For example, highly hydrophobic synthetic polymers such as polycaprolactone (PCL) and poly(lactic-co-glycolic acid) (PLGA) can be made wetable by the inclusion of collagen and gelatin.[33-35] Varying degrees of hydrophobicity can be achieved in poly-L-lactic acid (PLLA) matrix by incorporating varying quantities of glass particles.[36] Incorporation of bioglass (BG) in polyhydroxybutyrate-polyhydroxyvalerate (PHBV) rendered improvement in hydrophilicity of the composite.[37] In another study, the water-absorbing capability of chitosan was harnessed to improve hydrophilicity in composites prepared using polyester blends.[38] The ability to introduce hydrophilicity into a hydrophobic scaffold through a combination of materials enables the scaffold to take advantage of the desirable properties of hydrophobic polymers while simultaneously enhancing cellular activity on the scaffold, a prerequisite for successful tissue restoration.

Material solubility is an important physicochemical parameter that governs the biodegradability of the scaffold. A high or low solubility rate implies non-optimal performance by the scaffold in vivo. Therefore, controlling degradation kinetics is essential in materials used in regenerative medicine. Fine-tuned composite scaffolds have been created using materials with varying degrees of degradability to suit specific tissue regeneration applications. For hard-tissue engineering, such as bone, ceramic-polymer composites have vast applicability.[39] Fast degradable polymers are combined with bioceramics such as tri-calcium phosphate (TCP) and hydroxyapatite (HA) at varying ratios, yielding composite scaffolds with tuned degradability.[40] It has been reported that as the HA content in HA/PCL composite increases, the degradation rate also increases due to water infiltration into the scaffolds.[41] Comparison of the degradation profiles of PCL-TCP composite and PCL scaffolds in vitro and in vivo reveals that the degradation rate is faster for the composite, with increased average porosity in the in vivo environment.[42] Composite scaffolds with degradation rates desirable for cartilage regeneration have been fabricated by incorporating PHBV scaffolds with 20% BG.[37] Proteins such as gelatin are also used to tune degradability of polymers, as has been reported in the case of PLLA/gelatin composite scaffolds.[43] The presence of gelatin has been found to increase the rate of degradation of the composite.

Mechanical properties are an important consideration in the design of scaffolds, as the mechanics of the material may influence cell behavior.[44] For bone applications, there has been significant interest in polymer-ceramic combinations since bioceramics are stronger materials than polymers.[39] HA is most often used to improve mechanical properties in scaffolds composed of polymeric materials such as PCL, PLGA, and PLLA.[45-47] The use of TCP to form composite scaffolds with chitosan has shown improvements in compressive properties.[48] Wheeler et al.[49] have studied the use of carbon nanosphere chains to enhance mechanical stability in multicomponent composites that also included BG and collagen. Similarly, PLGA scaffolds containing carbon nanotubes display significantly enhanced mechanical properties compared to PLGA scaffolds alone.[50] Coating PLGA on an HA/TCP composite yields a final product with substantially enhanced compressive strength approximately 10-fold more than that obtained for HA/TCP without the PLGA coating.[43] The addition of BG to PLGA produces composite scaffolds with compressive modulus higher than that of PLGA alone.[51] Incorporation of gelatin with a PLGA/HA blend results in a high elongation ratio.[52] Additionally, HA/collagen composite scaffolds are reported to possess high mechanical stiffness as the ductile properties of collagen can aid in improving the fracture toughness of HA.[53,54] Apart from commonly used ceramics and polymers, proteins such as silk, known for its remarkable mechanical properties, are also being investigated for developing composite scaffolds.[55] Choi et. al.[56] have reported that composite structures composed of bacterial cellulose and silk have comparable mechanical strength to that of the human cortical bone (12.8–17.7 GPa). Such studies have demonstrated that a combinatorial approach using different materials with distinct physicochemical properties can lead to the development of new composite scaffold systems with fine-tuned attributes.

2.2.2 Biological Activity

A major challenge faced in tissue engineering is the identification of the appropriate material system that can elicit a desired biological/physiological effect. To a large extent, the physicochemical properties discussed in Section 2.2.1 govern the end biological effects. By utilizing natural polymers of the ECM as scaffold components, it is possible to trigger enhanced cellular activity in tissue engineering scaffolds.[57] Yan et al.[58] report a multicomponent composite scaffold composed of collagen, hyaluronic acid, and chitosan in an optimized ratio that exhibits significantly enhanced tissue formation response in in vitro static culture conditions when compared to that shown by collage matrix alone. The study also reveals that a majority of the cells seeded on the composite scaffold preserve their phenotypic integrity, indicating that the scaffold provides appropriate cues to seeded cells. Jiankang et al.[59] have found that a composite scaffold composed of gelatin and chitosan shows superior biocompatibility. Collagen/chitosan scaffolds proposed for dermal tissue regeneration showed good interactions with skin fibroblasts with enhanced cell proliferation and biological activity compared with that shown in monolayer cultures.[60] Composite scaffolds of collagen and elastin, key structural proteins found in the ECM, are found to be good substrates for cell attachment, differentiation, and subsequent mineralization.[61,62] Silk fibroin is another natural polymer that has been explored for composite scaffold development due to its biocompatibility.[63,64]

The combination of natural polymers with synthetic polymers allows the engineering of scaffolds that take advantage of the biological cues of natural polymers and the tunable properties of synthetic polymers. PCL scaffolds coated with gelatin promote nucleation and growth of calcium phosphate, a prerequisite for enhanced biological activity.[65] Composite scaffolds of PLA/silk fibroin/gelatin have been reported to be biocompatible and provide a cell-friendly environment for cell adhesion, spreading, and proliferation.[66] Elastin has been used with PCL to attain improved adhesion and proliferation of chondrocytes.[67]

Bioceramics confer a distinct set of advantages when used in composite scaffolds. For example, the incorporation of HA with PCL as well as with PCL-polydiisopropyl fumarate blend significantly improves cell biocompatibility and osteoconductivity.[68] Similarly, composite scaffolds of PCL/HA possess enhanced capability to express osteogenic differentiation markers in primary bone cells when compared to cells grown on PCL scaffolds.[69] Significant enhancement in the biomineralization rate in the case of PLGA/HA scaffolds was reported with increased biological activity in terms of cell viability, proliferation, and spreading.[70] Pang et al.[71] report that a PLGA/TCP composite scaffold covered with a collagen sponge and apatite shows improved proliferation and osteogenic differentiation of bone marrow stem cells. Xu et al.[72] prepared a composite scaffold based on bioglass-collagen-phosphotidylserine and found it to exhibit extensive osteoconductivity with host bone. The authors also report that seeding these scaffolds with mesenchymal stem cells results in dramatically increased new bone formation. Cheng et al.[73] have investigated the complex remodeling process of CaP/silk composite scaffolds implanted at osteoporotic defect sites and observed significantly increased bone formation and mineralization coupled with decreased osteoclast resorption.

2.3 Scaffold Architecture

Scaffold architecture is equally important as material choice for successful tissue regeneration. The inherent properties of the selected biomaterial and the applied scaffold fabrication technique are the major determinants of the overall architecture of the scaffold. However, architecture-related internal parameters such as porosity, pore size, pore geometry, pore interconnectivity, and structural dimensions of the pore wall can be controlled to a certain extent by fabrication technique. These internal parameters ultimately determine the mass transport, cell migration, and mechanical integrity of a given scaffold and its suitability for tissue regeneration applications.

2.3.1 Pore Parameters

Porosity is the percentage of void space in the bulk material.[74] Pores provide sites and space for the proliferation of incorporated cells, endogenous cell infiltration/migration, ECM deposition, and tissue formation. Generally, scaffold porosity of 90% or more is recommended in order to provide substantial surface area for cell–scaffold interaction, sufficient space for ECM deposition, and minimal diffusion constraints for in vitro cell-culture conditions.[75–77] Adequate pore size and interconnectivity are also necessary for sufficient supply of oxygen and nutrients throughout a scaffold for functional tissue regeneration.[76,78] Interconnected pores of sufficient size allow the infiltration and distribution of seeded cells throughout the scaffold and facilitate migration of the seeded cells and exogenous cells.[79–81] Lack of interconnections results in suboptimal gaseous and nutrient exchange within the scaffold and poor metabolic waste removal. Integration of the transplanted engineered construct with the host tissue can also be influenced by the porosity, pore size, and pore interconnectivity of the scaffold. Capillary in-growth from the surrounding tissue and vascularization of the scaffolds by migration of endothelial cells are affected by the pore-related parameters of the scaffolds.[81–83] In addition, pore-related parameters are directly correlated with the mechanical properties of the scaffolds. The pore size in the scaffold can be varied according to the scaffold fabrication technique in accordance with the desired mechanical properties of the scaffold.[84–85] Therefore, a balance between the interconnected porosity/pore size and the mechanical properties is essential for its use in tissue engineering applications.

It is important to remember that optimal porosity and pore size may not be the same for all tissue types. Pore sizes ranging from double the size of a cell (~20 µm) to 50 times the size of a cell (~500 µm) have been reported as optimal for different cell types. For example, significantly large number of cells showed chondrocyte morphology on collagen type-1 matrix with small pore diameter compared to large pore diameter at 3 hours, which suggests the sensitivity of cells to difference in pore diameter and pore wall thickness.[86] Murphy et al.[87] investigated the effect of mean pore size on cell attachment, proliferation, and migration on collagen-glycosaminoglycan scaffolds and found that scaffold mean pore size greatly affects cellular activity and even small changes in pore size can have significant effects. The effect of mean pore size ranging from 85 to 325 µm on osteoblast adhesion and proliferation up to 7 days after seeding was investigated, and results showed that the highest cell number in scaffolds occurred in scaffolds with the largest pore size (325 µm). The desired scaffold pore size is dependent on the type of tissue being engineered. In the case of osteoblasts, pores larger than 100 µm are reported to be optimal for bone formation, while pore sizes of 20–80 µm have been reported to be optimal for growing endothelial cells.

Pore shape has also been found to influence cell functions. Melchels et al.[88] compared the computer-designed gyroid architecture obtained by stereolithography with a random pore architecture resulting from salt leaching. Even though the scaffolds had comparable porosity and pore size values, the gyroid architecture showed more than 10-fold higher permeability, which has been attributed to the presence of pore interconnections adequately sized for cell distribution. This resulted in the homogenous distribution of cell population in the scaffold after dynamic seeding compared to the accumulation of cells in the scaffold periphery in the salt-leached scaffolds.

2.3.2 Nanostructured Scaffold Pore Walls

The scaffold pore wall can have nano- to macro-scale topography and particulate to fibrous features, depending upon the biomaterial and scaffold fabrication technique used. Scaffold matrices with nanoscale features have been found to provide a more favorable microenvironment for improved cell response than scaffold matrices with microscale structures. In anchorage-dependent cell types, anchorage with the immediate extracellular environment is an integral part of the cell's life cycle and cell processes.[89] Therefore, the ability of the scaffold to provide a favorable microenvironment for cell anchorage, with surface properties and structural dimensions similar to that of native ECM, is crucial for its applicability in tissue engineering. Recently, nanostructuring of the scaffold pore wall has become popular as a viable means for mimicking the structural dimensions and surface properties of native ECM.

There are several scaffold fabrication techniques available for fabrication of nanoscale scaffolds for tissue engineering purposes. Among them, self-assembly, phase separation, and electrospinning are commonly used for fabricating scaffolds with nanoscale fibrous structures.[90] Self-assembly is a bottom-up fabrication strategy that involves the interaction of pure molecules with one another, leading to the formation of complex assemblies with predefined nanoscale structures.[91] Self-assembly relies on weak noncovalent interactions to build nanofibers from engineered polymers, small molecules, proteins, peptides, and nucleic acids.[92] Even though this approach creates nanofibers of the smallest scale (5–8 nm in diameter), length of the resulting fibers is limited to one to several mm.[92]

In phase separation, selective enrichment and purification of a desired phase is performed in a controlled way to get nanostructured scaffold matrix. Porous polymer membranes and scaffolds are created by inducing the separation of a polymer solution into a polymer-poor phase and a polymer-rich phase.[93–94] This allows the creation of three-dimensional scaffolds with fibers in the submicron range.

Recently, electrospinning has gained popularity as a straightforward, cost-effective, and versatile technique for the fabrication of nano-featured scaffolds suitable for tissue engineering.[95–98] Electrospinning allows the fabrication of micro- to nano-scale diameter continuous polymeric fibres from a charged polymer droplet using high voltage.[95–98]

2.3.3 Protein Adsorption on Nanostructures

Protein–material interactions such as protein adsorption, desorption, diffusion, and conformational changes occur when scaffolds come in contact with biological fluids.[99,100] Protein–biomaterial interaction is crucial because the adsorbed protein layer on the biomaterial surface mediates cell adhesion to the scaffold.[101] When cells come in contact with the proteins on the material surface, interactions between the cell and proteins occur and are reflected as changes in cell behavior. These interactions occur on the nanoscale order.[102]

The high surface-to-volume ratio and favorable surface properties of nanostructures in the scaffold matrix have been found to influence the adsorbed protein behavior and cell response. It has been well documented that the adsorption and conformation of proteins can be significantly influenced through a combination of material surface properties such as chemical, electrostatic, van der Waals, and surface energy forces of materials.[101] For example, the adhesive protein fibronectin has been found to adhere to a greater extent on nanostructured scaffolds compared to scaffolds with solid pore walls or microscale features.[103,104] Moreover, the conformation of adsorbed fibronectin changes according to the surface properties. The fact that protein–material interactions can be influenced by the presence of nanoscale structures makes nanostructuring of scaffolds an important consideration in the development of tissue engineering scaffolds.

Several studies have reported the influence of nanostructures on protein adsorption. Significantly increased serum protein adsorption has been reported in scaffolds with nano-fibrous pore walls compared with solid pore wall scaffolds.[103] Selective enhancement in the adsorption of adhesive proteins such as fibronectin and vitronectin has also been reported in scaffold with nano-fibrous pore walls.[103,104] Ballard[105] observed that the secondary structures of fibronectin are different on small-diameter nanoparticles (4 nm or 20 nm) when compared to the unordered structure observed in the presence of 100 nm particles. However, vitronectin exhibited no change in secondary structures on small- or large-diameter particles. Vertegel et al.[106] investigated changes in the adsorbed protein confirmation and biological activity using lysozyme adsorbed on 4-, 20-, or 100-nm silica nanoparticles. Decreasing α-helicity and enzymatic activity of the adsorbed lysozyme with increased particle size was observed. Protein adsorption on nanostructured titania has been found to be low and randomly oriented on nanostructures of height 4 nm in contrast to high and parallel orientation on nanostructures of height between 1 and 2 nm.[107] These examples indicate the advantages of using nanostructured tissue engineering scaffolds to achieve desired interactions with the biological molecules.

2.3.4 Cell Interaction with Nanostructured Scaffolds

The influence of nanoscale features on cell behavior was reported by researchers as early as the 1960s.[108] Since then several studies have reported the influence of nanostructures, such as nanoparticles, nanocrystals, nanofibers, and nanofilms, on favorable cell–material interactions and improved cellular response.[109–113] Nanofibrous scaffolds have been largely applied in tissue regeneration studies, both in vitro and in vivo.[110–115] As shown in Figures 2.1 and 2.2,

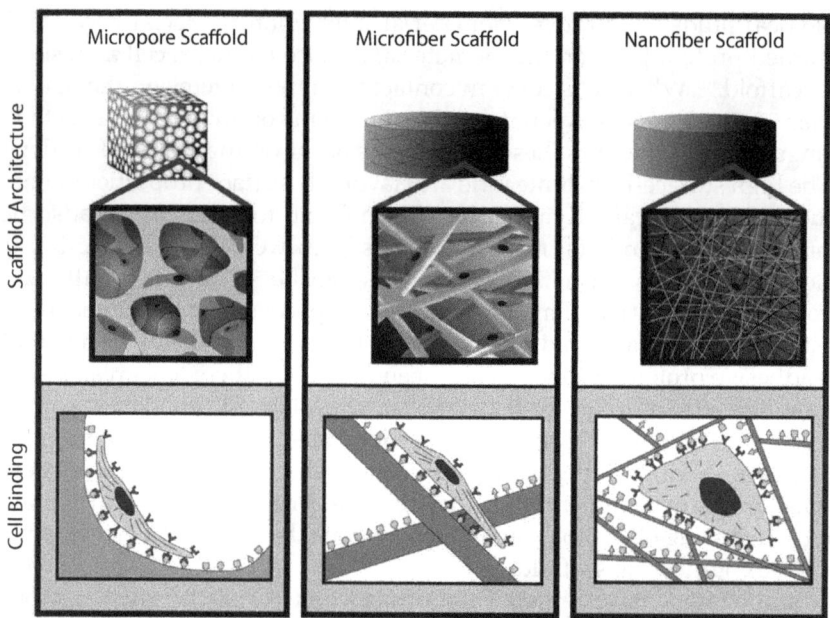

FIGURE 2.1
A pictorial representation showing the effect of scaffold architecture on cell binding and spreading. (Adapted from Stevens MM, George JH, *Science*, 310:1135–1138, 2005. With permission.)

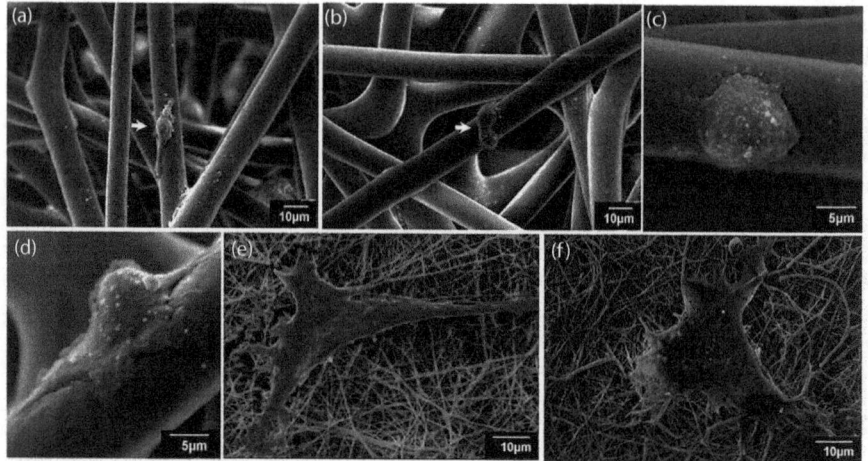

FIGURE 2.2
Scanning electron microscopic images of MSCs on both nano- and microfibers 12h after seeding. While microfibrous scaffolds show little cell spreading after 12 hours, (a, b, shown at low magnification and c, d, at high magnification), cell morphology is spread out on nano-fibrous scaffolds at the same time period (e, f). (Adapted from Binulal NS et al., *Tissue Eng Part A*, 16:393–404, 2010. With permission.)

nanoscale structural dimensions can positively influence the cell response, which may help to improve tissue regeneration.

Several investigators have explored nanofibrous scaffolds for regeneration of tissue types such as bone, cartilage, skin, vascular, bladder, neural, and cardiac tissues.[116,117] Yoshimoto et al.[118] report that MSCs seeded on electrospun PCL nanofibers and cultured under dynamic conditions penetrated into the nanofibers by 1 week and covered the nanofibers with multiple cell layers by 4 weeks. Mineralization and type I collagen deposition was also reported at 4 weeks. Li et al.[119–121] report that the nanofibrous structure of PLGA and PCL supports the attachment and proliferation of cultured fibroblasts, cartilage, and bone marrow–derived MSCs. It has also been reported that osteoblast adhesion, proliferation, alkaline phosphatase activity, and ECM secretion increases on carbon nanofibers as fiber diameter decreases in the range of 60–200 nm. The adhesion of other types of cells such as chondrocytes, fibroblasts, and smooth muscle cells was not influenced by fiber size in this range.[122,123] Increase in cell attachment, proliferation, and expression of matrix components has been reported in scaffolds with pore walls with increased nanoscale roughness.[124] Divya Rani et al.[125] report improved osteoblast response on nanomodified titanium implants.

Hsiao et al.[126] report that an aligned two-dimensional conductive nanofibrous mesh made of PLGA and polyaniline was able to induce elongated and aligned rat cardiomyocyte clusters with synchronous cell beating. Similarly, the differentiation capability of MSCs seeded on nanofibers was preserved, even after prolonged cell culture.[127] This is important because the decline of osteogenic potential of MSCs with increase in passage numbers can be a major limitation in MSC-related tissue regeneration approaches.[128,129]

Recent studies have demonstrated the use of nanofibrous scaffolds in the development of highly organized cell–scaffold constructs for improved tissue regeneration in a variety of tissue types. Exploiting the advantages of nanostructuring for the development of tissue engineering scaffolds without compromising scaffold architecture parameters, such as porosity and mechanical strength, may significantly enhance current tissue regeneration strategies.

2.4 Outlook

The key requirements of tissue engineering scaffolds can be fulfilled through an appropriate combination of biomaterials and scaffold development. Engineered scaffolds that mimic the structural and functional properties of natural ECM are a viable approach to facilitate improved tissue regeneration. Bicompatability, bioactivity, and biodegradability are material-driven properties that can be fine-tuned using various techniques. Porosity, pore geometry, pore size, pore interconnectivity, and structural dimensions of the matrix, which can be collectively termed as the architecture, are primarily governed by the scaffold fabrication technique. However, both material-driven properties and scaffold fabrication technique-driven properties can be influenced by each other. Nanostructuring of the matrix and use of biopolymeric hybrids and composites are strategies that have the potential to improve the outcome of the tissue regeneration. Nanostructuring the scaffold matrix can produce excellent cell culture results in the laboratory. However, it may not be wise to implement it in the tissue engineering scaffold at the expense of other scaffold architecture–related parameters such as porosity, pore size, and pore interconnectivity. For example, an electrospun wafer with aligned or non-woven nanofibers developed out of hybrid or composite biomaterials without sufficiently large enough pores cannot exploit the advantages of the biomaterial combination or nanostructures. Instead, a scaffold having large enough pore size, porosity, and interconnectivity with nanostructured pore walls may possibly get the advantages of both biomaterial combination and nanostructuring.

The role of hybrid and composite biomaterial scaffolds with optimal pore-related properties and nanostructured pore walls is an area which remains largely unexplored. Exploiting the advantages of nanotechnology and combinatorial biomaterial properties along with appropriate scaffold fabrication technique may improve the current tissue regeneration strategies. A careful evaluation of desired properties and prioritization of those properties is essential in the development of tissue engineering scaffolds.

References

1. Langer R, Vacanti JP. Tissue engineering. *Science* (New York, N.Y.) 1993; 260:920–926.
2. Vacanti CA. The history of tissue engineering. *J Cell Mol Med* 2006; 10:569–576.
3. Lanza R, Langer R, Vacanti JP. *Principles of Tissue Engineering* (2nd ed). San Diego, CA: Academic Press, 2000.
4. Chlupac J, Filováa E, Bacáková L. Blood vessel replacement: 50 years of development and tissue engineering paradigms in vascular surgery. *Physiol Res* 2009; Suppl. 2:S119–S139.
5. Blitch EL, Ricotta PJ. Introduction to bone grafting. *J Foot Ankle Surg* 1996; 35:458–462.
6. Khan SN, Cammisa FP, Sandhu HS, Diwan AD, Girardi FP, Lane JM. The biology of bone grafting. *J Am Acad Orthop Surg* 2005; 13:77–86.
7. Theoret C. Tissue engineering in wound repair: The three "R"s–repair, replace, regenerate. *Vet Surg* 2009; 38:905–913.
8. Finkemeier CG. Bone-grafting and bone-graft substitutes. *J Bone Joint Surg Am* 2002; 84:454–464.
9. Younger EM, Chapman MW. Morbidity at bone graft donor sites. *J Orthop Trauma* 1989; 3:192–195.

10. Laurencin C, Khan Y, El-Amin SF. Bone graft substitutes. *Expert Rev Med Devices* 2006; 3:49–57.
11. Ma Z, Kotaki M, Inai R. Potential of nanofiber matrix as tissue-engineering scaffolds. *Tissue Eng* 2005; 11:101–109.
12. Venugopal J, Low S, Choon AT, Ramakrishna S. Interaction of cells and nano-fiber scaffolds in tissue engineering. *J Biomed Mater Res B Appl Biomater* 2007; 8: 34–48.
13. Davis HE, Leach JK. Hybrid and composite biomaterials in tissue engineering. *Topics in Multifunctional Biomaterials and Devices* e-book, Vol. 1, N. Ashammakhi, (ed.), 2008.
14. O'Brien FJ. Biomaterials and scaffolds for tissue engineering. *Materials Today* 2011; 14:88–95.
15. Hutmacher DW. Scaffolds in tissue engineering bone and cartilage. *Biomaterials* 2000; 21:2529–2543.
16. Peter MX, Elisseeff J. *Scaffolding in Tissue Engineering.* Boca Raton, FL: CRC Press, Taylor & Francis Group, 2006.
17. Leong KF, Cheah CM, Chua CK. Solid free form fabrication of three-dimensional scaffolds for engineering replacement tissues and organs. *Biomaterials* 2003; 24: 2363–2378.
18. Freed LE, Vunjak-Novakovic G, Biron RJ, Eagles DB, Lesnoy DC. Biodegradable polymer scaffold for tissue engineering. *Biotechnology* (NY) 1994; 12:689–693.
19. Carson DD. Extracellular matrix: Forum introduction. *Reprod Biol Endocrinol* 2004; 7: 2:1.
20. Smith LA, Ma PX. Nano-fibrous scaffolds for tissue engineering. *Colloids Surf B Biointerfaces* 2004; 39:125–131.
21. Singh M, Kasper FK. and Mikos AG. Tissue engineering scaffolds. In: Ratner D. Hoffman AS, Schoen FJ, and Lemons JE, (eds.), *Biomaterials Science: An Introduction to Materials in Medicine*, (3rd ed). New York: Elsevier, 2013. pp. 1138–1159.
22. Frantz C, Stewart KM, Weaver VM. The extracellular matrix at a glance. *J Cell Sci* 2010; 123:4195–4200.
23. Fernandes H, Moroni L, van Blitterswijk C, de Boer J. Extracellular matrix and tissue engineering applications. *J Mater Chem* 2009; 19:5474–5484.
24. Flemming RG, Murphy CJ, Abrams GA, Goodman SL, Nealey PF. Effects of synthetic micro-and nano-structured surfaces on cell behaviour. *Biomaterials* 1999; 20:573–588.
25. Olsen BR. Matrix molecules and their ligands. In: Lanza R. Langer R. Chick W, (eds.). *Principles of Tissue Engineering*, Austin, TX: Academic Press, 1997. pp. 47–65.
26. Martins-Green M. Dynamics of cell-ECM interactions. In: Lanza RP, Langer RS, Vacanti JP, (eds.). *Principles of Tissue Engineering,* (2nd ed.) San Diego, CA: Academic Press, 2000. pp. 33–56.
27. Subia B, Kundu J, Kundu SC. Biomaterial scaffold fabrication techniques for potential TE applications. In Eberli D, (ed.), *Tissue Engineering*, Vienna, Austria: In-Tech, 2010. pp. 141–157.
28. Rickert D, Lendlein A, Peters I, Moses MA, Franke RP. Biocompatibility testing of novel multifunctional polymeric biomaterials for tissue engineering applications in head and neck surgery: An overview. *Eur Arch Otorhinolaryngol* 2006; 263:215–222.

29. Mikos AG, McIntire LV, Anderson JM, Babensee JE. Host response to tissue engineered devices. *Adv Drug Deliv Rev* 1998; 33:111–139.
30. Edalat F, Sheu I, Manoucheri S, Khademhosseini A. Material strategies for creating artificial cell-instructive niches. *Curr Opin Biotechnol* 2012; 23:820–825.
31. Armentano I, Fortunati E, Mattioli S, Rescignano N, Kenny JM. Biodegradable composite scaffolds: A strategy to modulate stem cell behaviour. *Recent Pat Drug Deliv Formul* 2013; 7:9–17.
32. Dowling DP, Miller IS, Ardhaoui M, Gallagher WM. Effect of surface wettability and topography on the adhesion of osteosarcoma cells on plasma-modified polystyrene. *J Biomater Appl* 2011; 26:327–47.
33. Zhang Y, Ouyang H, Lim CT, Ramakrishna S, Huang Z-M. Electrospinning of gelatin fibers and gelatin/PCL composite fibrous scaffolds. *J Biomed Mater Res* 2005; 72B:156–165.
34. Binulal NS, Natarajan A, Menon D, Bhaskaran VK, Mony U, Nair SV. PCL-gelatin composite nanofiberselectrospun using diluted acetic acid-ethyl acetate solvent system for stem cell-based bone tissue engineering. *J Biomater Sci Polym Ed* 2014; 25:325–340.
35. Li XK, Cai SX, Liu B, Xu ZL, Dai XZ, Ma KW, Lin SQ, Yang L, Sung KL, Fu XB. Characteristics of PLGA-gelatin complex as potential artificial nerve scaffold. *Colloids Surf B Biointerfaces* 2007; 57:198–203.
36. Navarro M, Engel E, Planell JA, Amaral I, Barbosa M, Ginebra MP. Surface characterization and cell response of a PLA/CaP glass biodegradable composite material. *J Biomed Mater Res A* 2008; 85:477–86.
37. Wu J, Xue K, Li H, Sun J, Liu K. Improvement of PHBV scaffolds with bioglass for cartilage tissue engineering. *PLoS ONE* 2013; 8:e71563.
38. Correlo VM, Pinho ED, Pashkuleva I, Bhattacharya M, Neves NM, Reis RL. Water absorption and degradation characteristics of chitosan-based polyesters and hydroxyapatite composites. *Macromol Biosci* 2007; 7:354–363.
39. Sahoo NG, Pan YZ, Li L, He CB. Nanocomposites for bone tissue regeneration. *Nanomedicine* 2013; 8:639–653.
40. Huang J, Ten E, Liu G, Finzen M, Yu W, Lee JS, Saiz E, Tomsia AP. Biocomposites of pHEMA with HA/β-TCP (60/40) for bone tissue engineering: Swelling, hydrolytic degradation, and in vitro behavior. *Polymer* 2013; 54:1197–1207.
41. Ang KC, Leong KF, Chua CK, Chandrasekaran M. Compressive properties and degradability of poly(epsilon-caprolatone)/hydroxyapatite composites under accelerated hydrolytic degradation. *J Biomed Mater Res A* 2007; 80:655–660.
42. Yeo A, Rai B, Sju E, Cheong JJ, Teoh SH. The degradation profile of novel, bioresorbable PCL-TCP scaffolds: An in vitro and in vivo study. *J Biomed Mater Res A* 2008; 84:208–218.
43. Feng S, Shen X., Fu Z., Shao M. Preparation and characterization of gelatin–poly(L-lactic) acid/poly(hydroxybutyrate-co-hydroxyvalerate) composite nanofibrous scaffolds. *J Macromol Sci Phys* 2010; 50:1705–1713.
44. Engler AJ, Sen S, Sweeney HL, Discher DE. Matrix elasticity directs stem cell lineage specification. *Cell* 2006; 126:677–689.
45. Calandrelli L., Immirzi B., Malinconico M., Luessenheide S., Passaro I., di Pasquale R, Oliva A. Natural and synthetic hydroxyapatite filled PCL: Mechanical properties and biocompatibility analysis. *J Bioact Compat Pol* 2004; 19:301–313.

46. Miao X, Tan DM, Li J, Xiao Y, Crawford R. Mechanical and biological properties of hydroxyapatite/tricalcium phosphate scaffolds coated with poly(lactic-co-glycolic acid). *Acta Biomater* 2008;4:638–645.
47. Charles LF, Kramer ER, Shaw MT, Olson JR, Wei M. Self-reinforced composites of hydroxyapatite-coated PLLA fibers: Fabrication and mechanical characterization. *J Mech Behav Biomed Mater* 2013; 17:269–277.
48. Hao R, Wang D, Yao A, Huang W. Preparation and characterization of β-TCP/CS scaffolds by freeze-extraction and freeze-gelation. *J Wuhan University of Technology-Mater Sci Ed* 2011; 26: 371–375.
49. Wheeler TS, Sbravati ND, Janorkar AV. Mechanical & cell culture properties of elastin-like polypeptide, collagen, bioglass, and carbon nanosphere composites. *Ann Biomed Eng.* 2013; 41:2042–55.
50. Cheng Q, Rutledge K, Jabbarzadeh E. Carbon nanotube-poly(lactide-co-glycolide) composite scaffolds for bone tissue engineering applications. *Ann Biomed Eng.* 2013; 41:904–916.
51. Miao X, Tan L-P, Tan L-S, Huang X. Porous calcium phosphate ceramics modified with PLGA-bioactive glass. *Mater Sci Eng C* 2007; 27:274–279.
52. Lee JB, Kim SE, Heo DN, Kwon IK, Choi B-J. In vitro characterization of nanofibrous PLGA/gelatin/hydroxyapatite composite for bone tissue engineering. *Macromol Res* 2010; 8: 1195–1202.
53. DA Wahl, JT Czernuszka. Collagen-hydroxyapatite composites for hard tissue repair. *Eur Cell Mater* 2006; 11: 43–56.
54. Yunoki S, Ikoma T, Tsuchiya A, Monkawa A, Ohta K, Sotome S, Shinomiya K, Tanaka J. Fabrication and mechanical and tissue ingrowth properties of unidirectionally porous hydroxyapatite/collagen composite. *J Biomed Mater Res B Appl Biomater* 2007; 80:166–173.
55. Keten S, Xu Z, Ihle B, Buehler MJ. Nanoconfinement controls stiffness, strength and mechanical toughness of β-sheet crystals in silk. *Nat Mater* 2010; 9:359–367.
56. Choi Y, Cho SY, HeoS, Jin H-J. Enhanced mechanical properties of silk fibroin-based composite plates for fractured bone healing. *Fibers and Polymers* 2013; 14: 266–270.
57. Badylak SF, Freytes DO, Gilbert TW. Extracellular matrix as a biological scaffold material: Structure and function. *Acta Biomater* 2009; 5:1–13.
58. Yan J, Li X, Liu L, Wang F, Zhu TW, Zhang Q. Potential use of collagen-chitosan-hyaluronan tri-copolymer scaffold for cartilage tissue engineering. *Artif Cells Blood Substit Immobil Biotechnol* 2006; 34:27–39.
59. Jiankang H, Dichen L, Yaxiong L, Bo Y, Hanxiang Z, Qin L, Bingheng L, Yi L. Preparation of chitosan-gelatin hybrid scaffolds with well-organized microstructures for hepatic tissue engineering. *Acta Biomater* 2009; 5:453–461.
60. Sun LP, Wang S, Zhang ZW, Wang XY, Zhang QQ. Biological evaluation of collagen-chitosan scaffolds for dermis tissue engineering. *Biomed Mater* 2009; 4:055008.
61. Rnjak-Kovacina J, Wise SG, Li Z, Maitz PK, Young CJ, Wang Y, Weiss AS. Electrospun synthetic human elastin: Collagen composite scaffolds for dermal tissue engineering. *Acta Biomater* 2012; 8:3714–3722.
62. Amruthwar SS, Janorkar AV. In vitro evaluation of elastin-like polypeptide-collagen composite scaffold for bone tissue engineering. *Dent Mater* 2013; 29: 211–220.

63. Ma X, Cao C, Zhu H. The biocompatibility of silk fibroin films containing sulfonated silk fibroin. *J Biomed Mater Res B Appl Biomater* 2006; 78:89–96.
64. Mobini S, Solati-Hashjin M, Peirovi H, Abu Osman NA, Gholipourmalekabadi M, Barati M, Samadikuchaksaraei A. Bioactivity and biocompatibility studies on silk-based scaffold for bone tissue engineering. *J Med Biol Eng*. 2012; 33: 207–214.
65. Li X, Xie J, Yuan X, Xia Y. Coating electrospunpoly(epsilon-caprolactone) fibers with gelatin and calcium phosphate and their use as biomimetic scaffolds for bone tissue engineering. *Langmuir* 2008; 24:14145–14150.
66. Gui-Bo Y, You-Zhu Z, Shu-Dong W, De-Bing S, Zhi-Hui D, Wei-Guo F. Study of the electrospun PLA/silk fibroin-gelatin composite nanofibrous scaffold for tissue engineering. *J Biomed Mater Res A* 2010; 93:158–163.
67. Annabi N, Fathi A, Mithieux SM, Martens P, Weiss AS, Dehghani F. The effect of elastin on chondrocyte adhesion and proliferation on poly (ε caprolactone)/elastin composites. *Biomaterials* 2011; 32:1517–1525.
68. Fernandez JM, Molinuevo MS, Cortizo MS, Cortizo AM. Development of an osteoconductive PCL-PDIPF-hydroxyapatite composite scaffold for bone tissue engineering. *J Tissue Eng Regen Med* 2011; 5:e126–135.
69. Chuenjitkuntaworn B, Inrung W, Damrongsri D, Mekaapiruk K, Supaphol P, Pavasant P. Polycaprolactone/hydroxyapatite composite scaffolds: Preparation, characterization, and in vitro and in vivo biological responses of human primary bone cells. *J Biomed Mater Res A* 2010; 94:241–251.
70. Lao L, Wang Y, Zhu Y, Zhang Y, Gao C. Poly (lactide-co-glycolide)/hydroxyapatite nanofibrous scaffolds fabricated by electrospinning for bone tissue engineering. *J Mater Sci Mater Med*. 2011; 22:1873–1884.
71. Pang L, Hao W, Jiang M, Huang J, Yan Y, Hu Y. Bony defect repair in rabbit using hybrid rapid prototyping polylactic-co-glycolic acid/β-tricalciumphosphate collagen I/apatite scaffold and bone marrow mesenchymal stem cells. *Indian J Orthop* 2013; 47:388–394.
72. Xu C, Su P, Chen X, Meng Y, Yu W, Xiang AP, Wang Y. Biocompatibility and osteogenesis of biomimetic bioglass-collagen-phosphatidylserine composite scaffolds for bone tissue engineering. *Biomaterials* 2011; 32:1051–1058.
73. Cheng N, Dai J, Cheng X, Li S, Miron RJ, Wu T, Chen W, Zhang Y, Shi B. Porous CaP/silk composite scaffolds to repair femur defects in an osteoporotic model. *J Mater Sci Mater Med*. 2013; 24:1963–1975.
74. Leon y Leon CA. New perspectives in mercury porosimetry. *Adv Colloid Interface Sci* 1998; 76–77:341–372.
75. Ge Z, Baguenard S, Lim LY, Wee A, Khor E. Hydroxyapatite–chitin materials as potential tissue engineered bone substitutes. *Biomaterials* 2004; 25:1049–1058.
76. Karageorgiou V, Kaplan D. Porosity of 3D biomaterial scaffolds and osteogenesis. *Biomaterials* 2005; 26:5474–5491.
77. Gomes ME, Holtorf HL, Reis RL, Mikos AG. Influence of the porosity of starch-based fiber mesh scaffolds on the proliferation and osteogenic differentiation of bone marrow stromal cells cultured in a flow perfusion bioreactor. *Tissue Eng* 2006; 12:801–809.
78. Kasten P, Beyen I, Niemeyer P, Luginbühl R, Bohner M, Richter W. Porosity and pore size of b-tricalcium phosphate scaffold can influence protein production and osteogenic differentiation of human mesenchymal stem cells: An in vitro and in vivo study. *Acta Biomater* 2008; 4:1904–1915.

79. Bai F, Wang Z, Lu JX, Liu JA, Chen GY, Lv R, Wang J, Lin K, Zhang J, Huang X. The correlation between the internal structure and vascularization of controllable porous bioceramic materials in vivo: A quantitative study. *Tissue Eng Part A* 2010; 16:3791–3803.
80. Chiu YC, Cheng MH, Engel H, Kao SW, Larson JC, Gupta S, Brey EM. The role of pore size on vascularization and tissue remodelling in PEG hydrogels. *Biomaterials* 2011; 32:6045–6051.
81. Choi SW, Zhang Y, Macewan MR, Xia Y. Neovascularization in biodegradable inverse opal scaffolds with uniform and precisely controlled pore sizes. *Adv Healthc Mater* 2013; 2:145–154.
82. Tsuruga E, Takita H, Itoh H, Wakisaka Y, Kuboki Y. Pore size of porous hydroxyapatite as the cell-substratum controls BMP-induced osteogenesis. *J Biochem* 1997; 121:317–324.
83. Feng B, Jinkang Z, Zhen W, Jianxi L, Jiang C, Jian L, Guolin M, Xin D. The effect of pore size on tissue ingrowth and neovascularization in porous bioceramics of controlled architecture in vivo. *Biomed Mater* 2011; 6:015007.
84. Guarino V, Causa F, Ambrosio L. Porosity and mechanical properties relationship in PCL porous scaffolds. *J Appl Biomater Biomech* 2007; 5:149–157.
85. Ikeda R, Fujioka H, Nagura I, Kokubu T, Toyokawa N, Inui A, Makino T, Kaneko H, Doita M, Kurosaka M. The effect of porosity and mechanical property of a synthetic polymer scaffold on repair of osteochondral defects. *Int Orthop* 2009; 33:821–828.
86. Nehrer S, Breinan HA, Ramappa A, Young G, Shortkroff S, Louie LK, Sledge CB, Yannas IV, Spector M. Matrix collagen type and pore size influence behaviour of seeded canine chondrocytes. *Biomoterials* 1997; 16:769–776.
87. Murphy CM, Haugh MG, O'Brien FJ. The effect of mean pore size on cell attachment, proliferation and migration in collagen-glycosaminoglycan scaffolds for tissue engineering. *Biomaterials* 2010; 31(3):461–466
88. Melchels FP, Barradas AM, van Blitterswijk CA, de Boer J, Feijen J, Grijpma DW. Effects of the architecture of tissue engineering scaffolds on cell seeding and culturing. *Acta Biomater* 2010; 6:4208–4217.
89. Hynes RO, Kenneth MY. *Extracellular Matrix Biology*. Cold Spring Harbor, NY: Cold Spring Harbor Laboratory, 2012.
90. Norman JJ, Desai TA. Methods for fabrication of nanoscale topography for tissue engineering scaffolds. *Ann Biomed Eng* 2006; 34:89–101
91. Zhang SG. Fabrication of novel biomaterials through molecular self-assembly. *Nat Biotechnol* 2003; 21:1171–1178.
92. Dahlin RL, Kasper FK, Mikos AG. Polymeric nanofibers in tissue engineering. *Tissue Eng Part B: Reviews* 2011; 17:349–364.
93. van de Witte P, Dijkstra PJ, van den. Berg JWA, Feijen J. Phase separation processes in polymer solutions in relation to membrane formation. *J Membr Sci* 1996; 117:1–31.
94. Mikos AG. Temenoff J. Formation of highly porous biodegradable scaffolds for tissue engineering. *Electron J Biotechnol* 2000; 3:114–119.
95. Jayaraman K, Kotaki M, Zhang Y, Mo X, Ramakrishna S. Recent advances in polymer nano-fibers. *J Nanosci Nanotechnol* 2004; 4:52–65.
96. Murugan R, Ramakrishna S. Nano-featured scaffolds for tissue engineering: a review of spinning methodologies. *Tissue Eng* 2006; 12:435–447.

97. Bhardwaj N, Kundu SC. Electrospinning: A fascinating fiber fabrication technique. *Biotechnol Adv* 2010; 28:325–347.
98. Rim NG, Shin CS, Shin H. Current approaches to electrospun nano-fibers for tissue engineering. *Biomed Mater* 2013; 8:014102.
99. Schmidt DR, Waldeck H, Kao WJ. Protein adsorption to biomaterials. In: Puleo DA, Bizios R, (eds.). *Biological Interactions on Materials Surfaces*. New York: Springer, 2009. pp. 1–18.
100. Latour RA. Biomaterials: protein–surface interactions. In: Wnek GE, Bowlin GL, (eds.). *The Encyclopedia of Biomaterials and Bioengineering*. New York: Informa Healthcare, 2008. pp. 270–284.
101. von Recum AF, Van Kooten. TG. The influence of micro-topography on cellular response and the implication for silicone implants. *J Biomater Sci Polym Ed* 1995; 7:181–198.
102. Ballard JD, Dulgar-Tulloch AJ, Siegel RW. Nanophase materials. In: *Wiley Encyclopedia of Biomedical Engineering*. New York: Wiley, 2006. pp. 2489–2507.
103. Woo KM, Chen VJ, Ma PX. Nano-fibrous scaffolding architecture selectively enhances protein adsorption contributing to cell attachment. *J Biomed Mater Res A* 2003; 67:531–537.
104. Binulal NS, Deepthy M, Selvamurugan N, Shalumon KT, Suja S, Mony U, Jayakumar R, Nair SV. Role of nanofibrous poly(caprolactone) scaffolds in human mesenchymal stem cell attachment and spreading for in vitro bone tissue engineering-response to osteogenic regulators. *Tissue Eng Part A* 2010; 16:393–404.
105. Ballard JD. Investigation of cell adhesion to silica nanoparticle-decorated surfaces and the associated protein mediated mechanisms. Ph.D. Dissertation, 2005, Rensselaer Polytechnic Institute, Department of Materials Science and Engineering, Troy, NY.
106. Vertegel AA, Siegel RW, Dordick JS. Silica nanoparticle size influences the structure and enzymatic activity of adsorbed lysozyme. *Langmuir* 2004; 20: 6800–6807.
107. Galli C, Coen MC, Hauert R, Katanaev VL, Wymann MP, Gröning P, Schlapbach L. Protein adsorption on topographically nanostructured titanium. *Surf Sci* 2001; 74:180–L184.
108. Rosenberg MD. Cell guidance by alterations in monomolecular films. *Science* 1963; 139:411–412.
109. Jäger M, Zilkens C, Zanger K, Krauspe R. Significance of nano- and micro-topography for cell-surface interactions in orthopaedic implants. *J Biomed Biotechnol* 2007; 8:69036.
110. Stevens MM, George JH. Exploring and engineering the cell surface interface. *Science* 2005; 310:1135–1138.
111. Andersson AS, Bäckhed F, von Euler. A, Richter-Dahlfors A, Sutherland D, Kasemo B. Nanoscale features influence epithelial cell morphology and cytokine production. *Biomaterials* 2003; 24:3427–36.
112. Ma Z, Kotaki M, Inai R, Ramakrishna S. Potential of nanofiber matrix as tissue-engineering scaffolds. *Tissue Eng* 2005; 11:101–109.
113. Li WJ, Chiang H, Kuo TF, Lee HS, Jiang CC, Tuan RS. Evaluation of articular cartilage repair using biodegradable nanofibrous scaffolds in a swine model: A pilot study. *Biomaterials* 2003; 24:2077–2082.

114. Shin M, Yoshimoto H, Vacanti JP. In vivo bone tissue engineering using mesenchymal stem cells on a novel electrospun nano fibrous scaffold. *J Tissue Eng Regen Med.* 2009; 3:1–10.

115. Jang JH, Castano O, Kim HW. Electrospun materials as potential platforms for bone tissue engineering. *Adv Drug Deliv Rev* 2009; 61:1065–1083.

116. R Vasita. DS Katti. Nanofibers and their application in tissue engineering. *Int J Nanomed* 2006; 1:15–30.

117. Shakhssalim N, Dehghan MM, Moghadasali R, Soltani MH, Shabani I, Soleimani M. Bladder tissue engineering using biocompatible nanofibrous electrospun constructs: Feasibility and safety investigation. *Urol J* 2012; 9:410–419.

118. Yoshimoto H, Shin YM, Terai H, Vacanti JP. A biodegradable nanofiber scaffold by electrospinning and its potential for bone tissue engineering. *Biomaterials* 2003; 24:2077–2082.

119. Li WJ, Laurencin CT, Caterson EJ, Tuan RS, Frank KK. Electrospunnano-fibrous structure: A novel scaffold for tissue engineering. *J Biomed Mater Res* 2002; 60:613–621.

120. Li WJ, Danielson KG, Alexander PG, Tuan RS. Biological response of chondrocytes cultured in three-dimensional nano-fibrous poly (caprolactone) scaffolds. *J Biomed Mater Res A* 2003; 67:1105–1114.

121. Li WJ, Tuli R, Okafor C, Derfoul A, Danielson KG, Hall DJ, Tuan RS. A three-dimensional nano-fibrous scaffold for cartilage tissue engineering using human mesenchymal stem cells. *Biomaterials* 2005; 26:599–609.

122. Price RL, Waid MC, Haberstroh KM, Webster TJ. Selective bone cell adhesion on formulations containing carbon nano-fibers. *Biomaterials* 2003; 24:1877–1887.

123. Elias KL, Price R.L, Webster TJ. Enhanced functions of osteoblasts on nanometer diameter carbon fibers. *Biomaterials* 2002; 23:3279–3287.

124. Pattison MA,Wurster S,Webster TJ, Haberstroh KM. Three-dimensional, nano-structured PLGA scaffolds for bladder tissue replacement applications. *Biomaterials* 2005; 26:2491–2500.

125. Divya Rani VV, Manzoor K, Menon D, Nair S. The design of novel nanostructures on titanium by solution chemistry for an improved osteoblast response. *Nanotechnology* 2009; 20:195101.

126. Hsiao CW, Bai MY, Chang Y, Chung MF, Lee TY, Wu CT, Maiti B, Liao ZX, Li RK, Sung HW. Electrical coupling of isolated cardiomyocyte clusters grown on aligned conductive nanofibrous meshes for their synchronized beating. *Biomaterials* 2013; 34:1063–1072.

127. Luong TH Nguyen, Susan Liao, Seeram Ramakrishna, Casey K Chan. The role of nanofibrous structure in osteogenic differentiation of human mesenchymal stem cells with serial passage. *Nanomedicine* 2011; 6:961–974.

128. Vacanti V, Kong E, Suzuki G, Sato K, Canty JM, Lee T. Phenotypic changes of adult porcine mesenchymal stem cells induced by prolonged passaging in culture. *J Cell Physiol* 2005; 205:194–201.

129. Colosimo A, Russo V, Mauro A, Curini V, Marchisio M, Bernabò N, Alfonsi M, Mattioli M, Barboni B. Prolonged in vitro expansion partially affects phenotypic features and osteogenic potential of ovine amniotic fluid-derived mesenchymal stromal cells. *Cytotherapy* 2013; 15:930–950.

3

Ceramic Composites for Bone Graft Applications

Joel D. Bumgardner, Carlos M. Wells, and Warren O. Haggard

CONTENTS

3.1 Introduction

The repair of bone defects from trauma or disease continues to be an active clinical need. This need is intensified when dental/craniofacial applications are considered. As a result, new products are continuously being researched and developed. Approximately six million bone fractures with bone loss occur in the United States each year.[1] This loss of bone in long bone fracture or dental procedures requires the use of some type of bone graft. Bone graft choices can be autograft, allograft, processed from natural materials, synthetic, or any combination of these with or without other biological agents or materials. Collagraft® bone graft substitute, PRO-DENSE®, the MASTERGRAFT® family of products, and STRUCSURE™ CP will be the products discussed herein. The chapter will address the reasons for the composite approach of these bone graft materials to help highlight their advantages for clinical use. The chapter goal is to acquaint the reader with some background and engineering for these representative bone graft composites.

3.2 Collagraft

Collagraft bone graft substitute was an early bone graft composite of collagen and hydroxyapatite developed and commercialized by Zimmer and Collagen Corporation. Collagraft was developed to partially simulate the major components in bone: collagen and hydroxyapatite. Collagraft received approval to market in 1993 by the U.S. Food and Drug Administration (FDA) through a Premarket Approval application.[2,3] Collagraft bone substitute is a composite of type 1 bovine dermal fibular collagen and a biphasic calcium phosphate ceramic, with each individual granule containing separate microdomains of hydroxyapatite (HA) and tricalcium phosphate (TCP) phases of a calcium phosphate ceramic. Collagraft created a combination of materials that were similar to bone and could have cells or other osteogenic materials/agents added to this synthetic graft.[4] The combination of collagen with fast and slow degrading bioceramics presents a bone graft scaffold that allows for new bone formation.[1] Multiple preclinical and clinical studies for bone graft repair reported the successful use of this bone graft composite with various biological agents and/or materials.[4–6] Collagraft was the initial approved composite bone graft substitute and thus laid a developmental outline for subsequent bone graft substitute composites. It was the first composite bone grafting material containing both a calcium phosphate ceramic and a collagen binder. Previous bone-grafting products were just loose ceramic granules while Collagraft's formulation provides a stable matrix for cells to attach to and deposit new bone within. Collagraft is no longer marketed/distributed through Zimmer; it is currently marketed/distributed through NeuColl, Inc. (Campbell, CA).

3.3 PRO-DENSE

3.3.1 General Information and Indications

Calcium sulfate (CS) has been used successfully as a bone void filler for over 120 years, but there have been reports of sterile effusion theorized to be due to the rapid dissolution of CS in vivo.[7] The osteogenic activity of each component combined with the crystalline phase-dependent dissolution rates (calcium sulfate > brushite > β-tricalcium phosphate) produce a novel resorbable bolus for the encouragement of a material-assisted therapy aimed at "creeping-substitution" bone healing. In comparison, products based on various calcium phosphate minerals have been shown to be osteoconductive and biocompatible, but often exhibit extremely slow in vivo dissolution profiles that prevent complete regeneration of bone. The injectable, in situ curing PRO-DENSE Bone Graft Substitute (Wright Medical Technology, Inc., Memphis, TN) cement has been engineered such that the physiochemical and osteoconductive properties of calcium sulfate and calcium phosphates are utilized in a complimentary manner which results in notable rates of osteogenesis within bone voids. The bone graft composite material is marketed in sterile kits which contain two vials (a precursor powder/β-tricalcium phosphate granule blend component and an aqueous liquid component), a vacuum mixing apparatus, and a syringe/Jamshidi® needle for minimally invasive delivery to a bone defect site.[8] By mixing the liquid and powder/granule components, two cement reactions are initiated and allowed to proceed in unison, forming a calcium sulfate dihydrate (gypsum) and calcium hydrogen phosphate dihydrate (brushite) matrix encompassing a distributed phase of β-tricalcium phosphate granules (see reaction formulas at the end of this section).[9,10] While in the preset paste form, the material can be syringe-loaded and injection-delivered via a large gauge needle; here, it can conform to defect site boundaries and harden in situ. Ultimately, after placement, the cured cement is a triphasic blend of calcium salts formed to the shape of a bone void. The cured product is a composite cement blend on a microscopic scale, largely consisting of gypsum with a lesser brushite component incorporating β-tricalcium phosphate granules (see Figure 3.1a).[10] Granules are mechanically incorporated chemically through the involvement of surface reactions with the brushite system, locking them into the phosphate matrix. An underlying dogma of composite science is to utilize the beneficial properties of multiple materials in a concerted effort such that in combination the resultant exhibits multifunctional and improved properties over those of the individual constituents, and such synergistic effects have been exhibited by PRO-DENSE as a bone void filler medical device.

Calcium sulfate hemihydrate to calcium sulfate dihydrate (gypsum) reaction:

$$2(CaSO_4 \cdot \tfrac{1}{2} H_2O) + 3H_2O \rightarrow 2(CaSO_4 \cdot 2H_2O)$$

Monocalcium phosphate monohydrate and beta-tricalcium phosphate to calcium hydrogen phosphate dihydrate (brushite) reaction:

$$Ca(H_2PO_4)_2 \cdot H_2O + 3Ca_3(PO_4)_2 + 7H_2O \rightarrow 4(CaHPO_4 \cdot 2H_2O)$$

3.3.2 Physical/Mechanical/Degradation Properties

The dissolution profile of PRO-DENSE's components combined with their microscopic structural integration appears to result in a mechanically supported dynamic structure in vivo, resulting in a resorption profile that greatly accommodates the multiple phases of osteogenesis across fractures, voids, and surgically created gaps. The fundamental steps associated with bridging such a defect have been generally described as overlapping stages of inflammation, repair, and remodeling.[11] The triphasic composition of PRO-DENSE has been shown to demonstrate tiered dissolution kinetics in vitro as faster dissolving calcium sulfate is released leaving behind a highly porous, slower resorbing calcium phosphate structure, which largely retains the original overall geometry of the initial set cement. Figures 3.1 and 3.2 show the results of an accelerated dissolution study in distilled water.

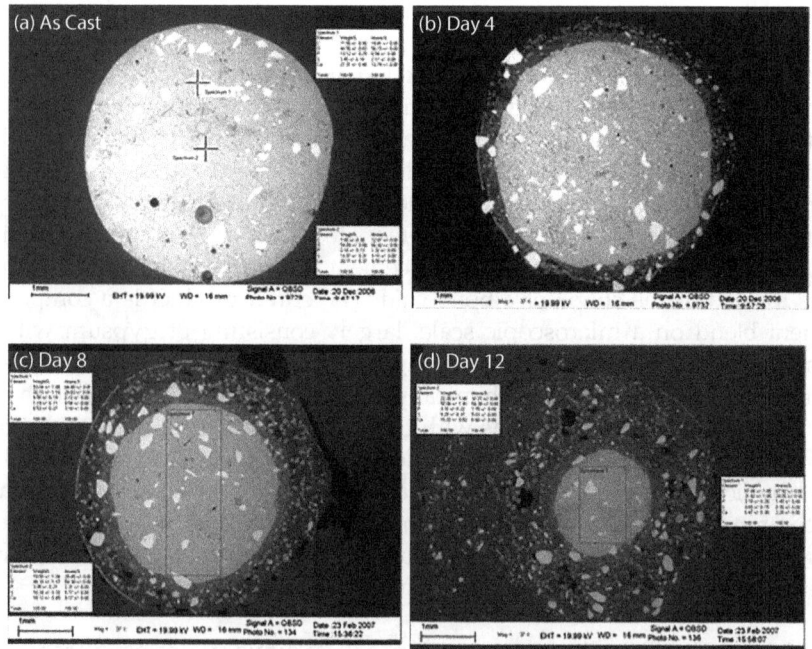

FIGURE 3.1

Exemplary micrographs of PRO-DENSE's staged dissolution profile are shown. Cast cylinders (3.3 x 4.8 mm OD) were exposed to an accelerated in vitro dissolution protocol using distilled water. Representative specimens at time points 0, 4, 8, and 12 days (frames a, b, c, and d, respectively) were withheld from further treatment for electron microscopy and electron dispersive spectroscopy processing (plastic embedded, polished, and cross-sections scanned). High-density β-tricalcium phosphate granules (white aggregate) can be seen throughout the continuous, composite matrix of gypsum ($CaSO_4 \cdot H_2O$) and brushite ($CaHPO_4 \cdot 2(H_2O)$) (light grey) in frame a. Consecutive frames (b-d) demonstrate the phosphate- and sulfate-staged dissolution of the composite. Note that as the faster dissolving sulfate component is dissolved, a highly porous yet structural osteoconductive brushite cement/β-tricalcium phosphate granule scaffold is left behind. Complete resorption of the material can be inferred through observation that the slowest dissolving granule/brushite components demonstrate an ever-reducing cross-sectional area with treatment time (a through d).[17]

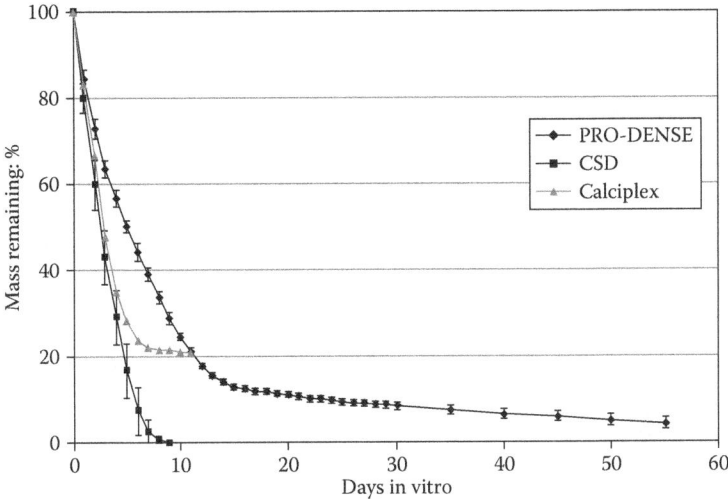

FIGURE 3.2

Results from an accelerated in vitro dissolution protocol are shown. Percent mass loss with time as a result of dissolving into distilled water has been monitored for pure calcium sulfate, pure calcium phosphate, and the composite PRO-DENSE material. PRO-DENSE's (diamond) tiered dissolution profile is demonstrated through comparison with faster dissolving pure calcium sulfate (CSD—square) and slower dissolving pure tricalcium phosphate (Calciplex— triangle). The composite nature of PRO-DENSE results in an extended yet ever-dissipating mass. Note—Continued monitoring of specimen masses was halted upon approaching steady state (PRO-DENSE's approach to complete dissolution). Calciplex was a blend of α- and β-tricalcium phosphate. It may be assumed that a majority of the α-tricalcium phosphate phase transformed to hydroxyapatite in the aqueous environment of the study, resulting in the 20% mass retention.[10]

Mass loss was measured as a function of time in vitro for cast pellets of PRO-DENSE, pure calcium sulfate, and pure calcium phosphate materials.[10] At selected time points, pellets were embedded in plastic, cross-sectioned, and polished to assess the morphology.[10] The early, more rapid dissolution kinetics of the calcium sulfate may harness the early stages of repair in which neovascularization penetrates and high-collagen-level woven bone is throughout a defect site in an inward-working fashion. The later, slower dissolution kinetics of the remaining phosphate compounds may support biomaterial-assisted remodeling of the immature bone through both osteoblast-assisted mineralization of woven bone to a high mechanical integrity state. Also, osteoclast-assisted resorption and dissolution of the final implant material will occur later. This theory of assisting in staged healing is supported by preclinical in vivo canine studies using critically sized defects, where histology identified bone cells and tissue types incorporated within the partially resorbed material.[12] PRO-DENSE has resulted in a statistically significant increased healing rate over that of autograft and pure calcium sulfate in critical defects based on biomechanical and histological findings (see Table 3.1 and Figures 3.3 and 3.4).[12]

TABLE 3.1

Biomechanical Tensile Test Data of Cored Trabecular Bone Specimens Are Presented.

Implant Material	In-Life Time (weeks)	Ultimate Compressive Strength $\pm$ SD (MPa); n	Modulus of Elasticity $\pm$ SD (MPa); n
		Compression Test Results of the Canine Proximal Humerus Osseous Preclinical Model	
PRO-DENSE®	13	5.29 ± 2.61; $n = 5$	283 ± 217; $n = 5$
PRO-DENSE®	26	2.19 ± 0.41; $n = 5$	150 ± 73.5; $n = 5$
Autograft	13	0.71 ± 0.31; $n = 8$	40.41 ± 21.72; $n = 10$
Normal healthy bone	NA	1.38 ± 0.66; $n = 8$	117 ± 71.5; $n = 8$

Source: Walsh WR, et al., *Clin Orthop Relat Res*, 375:258–266, 2000.

Note: Cored regions were from critically sized defects sites treated with either injectable PRO-DENSE® or autograft. Additionally, results of normal trabecular bone cores harvested from the same anatomical region are shown for comparison.

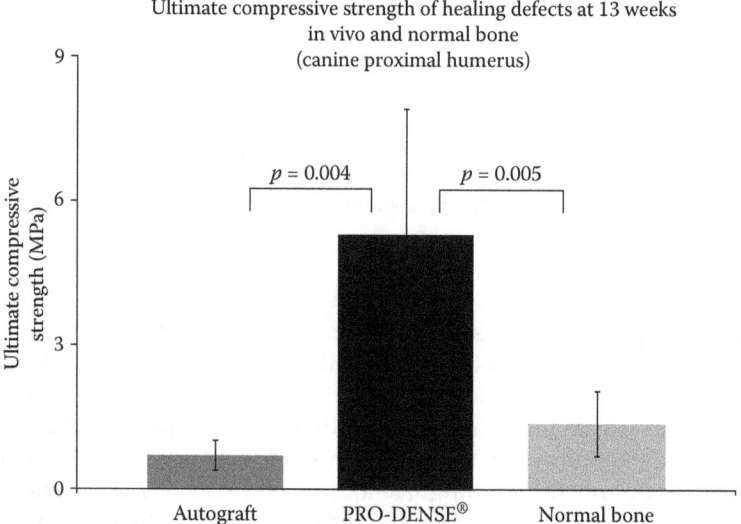

FIGURE 3.3

Ultimate compressive strength values associated with graft-assisted healing at the 13-week time point of a critically sized osseous canine proximal humerus in vivo preclinical model are shown. Additionally, values found for normal trabecular bone harvested from the same anatomical location is the comparison. Averages and standard deviations are shown. At 13 weeks, defects treated with PRO-DENSE demonstrated advanced healing over the autograft group based on a significant increase in ultimate compressive strength over the autograft group ($p = 0.004$). The increase in strength over that of normal bone seen for the PRO-DENSE groups decreased with time after 13 weeks, and biomechanical properties approached that of normal bone at a later 26-week time point.[12]

PRO-DENSE®   Autograft

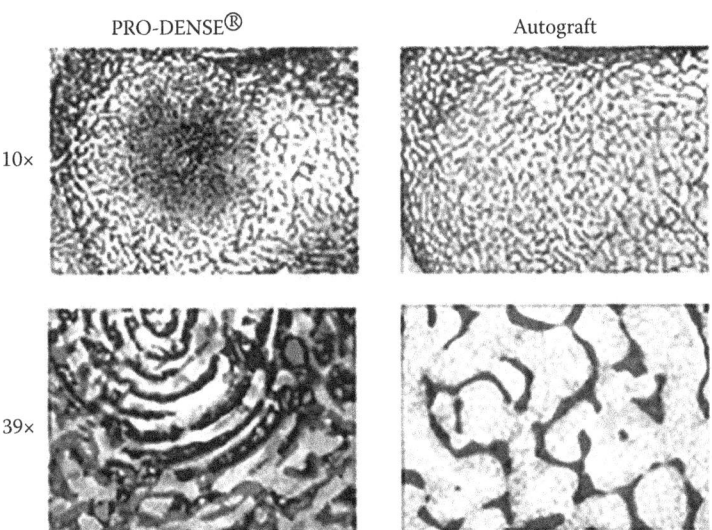

FIGURE 3.4
Plastic embedded, ground, and H&E stained section histology images are shown of canine proximal humerus critically sized defects treated with PRO-DENSE (left) and autograft (right) at the 13-week time point. PRO-DENSE images show increased new bone formation within the defect site in comparison to the remodeled defect of the autograft-treated site. A minor amount of PRO-DENSE material continues to be resorbed and can be seen as the dark material (gypsum/brushite) encompassing consolidated white material (β-tricalcium phosphate granules). Note the osteoconductivity of the PRO-DENSE material as new bone is well incorporated throughout the defect site and in contact with the highly porous matrix, which results from PRO-DENSE resorption.[12]

Such defects model highly compromised nonunion fractures, where treatment can be very challenging.[12] These studies, in combination with the known healing cascade, are suggestive of the potential benefit PRO-DENSE offers over more traditional, single-component bone graft substitutes which resorb through linear kinetics via an "outside-in" fashion, such as that of Wright Medical's comparatively faster resorbing pure calcium sulfate bone graft substitutes. The bulk materials of the composite PRO-DENSE demonstrate comparatively slower resorption, such as found in commercially available hydroxyapatite cements.[13,14] Clinical complications have been associated with the faster resorbing materials; sterile exudates and delayed mineralization have been noted within the literature.[15,16]

3.3.3 Biological/Preclinical Studies

Supplementing the passive, yet favorable, nature of PRO-DENSE's multiphase dissolution in vivo is the bioactive phenomenon of a well-orchestrated relationship between protein adsorption and desorption on the material's surface and the beneficial cellular activities that emanate on and are adjacent to the composite cement as a result of these dynamic processes. In vitro protein adsorption/desorption studies have demonstrated that osteogenesis-related chemotactic agents, angiogenic factors, and differentiation factors exhibit a higher affinity for PRO-DENSE versus pure calcium sulfate. Bone morphogenetic protein-2 (BMP-2) and vascular endothelial growth factor (VEGF) have demonstrated preferential absorption onto the surface of PRO-DENSE over pure calcium sulfate.[17] Preservation of protein functionality has been demonstrated through release of absorbed VEGF from PRO-DENSE's surface. PRO-DENSE specimens exposed to VEGF-containing buffer solutions for various times passively desorbed protein into fresh solutions where chemotactic bioactivity was shown to be retained in vascular endothelial cells (see Figure 3.5). The novel addition of calcium phosphate cement and granules with calcium sulfate cement results in a more bioactive composite over calcium sulfate alone and may explain the enhanced tissue healing response associated with PRO-DENSE over that of pure calcium sulfate and autograft treatment seen in preclinical canine models.[12]

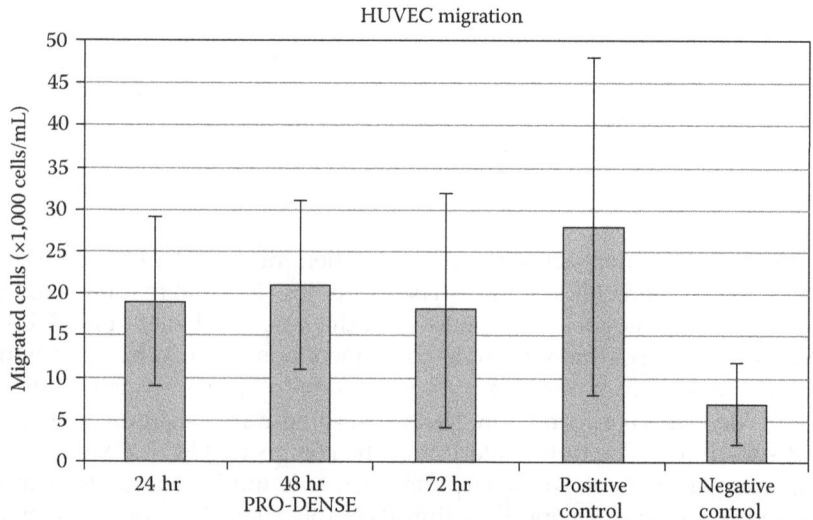

FIGURE 3.5
Chemotaxis results (average cell count and standard deviation) from an in vitro study in which human umbilical vein endothelial cells (HUVECs) migrated through transwell plate filters are shown, demonstrating PRO-DENSE's angiogenic potential. PRO-DENSE demonstrated the ability to sustain release of VEGF over a 72-hour period in vitro, inferring absorption of the protein as well. VEGF-containing eluates, derived from a protein absorbtion/desorption protocol from PRO-DENSE surface, were used for the experimental conditions shown. Desorption was allowed for the times shown (24, 48, and 72 hours). The positive and negative controls were 40 ng/mL VEGF in phosphate buffer and buffer alone, respectively.[17]

3.3.4 Clinical Studies

This composite bone graft substitute has been used with large success in U.S. clinics since its FDA marketing approvals in 2007 as a bone void filler and a core decompression material for the osteonecrotic femoral head.[18,19] Clinical studies have largely reported positive findings with use of the injectable graft. In retrospective studies, a 24 patient population with benign primary bone tumors was successfully treated with PRO-DENSE.[20,21] In 21 of 24 patients bone void repair was achieved with early return to load bearing activity.[20,21] There were two tumor recurrences and one infection in this small series after wound break-down events.[20,21] Another large retrospective study on PRO-DENSE's treatment of benign tumors was conducted by Fillingham, et al. where 56 patients' records were reviewed with a high degree of treatment benefit. In this study, the following adverse events were observed: three recurrences (successfully treated through an additional administration of PRO-DENSE or curettage), two post-op fractures (treated through closed technique), and two cases of wound complications that did not require graft retrieval.[22] Backfilling of the surgical site and replacement of the necrotic bone space in hip core decompression surgeries was prospectively evaluated by Civinini et al. The treatment of 37 enrolled patients' hips revealed the following clinical observations: a statistically significant increase in average Harris hip score (68 to 86), either radiographic improvement or the absence of further collapse in 29 (78.4%) of these hips, and disease progression to the stage that arthroplasty was required in three hips.[23] These mostly successful clinical experiences with the use of PRO-DENSE reflect positive effects that can be achieved with the innovative design of this composite bone graft substitute.

Collectively, the aforementioned work illustrates PRO-DENSE to be a novel composite from material and biologic perspectives, and a biomaterial with a unique blend of physiochemical and bioactive functionality that has proven efficacious in the treatment of clinically demanding bone voids.

3.4 MASTERGRAFT Family of Products

3.4.1 General Information and Indications

In the United States, the MASTERGRAFT family of products includes MASTERGRAFT Granules, MASTERGRAFT Mini Granules, MASTERGRAFT Putty, MASTERGRAFT Strip, and MASTERGRAFT Matrix EXT. The Granules (diameter 1.6–3.2 mm) and Mini Granules (diameter 0.5–1.6 mm) are biphasic calcium phosphate (BCP) ceramic bone void fillers composed of 85% beta-tricalcium phosphate (β-TCP) and 15% hydroxyapatite (HA) by mass.[24,25] This ratio falls within the range described in the literature as an optimal ratio for use in vivo.[26–28] These ceramic granules have an interconnected porous structure that facilitates bone ingrowth.[29] The Putty, Strip, and Matrix EXT products are composite materials that combine the BCP ceramic granules with bovine type I collagen.

The MASTERGRAFT Granules and Mini Granules (Figures 3.6 through 3.8) are indicated for filling of bony voids or gaps not intrinsic to the

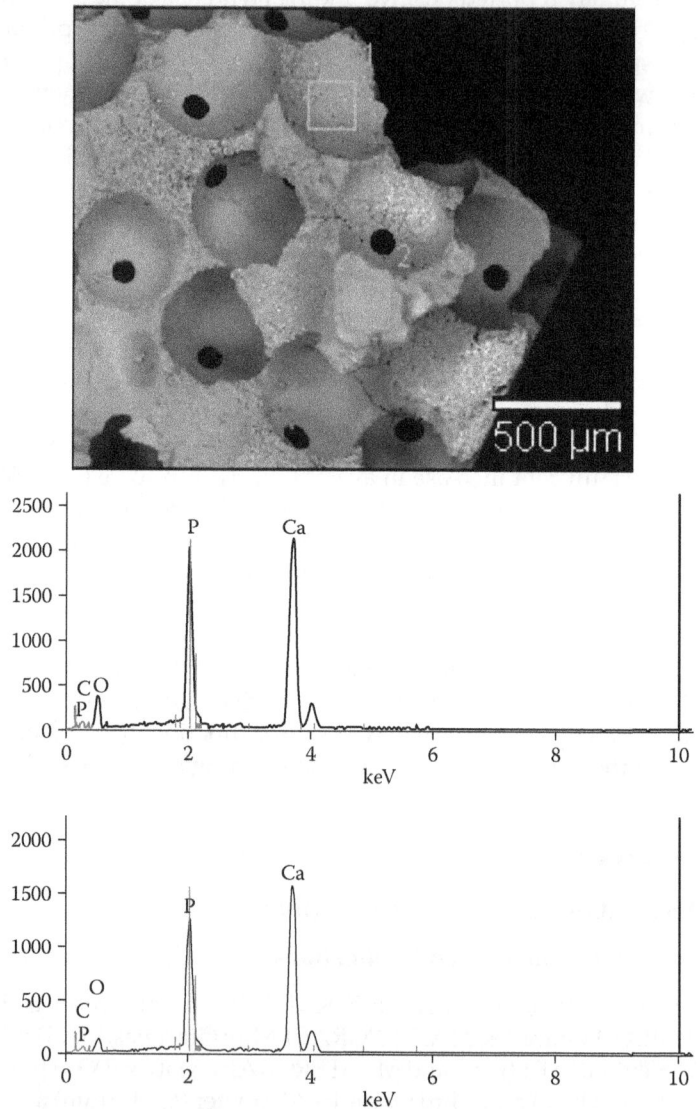

FIGURE 3.6

Top: Scanning electron microscopy (SEM) image of MASTERGRAFT Granules. The porous struc-ture of the ceramic granule can be seen. Middle: Energy Dispersive X-ray Spectroscopy (EDS) spectrum of Region 1 in the SEM. Peaks representing calcium and phosphorus are seen. Bottom: EDS spectrum of Region 2 in the SEM. Peaks representing calcium and phosphorus are seen.

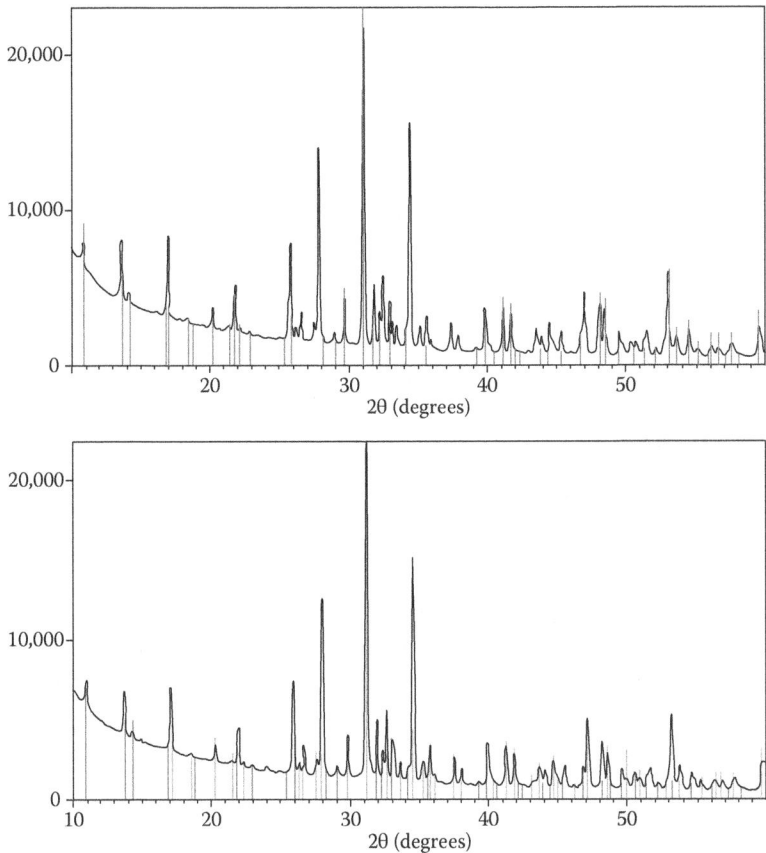

FIGURE 3.7
X-ray diffractograms (XRD). Top: XRD showing the crystal structure of MASTERGRAFT Granules. Bottom: XRD showing the crystal structure of MASTERGRAFT Strip. Note that the same peaks are present for both materials.

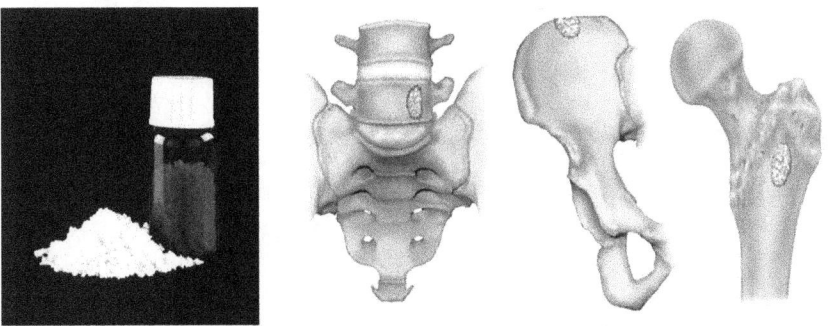

FIGURE 3.8
MASTERGRAFT Granules. Left: Photograph of Granules. Right: Schematic showing bone voids filled with Granules.

stability of the bony structure including the extremities, pelvis, ilium, and posterolateral spine.[24] They are also indicated for use in oral/maxillofacial applications including filling of dental extraction sockets and cystic defects.[25] The smaller size of the Mini Granules allows them to be used for the filling of periodontal defects, sinus lifts, and alveolar ridge augmentation.[25] The ability of MASTERGRAFT Granules to promote osseous filling of alveolar extraction sockets and backfilling of iliac crest defects has been demonstrated.[30,31]

MASTERGRAFT Putty (Figures 3.9 and 3.10) is a composite material indicated for filling of bony voids or gaps not intrinsic to the stability of the bony structure and also for oral/maxillofacial applications. MASTERGRAFT Putty contains BCP particles (diameter 0.5–1.6 mm) uniformly distributed throughout bovine type I collagen for enhanced handling characteristics.[32,33] The collagen is a combination of 70% insoluble fibrous collagen and 30% soluble collagen.[29] Putty is supplied dry and becomes moldable when hydrated with autogenous bone marrow aspirate or sterile water.[32,33]

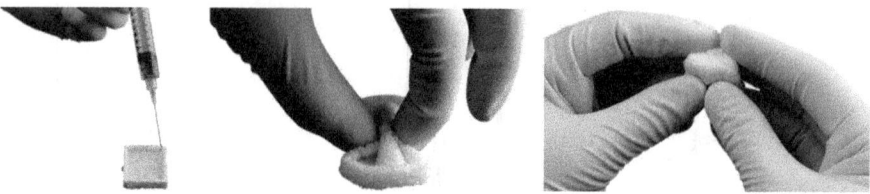

FIGURE 3.9
MASTERGRAFT Putty. Left: MASTERGRAFT Putty being hydrated with sterile water. Middle: The Putty is malleable after being hydrated. Right: Putty being manipulated after hydration.

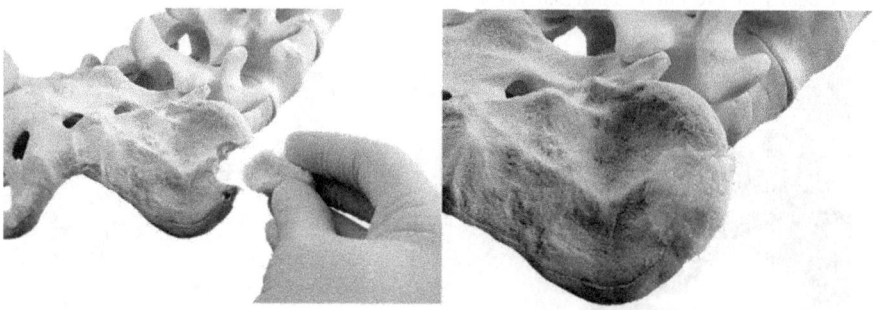

FIGURE 3.10
MASTERGRAFT Putty. Left: Example of Putty being placed into a bone void. Right: Close-up of Putty in bone void demonstrating the ability of Putty to conform to geometry of defect space.

MASTERGRAFT Strip (Figures 3.11 through 3.14) and Matrix EXT must be combined with autogenous bone marrow aspirate and are indicated for filling of bony voids or gaps not intrinsic to the stability of the bony structure. Strip and Matrix EXT are similar to Putty in that they contain BCP ceramic particles (diameter 0.5–1.6 mm) dispersed throughout bovine type I collagen; however, all of the collagen is insoluble and the mineral:collagen ratio is increased compared to that of Putty.[34,35] This formulation allows the products to be both flexible and compression-resistant. The ability to resist compression by the surrounding tissue and muscles maintains space at the defect site, facilitating complete bone healing in challenging applications such as posterolateral spine arthrodesis. Additionally, the geometry (2.0 cm wide, 0.6 cm thickness, and 10 cm or 36 cm lengths) and flexible nature of Strip allows a single implant to span multiple spinal levels. For instance, the 36-cm-long Strip can be used to fill the bony voids associated with scoliosis reconstructions.

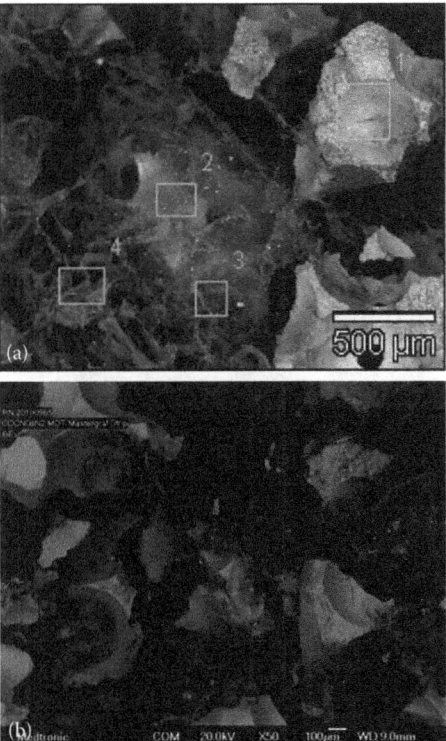

FIGURE 3.11
(a and b) SEM images of MASTERGRAFT Strip. The collagen and ceramic components of the composite can be seen. *(Continued)*

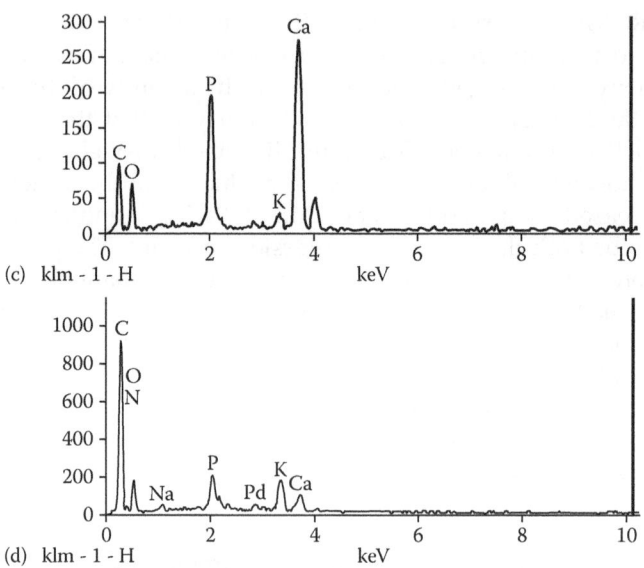

FIGURE 3.11 (*Continued*)
(c) Energy dispersive x-ray spectroscopy (EDS) spectrum of Region 1 in the SEM on the left. Peaks representing high levels of calcium and phosphorus indicative of ceramic are seen. (d) EDS spectrum of Region 4 in the SEM on the left. Peaks corresponding to high levels of carbon, nitrogen, and oxygen indicative of collagen are present.

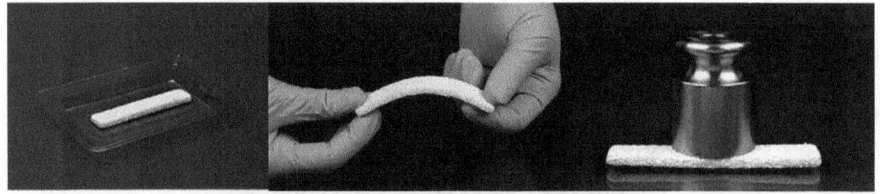

FIGURE 3.12
MASTERGRAFT Strip. Left: Strip in plastic tray. Middle: The flexibility of Strip is being demonstrated. Right: The compression resistance of Strip is shown.

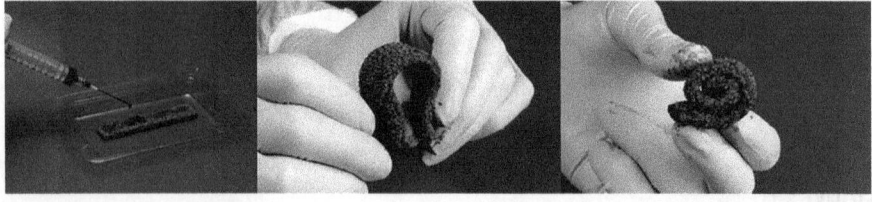

FIGURE 3.13
MASTERGRAFT Strip. Left: Strip is being hydrated with BMA. Middle and right: The Strip is extremely flexible after hydration.

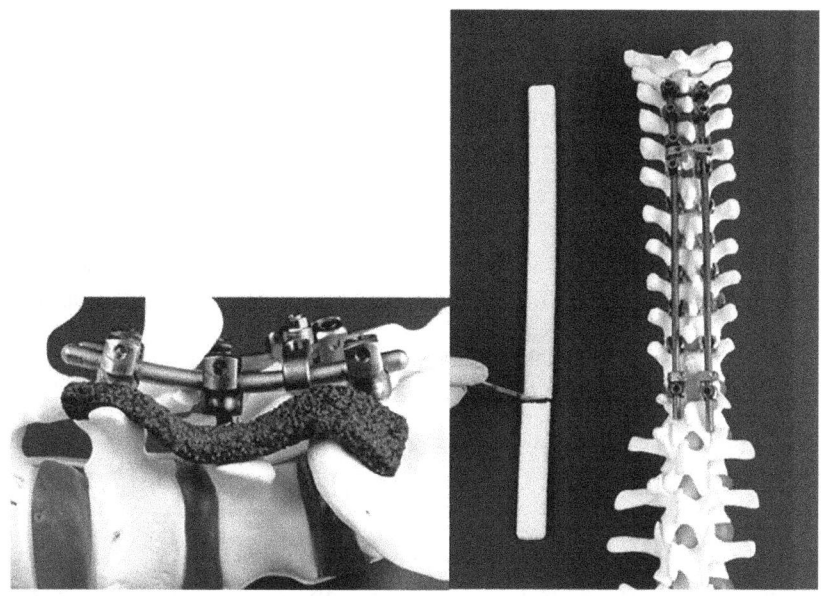

FIGURE 3.14

MASTERGRAFT Strip. Left: Demonstration of Strip being placed on the transverse processes of the spine. Right: The 36 cm long Strip is capable of spanning multiple spinal levels.

Since the MASTERGRAFT materials do not possess sufficient mechanical strength to support reduction of a defect site prior to soft and hard tissue ingrowth, rigid fixation methods are recommended as needed to ensure stabilization of the defect. If desired, autograft bone can be used in conjunction with the MASTERGRAFT products.[24,25,32–35] In rabbit posterolateral fusion studies, MASTERGRAFT Strip and Putty were successfully used as autograft extenders.[36,37] The advantage of these composites is that the addition of collagen to the BCP granules yields products with improved handling characteristics and reduces the possibility of granule migration from the defect site. The MASTERGRAFT family of products provides options for surgeons when selecting the proper bone void filler (Table 3.2).

3.5 STRUCSURE CP Cement

3.5.1 General Information and Indications

STRUCSURE CP cement from Smith & Nephew Inc. (Memphis, TN) is an injectable, self-setting bone graft substitute that incorporates hydroxypropyl methylcellulose (HPMC) into the formulation. This polymer/ceramic formulation allows greatly improved mixing and handling characteristics.

TABLE 3.2

The MASTERGRAFT Family of Products

Product	Composition	Description of Composite	Indication
MASTERGRAFT Granules and Mini Granules	Biphasic calcium phosphate (BCP) granules	N/A	Oral/maxillofacial bony tissue + bony voids or gaps of the skeletal system
MASTERGRAFT Putty	BCP granules + collagen (70% insoluble, 30% soluble)	Malleable	Oral/maxillofacial bony tissue + bony voids or gaps of the skeletal system
MASTERGRAFT Strip and Matrix EXT	BCP granules + insoluble collagen	Flexible and compression resistant	Bony voids or gaps of the skeletal system

The addition of the polymer provides multiple benefits including enhanced viscosity during curing, improved cohesion, and permeability of the cement. This improved rheological behavior allows the cement to be mixed and delivered from the syringe. The addition of a gun to hold the syringe allows a simple, one-handed delivery system.

3.5.2 Physical/Mechanical/Degradation Properties

Calcium phosphate cements are useful materials to replace or augment bone loss in orthopedic surgery.[38] Traditionally, these materials have required the materials engineer to balance a range of competing properties in the formulation selection. For example, increasing the viscosity of the cement to improve its injectability would also significantly decrease the set time of the final product. Early injectable cement systems had a viscosity that was initially very low and would increase with time as the setting reaction progressed. This would make the injection inconsistent throughout the delivery of the product. The initial, low viscosity of the product (similar to water) would make it difficult for the injected material to stay in place when injected. As the curing reaction progresses, the viscosity of the cement increases allowing the cement to be used; eventually, the viscosity becomes too high and the cement is no longer injectable. In some cases, this can result in the material setting before it can be injected. Another common issue with early products was a phenomenon called "filter press," which is a form of phase separation of the liquid and powder ingredients during mixing.[39] This can prematurely plug the tip of the syringe, thus preventing full use of the product.

By moving to a composite system, the trade-offs of a simple powder-liquid system were greatly changed, allowing for improved products to be developed. The components of the STRUCSURE CP cement system are shown in Figure 3.15. The inclusion of the polymer provides a more consistent viscosity throughout the injection of the cement. This is shown in Figure 3.16, which illustrates the force required to deliver STRUCSURE from a 10 mL syringe as a function of displacement. The test was conducted at a rate of 1 mm/min.

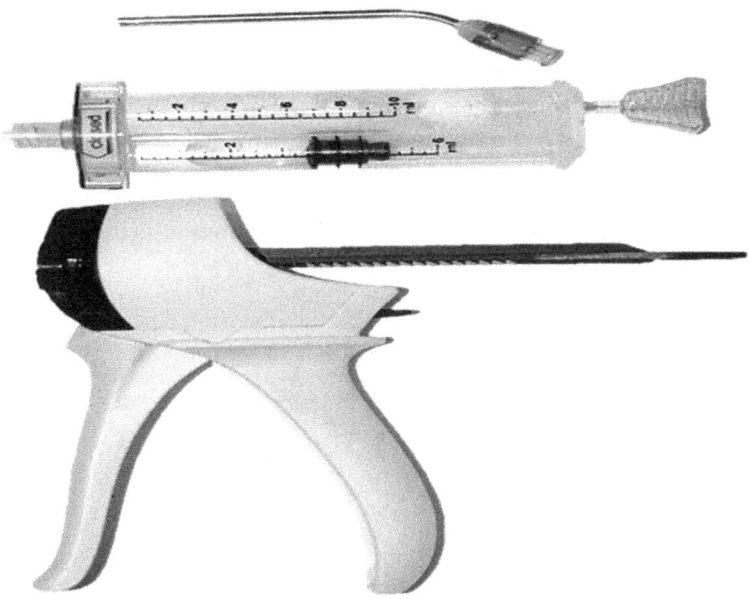

FIGURE 3.15
Components of the STRUCSURE CP delivery system. Top: Cannula. Middle: Mixing syringe pre-loaded with the powder and liquid components. Bottom: Delivery gun into which the syringe is placed after mixing. This allows a one-handed delivery of the mixed cement.

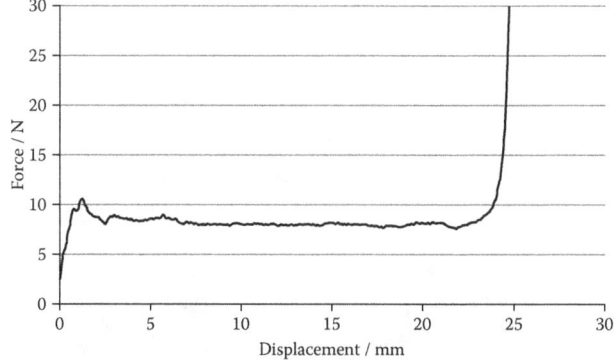

FIGURE 3.16
Injection force vs. displacement for the STRUCSURE CP cement. The force required to inject the cement is almost constant until the end of the syringe is reached at ~25mm displacement.[40]

The graph in Figure 3.16 shows an almost constant injection force for the cement, even though the setting reaction is ongoing. The cohesion of the material is also improved as the polymer acts to hold together the powder as it reacts and cures. These improved rheological and cohesive properties also allow the cement to stay in place, allowing the surgeon to have great control over the location of the material. This also allows the cement to be drilled and hardware (e.g., screws) to be inserted into the cement before it is fully cured.[41] The improved cohesion of the cement means it will not fracture or sag when a hole is drilled into the material (Figure 3.17). Figure 3.18 shows a cross-section of the cement after placement of hardware through the cement.

Finally, the water-soluble polymer will dissolve out of the cement in the first few days after implantation; this space vacated by the polymer will be replaced with the patient's extracellular fluids (interstitial fluid and blood plasma). This inclusion of extracellular fluids improves the biocompatibility and osteoconductivity of the implanted cement.

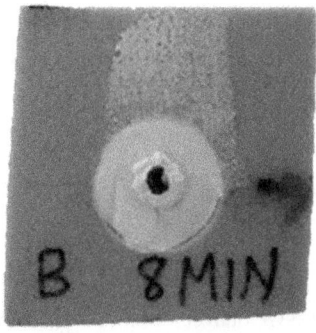

FIGURE 3.17
Photograph of STRUCSURE cement which was drilled 8 minutes after injection.

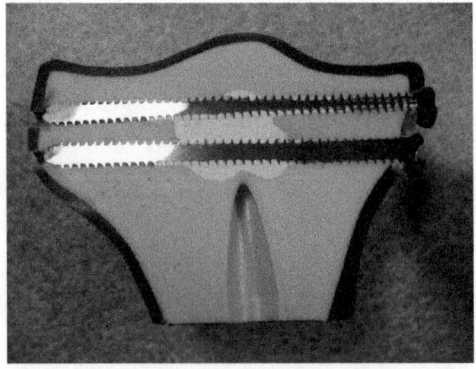

FIGURE 3.18
Sectioned Sawbone after insertion of hardware through cement.

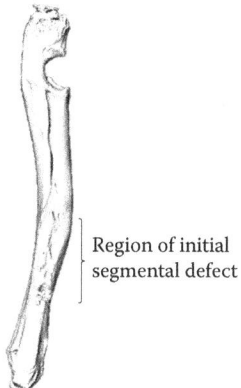

Region of initial
segmental defect

FIGURE 3.19
A micro-CT image showing the regenerated bone after 8 weeks. The segmental defect, which
was in the distal portion of the radius, is mostly filled with new bone.

3.5.3 Biological/Preclinical Study

STRUCSURE CP cement was evaluated in an in vivo model for its biocompatibility and osteoconductivity.[42] The cement was placed into 2 cm segmental defects made in the distal radius of New Zealand white rabbits. The performance of the STRUCSURE material was evaluated through radiological scoring and histological analysis, including measuring the percentage of bone in the defect at 4 and 8 weeks post-operatively. In all of these measures, the performance of the tested cement was compared to morselized autograft, the gold standard in scaffolds for bone regeneration. In this study, the STRUCSURE CP material behaved similarly to the autograft group. The STRUCSURE CP material was statistically equivalent to autograft in all measures at all time points apart from the amount of bone formed at 4 weeks as measured from the radiographs. No inflammatory response was seen in any of the animals. A micro-CT image of the treated defect, at 8 weeks, is shown in Figure 3.19.

3.6 Summary

With this chapter, several bone graft composites were discussed, while outlining the reasons for their composite approach. The clinical need for bone graft in musculoskeletal and dental/craniofacial applications continues to expand. Composite approaches to bone grafting, while currently clinically successful, may offer improved bone restoration outcomes in the future with further scientific and technical refinements.

Acknowledgements

The authors would like to thank Jonathan McCanless, Jon Moseley, John Rose, Ben Reeves, and Cheyenne Rhodes for their support and assistance with this book chapter.

References

1. Johnson EN, Burns TC, Hayda RA, Hospenthal DR, Murray CK. Infectious complications of open type III tibial fractures among combat casualties. *Clin Infect Dis*, 2007; 45(4):409–415.
2. FDA, COLLAGRAFT(TM) BONE GRAFT SUBSTITUTE, Docket # 93M-0210, PMA # P900039. NEUCOLL, INC, 05/28/1993.
3. FDA, COLLAGRAFT(TM) BONE GRAFT SUBSTITUTE, PMA # P900039, Supplement # S002. COLLAGEN CORP., 08/05/1993.
4. Grimes JS, Bocklage TJ, Pitcher JD. Collagen and biphasic calcium phosphate bone graft in large osseous defects. *Orthopedics* 2006; 29(2):145–148.
5. Cornell CN, Lane JM, Chapman M, Merkow R, Seligson D, Henry S, Gustilo R, Vincent K. Multicenter trial of Collagraft as bone graft substitute. *J Orthop Trauma* 1991; 5(1):1–8.
6. Walsh WR, Harrison J, Loefler A, Martin T, Van Sickle D, Brown MK, Sonnabend DH. Mechanical and histologic evaluation of Collagraft in an ovine lumbar fusion model. *Clin Orthop Relat Res* 2000; 375:258–266.
7. Dressman H. Ueber knockenplombierung bei hohlenformigen defekten des knochens. *Biert Klin Chir* 1892; 9:804–810.
8. Griffin M, Hindocha S, Jordan D, Saleh M, Khan W. An overview of the management of flexor tendon injuries. *Open Orthopaedics J* 2012; 6:28–35.
9. Moseley J, McCanless JD, Urban J, Turner T, Hall D, Carroll M. In vitro and in vivo evaluation of a slower resorbing calcium sulfate cement. Presentation 1715, *Transactions Vol 31 of 52nd Annual Meeting of the Orthopaedic Research Society*, Chicago, IL, 2006.
10. Moseley JP, Scholvin D, McCanless J, Burgess A, Morris L. Dissolution kinetics of composite calcium sulfate, calcium phosphate cement. Presentation 1714, *Transactions Vol 33 of 54th Annual Meeting of the Orthopaedic Research Society*, San Fransisco, CA, 2008.
11. Phillips A. Overview of fracture healing cascade. *Injury* 2005; 36 (Suppl 3):S5–S7.
12. Urban RM, Turner TM, Hall DJ, Inoue N, Gitelis S. Increased bone formation using calcium sulfate-calcium phosphate composite graft. *Clin Orthop Relat Res* 2007; 459:110–117.
13. Kim JH, Oh JH, Kim HS, Chung SW. Grafting using injectable calcium sulfate in bone tumor surgery: Comparison with demineralized bone matrix-based grafting. *Clin Orthop Surg* 2011; 3(3):191–201.
14. Larsson S, Bauer TW. Use of injectable calcium phosphate cement for fracture fixation: A review. *Clin Orthop Relat Res*, 2002(395):23–32.

15. Hak DJ. The use of osteoconductive bone graft substitutes in orthopaedic trauma. *J Am Acad Orthop Surg* 2007; 15(9):525–536.
16. McKee MD. Management of segmental bony defects: the role of osteoconductive orthobiologics. *J Am Acad Orthop Surg* 2006; 14(10 Spec No.):S163–S167.
17. McCanless, JD, Chesnutt B, Slack S, Bumgardner JD, Haggard WO. Comparison of bone graft substitutes through protein absorption and cellular response. Presentation 0995, *Transactions Vol 33 of 54th Annual Meeting of the Orthopaedic Research Society*, San Franscisco, CA, 2008.
18. FDA 510(k) approval summary letter K070437. PRO-DENSE™ Bone Graft Substitute, May 9, 2007.
19. FDA 510(k) approval summary letter K072597. PRO-DENSE™ Core Decompression Procedure Kit, October 15, 2007.
20. Evanview N, Tan V, Parasu N, Juriaans E, Finlay K, Deheshi B, Ghert M. Use of a calcium sulfate-calcium phosphate synthetic bone graft comosite in the surgical management of primary bone tumors. *Orthopedics* 2013; 36(2):e216–e222.
21. Kotnis NA, Parasu N, Finlay K, Juriaans E, Ghert M. Chronology of the radiographic appearances of the calcium sulphate-calcium phosphate synthetic bone graft composite following resection of bone tumours: A preliminary study of the normal post-operative appearances. *Skeletal Radiol* 2011; 40(5):563–570.
22. Fillingham YA, Lenart BA, Gitelis S. Function after injection of benign bone lesions with a bioceramic. *Clin Orthop Relat Res* 2012; 470(7):2014–2020.
23. Civinini R, De Biase P, Carulli C, Matassi R, Nistri L, Capanna R, Innocenti M. The use of an injectable calcium sulphate/calcium phosphate bioceramic in the treatment of osteonecrosis of the femoral head. *Int Orthop* 2012; 36(8):1583–1588.
24. MASTERGRAFT® Granules IFU-0381438 Rev. C.
25. MASTERGRAFT® Granules IFU-0381416 Rev. C.
26. Arinzeh TL, Tran T, Mcalary J, Daculsi G. A comparative study of biphasic calcium phosphate ceramics for human mesenchymal stem-cell-induced bone formation. *Biomaterials* 2005; 26(17):3631–3638.
27. Jensen SS, Bornstein MM, Dard M, Bosshardt DD, Buser D. Comparative study of biphasic calcium phosphates with different HA/TCP ratios in mandibular bone defects. A long-term histomorphometric study in minipigs. *J Biomed Mater Res B Appl Biomater* 2009; 90(1):171–181.
28. Ripamonti U, Richter PW, Nilen RW, Renton L. The induction of bone formation by smart biphasic hydroxyapatite tricalcium phosphate biomimetic matrices in the non-human primate Papio ursinus. *J Cell Mol Med* 2008; 12(6B):2609–2621.
29. Biohorizons. MASTERGRAFT® Family of Products. [Web] [cited June 6, 2014]; Available from: http://www.biohorizons.com/mastergraft.aspx.
30. Wakimoto M, Ueno T, Hirata A, Iida S, Aghaloo T, Moy PK. Histologic evaluation of human alveolar sockets treated with an artificial bone substitute material. *J Craniofac Surg* 2011; 22(2):490–493.
31. Burton DC, Carlson BB, Johnson PL, Manna BJ, Riazi-Kermani M, Glattes RC, Jackson RS. Backfilling of iliac crest defects with hydroxyapatite-calcium triphosphate biphasic compound: A prospective, randomized computed tomography and patient-based analysis. *The Spine Journal*, 2013; 13(1):54–61.
32. MASTERGRAFT® Putty IFU-M708348B119 Rev. B.
33. MASTERGRAFT® Putty IFU-M708348B115 Rev. B.
34. MASTERGRAFT® Matrix EXT IFU-M708348B371 Rev. A.
35. MASTERGRAFT® Strip IFU-M708348B118 Rev. B.

36. Smucker JD, Petersen EB, Nepola J, Fredericks DC. Assessment of MASTERGRAFT® STRIP with bone marrow aspirate as a graft extender in a rabbit posterolateral fusion model. *The Iowa Orthopaedic Journal* 2012; 32:61–68.
37. Smucker JD, Petersen EB, Fredericks DC. Assessment of MASTERGRAFT PUTTY as a graft extender in a rabbit posterolateral fusion model. *Spine* 2012; 37(12):1017–1021.
38. Jeng L, Moore C, Rose J. The efficacy of synthetic bone graft substitutes. *Bone & Joint Science* 2011; 02(8):1–4.
39. Bohner M. Design of ceramic-based cements and putties for bone graft substitution. *Eur Cell Mater* 2010; 20:1–12.
40. Private Communication with J-M Bouler. Graftys, France.
41. Granberry L, Ewing M, Rose J, Jeng L. Evaluation of Hardware Use with STRUCSURE CP Macroporous Calcium Phosphate Bone Graft Substitute. *Bone & Joint Science* 2012; 03(10):1–4.
42. Jennings JA, Reves BT, Smith R, Rose J, Bumgardner JD, Haggard WO. In vivo evaluation of STRUCSURE CP for augmentation of segmental defect healing. Society for Biomaterials Annual Meeting and Exposition, 2014, Denver, CO, April 16–19, 2014.

4

Commercial Non-Allograft Bone Graft Products

James W. Poser

CONTENTS

4.1 Introduction

Bone graft substitutes and autograft extenders have been in clinical use since the late 1800s.[1] Years of research and refinement, with amazing advances in material science and medicine, have produced a fundamental understanding of the material properties that contribute to the effectiveness of a bone graft substitute. Nonetheless, a synthetic bone graft material that is a true alternative to autologous bone, with an established clinical evidentiary base, remains elusive. That does not diminish the clinical need or commercial opportunity for products that are intended to augment or replace autologous bone.

The bone graft substitutes on the market share a number of common attributes. They are osteoconductive and will support bone repair and regeneration, biocompatible, often osseointegrate with the surrounding bone, and remodel into viable bone. The length of time and precise mechanism by which these events occur is not the same for all bone graft substitutes and that may be their defining difference.

The present review will discuss current commercial synthetic and semi-synthetic bone graft substitutes that are intended for use as bone void fillers for filling voids or gaps of the skeletal system including extremities, pelvis and spine (where specifically approved). Virtually all these products are classified as bone void fillers and are composed of some combination of calcium salts, substituted calcium salts, xenogeneic collagen, or resorbable natural and synthetic polymers. One of the objectives in this chapter is to highlight the similarities and clarify the important differences between these products that contribute more or less to their commercial success.

The term bone graft substitute also includes allograft tissues, growth factor, and cell-based products that are used clinically for bone grafting. These are outside of the scope of this review and the reader is directed to Chapters 8 through 10 in this book for information on these materials, and reviews on the subject cited here.[2–5]

4.2 Commercially Available Non-Allograft Bone Graft Substitutes

Table 4.1 is a compilation of several non-allograft bone graft substitutes commercially available in the United States at the time of this writing. Without exception, these products have been approved for sale in the United States as Class II Resorbable Calcium Salt Bone Void Filler Devices under regulation number 21 CFR 888.3045 and are cleared for commercial sale under the 510(k) notification process. The total U.S. sales for non-allograft, non-growth factor bone graft substitutes in 2010 was $297 million.[6]

All products in Table 4.1 have satisfactorily passed the biocompatibility testing required at the time of 510(k) submission, and where necessary to support specific labeling and clinical use they have been evaluated in appropriate animal models (e.g., posterolateral spinal fusion). None of the products are classified as osteoinductive as they have not been shown to induce pluripotential stem cells to become competent osteoblasts. Nor are they osteogenic as there are no viable, functional osteoblasts in the products as sold. Only autograft is osteoconductive, osteoinductive, and osteogenic and for that reason it is the standard against which all graft materials are compared.

Promulgated in part by guidance from the FDA and the International Organization for Standardization (ISO), and in part by a competitive marketplace, most of the current commercially available bone graft substitutes are osteoconductive, biocompatible, non-fibrotic, and remodel or resorb in a

TABLE 4.1

Summary of Typical Non-Allograft Bone Graft Substitutes Commercially Available in 2013

Company	Product	Composition	Product Form	510(k) Clearance
Baxter International	ActiFuse® ABX	Silicate substituted CaP	Granules	BVF
Berkeley Advanced Biomaterials	Bi-Ostetic™	60% HA 40% β-TCP	Granules, blocks	BVF
	Bi-Ostetic™ Foam	HA β-TCP Bov Type I collagen	Granules, blocks	BVF
	Cem-Ostetic®	Nanocrystalline HA Calcium salts	Granules	BVF
	GenerOs™	β-TCP	Granules	BVF
Biocomposites	Allogran-R®	β-TCP	Granules	BVF
	Genex® putty	β-TCP Ca sulfate	Putty	BVF
	Genex® ZPG	Biphasic Ca salt	Injectable	BVF
	Stimulan®	Ca sulfate	Pellets, injectable, moldable putty	BVF
BioMet	Calcigen® PSI	Ca P	Granules, cubes, blocks	BVF
	Calcigen® S	Ca sulfate	Moldable putty	BVF
	ProOsteon® 500R, 200R	HA Ca carbonate	Granules, blocks	BVF
Collagen Matrix	OssiMend™	Anorganic bov bone Bov Type I collagen	Granules, strips, pads	BVF
DePuy Synthesetex	chronOS®	β-TCP	Granules	BVF CMF
	Healos® Bone Graft Replacement	HA Bov Type I collagen	Strips	BVF
	Norian® SRS, CRS Rotary Mix	Carbonated CPC	Injectable hard setting paste	BVF CMF
	Norian® SRS, CRS Fast Set Putty	Carbonated CPC	Moldable hard setting putty	BVF CMF
	Norian® SRS Drillable	Fiber reinforced CPC	Injectable paste	BVF

(Continued)

TABLE 4.1 (*Continued*)

Summary of Typical Non-Allograft Bone Graft Substitutes Commercially Available in 2013

Company	Product	Composition	Product Form	510(k) Clearance
Etex	Beta-bsm®	Poorly crystalline apatite CPC	Injectable paste	BVF
	CarriGen®	Poorly crystalline apatite CPC	Injectable, moldablehard setting putty	BVF
	Gamma-bsm®	Poorly crystalline apatite CPC	Moldable hard setting putty	BVF
Exactech	OpteMX®	60% HA 40% β-TCP	Granules, Sticks, Wedges, Cylinders	BVF
Integra Orthobiologics	Mozaik®	80% β-TCP 20% Bov Type I collagen	Strips, Putty, Moldable morsels	BVF
	OsSatura TCP®	β-TCP	Granules	BVF
IstoTechnologies	InQu® Matrix	PLGA Hyaluronic acid	Strips	BVF
	InQu® Paste Mix Plus	PLGA Hyaluronic acid	Putty	BVF
Medtronic Spinal & Biologics	MasterGraft® Granules	85% β-TCP 15% HA	Granules	BVF
	MasterGraft® Matrix	85% β-TCP 15% HA Bov Type I collagen	Block	BVF
	MasterGraft® Putty	85% β-TCP 15% HA Bov Type I collagen	Moldable putty	BVF BGE
	MasterGraft® Strip	85% β-TCP 15% HA Bov Type I collagen	Strips	BVF
NovaBone	NovaBone®	Silicate substituted CaP	Granules, Putty	BVF
Olympus Terumo Biomaterials	OSferion60	β-TCP	Wedges	BVF
Pioneer Surgical	nanOss® Bioactive	Nano-structured HA Porcine gelatin	Granules	BVF
	nanOss® Bioactive 3D	Nano-structured HA Porcine gelatin	Strips	BVF

(*Continued*)

TABLE 4.1 (*Continued*)

Summary of Typical Non-Allograft Bone Graft Substitutes Commercially Available in 2013

Company	Product	Composition	Product Form	510(k) Clearance
Skeletal Kinetics	Callos® Skaffold™	CPC	Moldable putty	BVF BGE
Smith & Nephew	JAX®	Ca sulfate Hydrogel	Granules	BVF
	JAX® TCP	β-TCP	Granules	BVF
	Truegraft™	PLGA, PGA Ca sulfate Surfactant	Granules	BVF
Stryker	BoneSave®	80% β-TCP 20% HA	Granules	BVF
	BoneSource®	CaP cement	Injectable hard setting paste	BVF CMF
	HydroSet®	CaP cement	Injectable hard setting paste	BVF CMF
	Vitoss®	β-TCP	Granules	BVF
	Vitoss® Foam	80% β-TCP 20% bov Type I collagen	Strips, Injectable Moldable putty	BVF
	Vitoss® BA & BA2X Foam	β-TCP Bioactive glassbov Type I collagen	Strips, Moldable putty	BVF
Wright Medical Technology	MIIG® X3	Ca sulfate	Injectable paste	BVF
	Osteoset®	Ca sulfate	Pellets	BVF
	PRO-DENSE®	75% Ca sulfate 25% CaP	Injectable paste	BVF
Zimmer	CopiOs®	CaP bov Type I collagen	Sponge, paste	BVF

Abbreviations: β-TCP, β-tricalcium phosphate; CaP, calcium phosphate; CMF, craniomaxillofacial; CPC, calcium phosphate cement; BGE, bone graft extender; BVF, bone void filler; PGA, polyglycolic acid; PLGA, poly(lactide-co-glycolide); HA, hydroxyapatite.

time frame that is consistent with the formation of new bone at the site they are placed. Since they are approved for use as bone void fillers and/or autograft extenders these materials are intended to augment the bone formation process, maintain space, and provide an environment that is cell friendly. Bone graft substitutes are neither intended nor approved for providing structural support. A notable exception is some of the calcium phosphate (CaP) cements that are specifically indicated for use in applications where they provide internal stabilization of fractures.

This review includes only commercial products approved for sale in the United States. Many of these products, often under a different brand name, are approved for sale outside of the United States. The focus is on bone void fillers for orthopedic and spinal indications. Products cleared for use in craniofacial surgery and craniomaxillofacial trauma are also identified.

Bone graft materials intended for use in the extremities, pelvis, and spine require separate approvals from materials for dental or craniofacial applications. Clearance of materials for these non-orthopedic indications can be found by searching the FDA Medical Device website at http://www.fda.gov/medicaldevices/productsandmedicalprocedures/deviceapprovalsandclearances/510kclearances/default.htm.

4.2.1 Calcium Sulfate

Calcium sulfate (plaster of Paris) has a long history of use in orthopedic medicine. Initially used for fracture stabilization as a hardening agent in external bandages, Peltier is most often cited as introducing the widespread use of calcium sulfate for treating osseous defects.[7] It is regarded as an osteoconductive matrix that promotes vascular ingrowth and creates an environment that supports the proliferation and growth of osteogenic cells. When implanted into an osseous defect calcium sulfate in pelletized form is removed by dissolution and is completely resorbed within 6 months.[8] The relatively short length of time that they persist at the site of implantation makes 100% calcium sulfate products suitable for use as bone void fillers or bone graft extenders, and not the preferred choice for applications where the graft is expected to provide sustained structural support.[9] Rapid resorption of calcium sulfate may be an advantage, however, when it is used for drug delivery. As can be seen in Table 4.1, a number of companies sell products containing medical grade calcium sulfate, including Osteoset® from Wright Medical Technology, JAX® from Smith & Nephew, and Stimulan® from Biocomposites.

4.2.2 Calcium Phosphates

Calcium phosphates (CaPs) are by far the largest category of synthetic bone graft materials. Their popularity as bone void fillers is based on their long history of safe and effective use in virtually all orthopedic indications. Depending on their chemical composition, crystallinity, and the sintering processes used in manufacturing, CaPs will have wide range of dissolution, degradation, and clearance properties. They can be visible radiographically for as little as a few months to over 10 years post implantation. Included within the category of CaPs are β-tricalcium phosphate (β-TCP), hydroxyapatite (HA), combinations of β-TCP and HA, CaP cements (CPCs), CaP collagen composites, and ion-substituted CaPs.

4.2.2.1 β-*Tricalcium Phosphate*

β-TCP is the most widely used CaP bone void filler. It is provided in porous granules and blocks by several companies. Examples include Biocomposites' Allogran-R®, DePuy Synthes' chronOs®, and JAX® TCP from Smith & Nephew. All are osteoconductive materials that undergo degradation by dissolution and fragmentation. Typically it takes between 2 to 18 months for β-TCP to fully degrade in an osseous defect. Depending on the size and vascularity of the defect, the resorption rate of β-TCP may be too fast, which is why the volume of bone that forms in defects filled with β-TCP is often less than the volume of graft material initially placed into the defect. This is mitigated to some extent by combining HA and β-TCP.

4.2.2.2 *Hydroxyapatite*

Hydroxyapatite (HA) is the principal mineral component in bone. Synthetic HA in the form of granules or blocks was introduced as a bone graft substitute in the 1970s. More easily tailored by varying the porosity and degree of sintering, HA has a slower resorption rate and in denser forms retains volume better than β-TCP.

A number of commercial CaP products combine β-TCP with sintered HA to slow the overall resorption rate of the graft. Compositions range from 15% HA in MasterGraft® to 60% HA in OpteMX® and Bi-Ostetic™. There is a small number of differentiated products that incorporate or present HA in a unique manner. BioMet's ProOsteon® 500R and 200R, and DePuy Synthes' Healos® Bone Graft Replacement are two very different products containing HA that has been formed on a substrate. The HA in ProOsteon® is formed through the low temperature conversion of $CaCO_3$ to HA on the surface of a coral exoskeleton. Healos® is formed by the accretion of HA on the surface of collagen fibrils. Both products present an osteoconductive microcrystalline HA surface as a substrate for bone formation. Pioneer Surgical's nanOss® Bioactive and Bioactive 3D contain nanocrystalline HA that is purported to be dimensionally and chemically similar to the HA that occurs naturally in bone.

4.2.2.3 *Calcium Phosphate Cements (CPCs)*

CPCs are injectable or moldable bone void fillers that harden in situ. Bioabsorbable CPCs like Norian® Skeletal Repair System (SRS) from Depuy Synthes represent a minimally invasive approach to filling voids in bone or augmenting fracture repair. Norian® SRS cement has crystallinity and composition similar to the mineral phase of bone and remodels into structural bone over several months. Etex's βBeta- and γGamma-bsm® CPCs employ the company's "nanocrystalline technology" to produce a poorly crystalline apatite that sets slowly at room temperature but quickly hardens at body temperature. βBeta- and γGamma-bsm® also undergo cellular remodeling over a few to several months and are ultimately replaced by structural bone. CPCs share similar mechanical properties. They are resistant to compression but lack shear strength and undergo mechanical failure in distraction.

CPCs are widely used in craniomaxillofacial reconstruction, notably filling neurosurgical burr holes, contiguous craniotomy cuts, and other cranial defects, as well as in the augmentation or restoration of bony contour in the craniofacial skeleton. Norian® CRS Fast Set Putty and Stryker's HydroSet® are specifically approved and sold for these applications.

4.2.2.4 CaP Collagen Composites

A major motivation behind innovation in bone graft substitutes has been to improve their intraoperative handling. Desirable attributes include rapid and predictable hydration, cell retention, and favorable handling and packing properties. Collagraft® (Collagen Corporation, Palo Alto, CA) was the first HA/β-TCP/bovine dermal collagen composite bone graft material approved in the United States. The FDA approved Collagraft® in 1993 as a Class III device that required prospective clinical studies and a Premarket Approval (PMA). Since that time xenogeneic collagen/ceramic composites for bone grafting have been downclassified and are now Class II devices subject to Premarket Notification and clearance via the 510(k) process.

Several examples of collagen/ceramic composites are presented in Table 4.1. Based on annual sales at the time of this writing, the most successful commercial product is Stryker's Vitoss® Foam which is a composite of 80% β-TCP/20% bovine Type I collagen. Integra's Mozaik®, shown in Figure 4.1, has a similar β-TCP/collagen composition and enjoys significant commercial success.

Mozaik® has very good wicking properties, readily adsorbing and retaining blood or bone marrow aspirate. The integrity and favorable intraoperative handling characteristics of Mozaik® are product attributes widely

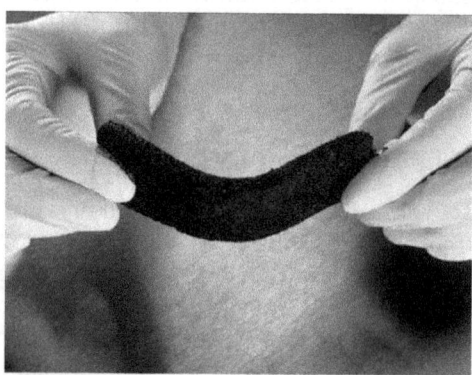

FIGURE 4.1
Mozaik® following addition of bone marrow aspirate. When wet the matrix is bendable and moldable, and resists compression while retaining its original volume.

appreciated by surgeons. Other xenogeneic collagen/CaP composites include Berkeley's Bi-Ostetic™ Foam, Collagen Matrix's OssiMend™, and the MasterGraft® Matrix, Putty, and Strips from Medtronic.

Two uniquely different HA/collagen composites worth noting are Healos® Bone Graft Replacement from DePuy Synthes and Pioneer Surgical's nanOss® Bioactive 3D. Healos® is an open cell sponge strip comprised of a mineralized bovine Type I collagen where the surfaces of the collagen fibrils have been coated with HA. NanOss® Bioactive 3D is comprised of nano-structured HA particles combined with porcine gelatin. Both claim to be tailored for optimized cell infiltration and adsorption, and provide an in situ environment that is ideal for bone formation.

4.2.2.5 Substituted Apatites

The mineral phase in bone is not pure hydroxyapatite. Products like Collagen Matrix's Ossimend™ and the DePuy Synthes Norian® SRS cements incorporate carbonated apatite which is purported to undergo more physiologic remodeling and recapitulate a natural bone healing environment, resulting in direct bone apposition onto the mineral component of the graft material.[10]

4.3 Bioactive Materials That Change the Regenerative Microenvironment

Effective bone graft substitutes must be cell friendly. It is implicit that they should not elicit a significant cytotoxic response. Materials (e.g., CPCs) should not be exothermic to the extent it results in thermal necrosis of the cells and tissue at the site of implantation. Other than the more occlusive CPCs, most products listed in Table 4.1 will adsorb and retain cells. Materials that retain cells, and those with the potential to directly influence cellular expression, have been called "osteostimultory." Importantly, they may act synergistically with cells to create a regenerative microenvironment.

4.3.1 Bioactive Glass

NovaBone® contains 45S5 Bioglass® (46.1% SiO_2, 26.9% CaO, 24.4% Na_2O, and 2.6% P_2O_5), which following implantation releases Ca^{2+} and PO_4^- ions, along with soluble silica, forming a gel with a carbonated apatite surface layer that proteins adhere to and create sites for cellular attachment.[11] Furthermore, the local environment created by 45S5 Bioglass® is reported to be uniquely favorable to osteoblasts and osteoprogenitor cells.[12] The FDA has allowed the use of the term "osteostimulatory" to describe this cellular response and is the justification for describing silicate-substituted bone graft materials as "bioactive." In 1993 NovaBone® received 510(k) clearance for PerioGlas®, a 45S5 Bioglass® particulate for restoring bone loss due to periodontal disease.

Vitoss® BA and BA2X contain bioactive glass, β-TCP, and bovine Type I collagen. These ternary composites appear to have the components to meet customer demands in today's commercial products: a resorbable CaP ceramic, an "osteostimulatory" component, and collagen to enhance cell retention and handling. It is perhaps understandable that at the time of this writing the Vitoss family of products is the number one selling synthetic bone graft substitute in the world.[13]

4.3.2 Ion-Substituted Ceramics

There is a strong interest in the potential to enhance the bioactivity of ceramics by incorporating non-physiologic impurities into their crystal structure. Baxter's ActiFuse® is a silicate-substituted calcium phosphate (Si-CaP) where 0.8 wt% of the PO_4^{3-} has been substituted with SiO_4^{4-}. This level of silicate substitution reportedly creates an optimal anionic charge on the surface of the apatite, enhancing protein adsorption and cell adhesion, and accelerating bone formation.[14]

4.3.3 Hyaluronic Acid

InQu® from ISTO Technologies is a unique bone graft material. It is a composite of hyaluronic acid (HyA) and poly(lactide-co-glycolide) (PLGA), which have been comingled into a compression-resistant open cell structure that is believed to create a microenvironment that is conducive to new bone formation (Figure 4.2a).

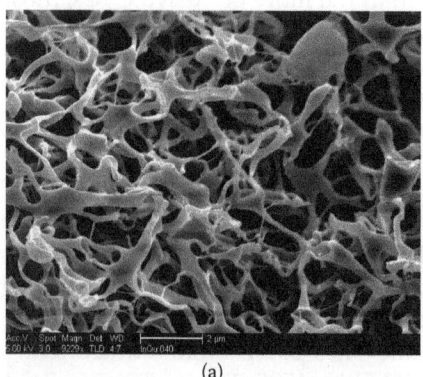
(a)

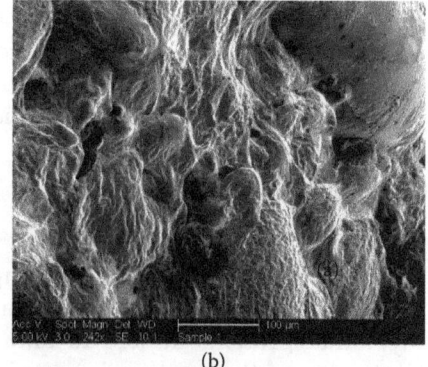
(b)

FIGURE 4.2
(a) SEM of InQu showing 75%–90% porosity and 1–300 μm diameter pores. (b) SEM of InQu® co-cultured with viable human cancellous bone showing osteoblastic outgrowth.

PLGA serves to create and retain the porous architecture of InQu® where the HyA is believed to facilitate angiogenesis[15] and cell attachment.[16] In vitro studies have demonstrated that InQu® promotes osteoblastic cell migration, growth, and attachment, and extracellular matrix deposition as shown in Figure 4.2b.

4.4 Conclusion

The decision on which bone graft substitute is the best option for a specific patient or clinical indication can be a daunting task. Surgeons, scientists, hospital purchasing agents, and patients are understandably confused by the reams of information available about bone graft substitutes. Products listed in this chapter have all gone through the same 510(k) Premarket Notification process. As promulgated by the FDA, clearance via 510(k) requires the declaration that a product is substantially equivalent to other products approved for the same indicated use. Apparently identical products are often represented as having vastly different performance properties and patient benefits. While products have evolved based on customer input and market demands, within each class of products the physical, chemical, and functional characteristics are quite similar and not well differentiated. This is not for lack of creativity on the part of the product developers. It is rather a reflection of the regulatory requirements to gain approval to place a product in commerce, and once in commerce what a company is legally allowed to claim regarding the attributes of the product.

It is implicit that bone graft substitutes must satisfy customer expectations to achieve commercial success. Acceptable performance generally implies that when used in accordance with the instructions for use provided by the company the product consistently results in favorable clinical outcomes for their patients. It often takes 2 or 3 years following product introduction for surgeons to develop sufficient clinical experience to establish whether a graft material performs as advertised and their mid- to long-term patient outcomes meet expectations. Products that survive these initial years of vetting in the market are regarded as having met the performance standard.

Like most consumer products, once a bone graft substitute has been accepted in the market, access to customers drives product sales. In 2010 nearly 50% of the synthetic bone graft substitute sales in the United States were attributed to two product families: Stryker's Vitoss® and Medtronics MasterGraft® family of products.[6] There are several products similar to Vitoss® and MasterGraft® that are also FDA-approved for sale, but these two brands dominate the market because of history, customer access, and loyalty.

However the dynamics of product choice are changing. In their diligent efforts to control costs and reduce the number of redundant products on the shelf, hospitals are becoming emboldened and mandating which bone graft substitutes physicians will be allowed to use. Once minimal standards of product performance have been established, hospital purchase and stocking decisions are made on a cost basis, oftentimes irrespective of physician preference.

Synthetic bone graft substitutes that incorporate new materials, act through a cellular or systemic mechanism, or for which new and beneficial performance is claimed will be subject to a more onerous regulatory review and approval process where scientific and clinical data must be provided to support product safety and efficacy. Regardless of the potential for improved clinical outcomes, progressive companies developing truly innovative bone graft substitutes will continue to experience significant barriers to market entry. In addition to the regulatory restrictions, downward pressure to reduce health care costs and capitation on reimbursement will weigh heavily on business decisions to invest in new product development. Even with these uncertainties, a look at the bone graft substitutes that have been introduced into the market over the last 5 years provides a glimpse into what the future may hold.

Synthetic bone grafts were originally designed to mimic the inorganic phase of bone and engineered to match the architecture and mechanical properties of the bone they were intended to replace. That inexorably led to the use of CaP salts in various forms and crystallinity. Developers of CaP-based materials have focused on material purity, biocompatibility, mechanical properties, resorption rate, and bony integration. These are all important, but for the most part do not address how to direct a bone graft substitute to favorably influence the biology of bone formation.

In orchestrating skeletal tissue repair and regeneration bone graft substitutes should play the principal supporting role in establishing a regenerative microenvironment. The surface of a material and the local milieu it generates are important determinants of a successful clinical outcome. For example, increased surface area or anionic charge density and distribution have been shown to enhance the binding of the cell adhesive proteins fibronectin and laminin, thereby providing a means to enhance cell adherence at the site of skeletal repair.[17–19] It is not a stretch to envision how nanotechnology can provide the tools to make CaP nanoparticles of exquisitely defined surface chemistry and topography, and to selectively combine elements that will enhance cell migration while improving mechanical strength of the material.[20] If the effort to develop these materials is rewarded with improved patient outcomes then health care providers and payers will acknowledge the clinical and cost benefit, and it is reasonable to anticipate that companies will make the business decision to invest in development of the next-generation bone graft products.

References

1. Dreesmann H. Ueber knockenplombierung bei hohlenformigen defekten des knochens. *Bietr Klin Chir* 1892; 9:804–810.
2. Giannoudis PV, Dinopoulos H, Tsiridis E. Bone substitutes: An update. *Injury* 2005; 36(Suppl 3):S20–S27.
3. Laurencin C, Khan Y, El-Amin SF. Bone graft substitutes. *Expert Rev Med Devices* 2006; 3(1):49–57.
4. Pryor LS, Gage E, Langevin C-J, Herrera F, Breithaupt AD et al. Review of bone substitutes. *Craniomaxillofac Trauma Reconstr* 2009; 2(3):151–160.
5. Brydone, AS, Meek D, Maclaine S. Bone Grafting, orthopedic biomaterials, and the clinical need for bone engineering. *J Engineering in Med* 2010; 224(12):1329–1343.
6. Mendenhall S. Bone grafts and bone substitutes. *Orthopedic Network News* 2010; 21(4):16–19.
7. Peltier LF. Use of Plaster of Paris to fill defects in bone. *Clin Orthop Relat Res* 1961; 21:1–31.
8. Kelly CM, Wilkins RM, Gitelis S, Hartjen C, Watson JT and Kim PT. The use of a surgical grade calcium sulfate as a bone graft substitute: Results of a multi-center trial. *Clin Orthop Telat Res* 2001; 382:42–50.
9. Hak DJ. The use of osteoconductive bone graft substitutes in orthopedic trauma. *J Am Acad Orthop Surg* 2007; 15(9):525–536.
10. Oguz A, Lehmicke M, Aberman H, Toms D, Hollinger JO, Fulmer M. Bone healing response to an injectable calcium phosphate cement with enhanced radiopacity. *J Biomed Mater Res* 2008; 86B(1):56–62.
11. Hench LL, Polak J. A genetic basis for design of biomaterials for in situ tissue regeneration. *Key Engineering Mater* 2008; 377:151–166.
12. Hench LL. Genetic design of bioactive glass. *J Eur Ceramics Soc* 2009; 29:1257–65.
13. Stryker Orthobiologics Internal Sales Data (April 2012).
14. Hing KA, Revell PA, Smith N, Buckland T. Effect of silicon level on rate, quality and progression of bone healing within silicate-substituted porous hydroxyapatite scaffolds. *Biomater* 2006; 27(29):5014–5026.
15. West DC, Hampson IN, Arnold F, Kumar S. Angiogenesis induced by degradation products of hyaluronic acid. *Science* 1985; 228(4705):1324–1326.
16. Chen WY, Abatangelo G. Functions of hyaluronan in wound repair. *Wound Rep Regen* 1999; 7(2):79–89.
17. Anselme K. Osteoblast adhesion on biomaterials. *Biomater* 2000; 21(7):667–681.
18. Ohgaki M, Kizuki T, Katsura M, Yamashita K. Manipulation of selective cell adhesion and growth by surface charges of electrically polarized hydroxyapatite. *J Biomed Mater Res* 2001; 75(3):366–373.
19. Guth K, Campion C, Buckland T, Hing KA. Effect of silicate-substitution on attachment and early development of human osteoblast-like cells seeded on microporous hydroxyapatite discs. *Adv Engineering Mater* 2010; 12(4):B77–B82.
20. Harvey JH, Henderson JE, Vengallatore ST. Nanotechnology and bone healing. *J Orthop Trauma* 2010; 24(3):S25–S30.

5

Demineralized Bone Matrix (DBM) and Bone Grafts

Su-Gwan Kim and Ji-Su Oh

CONTENTS

5.1 Introduction

Osteogenic cells, scaffolds, growth factors (bone morphogenic proteins [BMP], transforming growth factor-ß [TGF-ß], insulin-like growth factor [IGF]-II, platelet-derived growth factor [PDGF])[1] and mechanical stability are essential in bone healing.[2] Although an autologous bone graft has all of these factors, it also displays various results and unpredictable resorption in several cases. In addition, the morbidity of the donor site for the harvest of autologous bone has caused practitioners to seek other methods to enhance healing using bone graft substitutes (Table 5.1).[3]

5.2 Allograft

Osteoinduction is the process by which some factor or substance stimulates an undifferentiated osteoprogenitor stem cell to differentiate into an

TABLE 5.1

Current Requirements for Ideal Bone Substitutes

Biocompatibility	Resorbability/degradability
Osteoinduction and osteopromotion/ osteoconduction	Plasticity
Porosity	Sterility
Stability under stress	Stable and long-term integration of implants

Source: Kolk A et al., *J Craniomaxillofac Surg*; 40(8):706–718, 2012.

osteogenic cell. This process is mediated by numerous growth factors found within the bone matrix itself.[5] Thus, any material that induces this process can be considered osteoinductive.[3]

The allograft bone obtained from the donor bones of cadavers has both variable osteoinductive (released bone morphogenic proteins that act on bone cells) and osteoconductive properties, but these bones lack osteogenic properties due to the absence of viable cells, such as osteoblasts and precursors (Table 5.2).[2] In addition, an allograft demonstrates good osteointegrative capability at the host–recipient interface.[6]

An allograft is available in many forms: mineralized (frozen or freeze-dried chips of cancellous or cortical bone), demineralized bone matrix (DBM), osteochondral and whole-bone segments.[7] The osteoinductive property varies depending on the preparation of the allograft. The mineralized frozen allografts are mechanically stable, whereas mineralized freeze-dried bone is mechanically less resistant and exhibits less osteoinductive capability but can be vacuum packed at room temperature.[2,6] DBM has a higher osteoinductive property than mineralized allografts.

5.3 Demineralized Bone Matrix (DBM)

DBM consists of sponge-like collagen obtained from human, bovine, or equine origin, which has undergone decalcification and sterilization and thus can be classified as an allogenic or xenogenic material depending on the origin, although most DBM consists of commercially allogenic bone.[4] Depending on how the bone is constructed and processed, different preparations can consist of granules, strips of interwoven fibers, or putty-like preparations.[7] The organized scaffold of DBM serves as an osteoconductive component.

Calcium phosphate may arrest bone morphogenesis.[8] Removal of the mineral phase of the allograft improves the potential, albeit variable,

TABLE 5.2

Modification of Laurencin's Classification

Bone Grafts and Substitutes			OG	OI	OC	SS	Cost
Autograft			+	+	+	+[a]	+++/++++[b]
Allograft			−	+	+	+[a]	+/++
Substitutes	Biologic	Coral	−	+	+	−	++/+++
		Collagen type 1	−	+	+[c]	−	(No studies on DRFx)
		Demineralized bone matrix	−	±	+	−	+/++
	Synthetic	Factor-based (TGF-ß, PDGF, EGF, BMP)	−	+	±	−	+++/++++[d]
		Cell-based (mesenchymal stem cells)	+	−	+[c]	−	(No studies on DRFx)
		Ceramic-based (calcium HA, tricalcium phosphate, calcium phosphate cement)	−	−	+	+	+/++
		Polymer-based	−	−	+	−	(No studies on DRFx)

Source: Ozer K, Kevin CC, *Hand Clinics*; 28(2):217–223, 2012. With permission.

Abbreviations: BMP, bone morphogenic proteins; DRF, distal radius fracture; FGF, fibroblast growth factor; HA, hydroxyapatite; OC, osteoconductive; OG, osteogenic; OI, osteoinductive; SS, structural support; TGF, transforming growth factor.

[a] If the graft includes cortical bone.

[b] Including direct and indirect costs, data based on studies of spinal fusion and tibial nonunions.

[c] If used with a carrier.

[d] Only Rh-BMP is tested on distal radius fractures.

availability of osteoinductive growth factors.[6] Thus, DBM promotes the differentiation of stem cells into bone-forming cells. The mechanism underlying DBM stimulation of new bone formation is affected by residual calcium levels, degradation of the organic matrix, release of growth factors, and preparation of the matrix.[8] It provides no structural stability to the articular surface and thus is commonly used in structurally stable bone defects to stimulate bone healing.[9] It is mainly used as a "bone graft extender" (Table 5.3).[4]

TABLE 5.3

Properties and Functions That Determine Bone Graft Efficacy

Properties of bone graft materials	*Osteoconductive* The donation of biocompatible scaffolding material that provides mechanical structure upon which new bone formation takes place	*Osteogenic* The contribution of whole cells which are along the spectrum of osteoblastic differentiation (osteoprogenitor cells) and participate directly in bone synthesis	*Osteoinductive* The recruitment of stem cells and promotionof their osteoblastic differentiation by thedonation of signaling molecules and growthfactors
Mechanisms of bone graft alternatives	*Graft extender* Stimulates bone formation and can becombined with a limited supply of autologous bone to decrease the amount needed in achieving a comparable fusion rate or combined with a standard allotment of autologous graft to allow the fusion of a greater number of levels	*Graft enhancer* Enhances the fusion rate when combined with a standard allotment of autologous bone or allows comparable fusion rates in patients with a poor or limited supply,i.e. re-harvest, adolescent, or requiring multi-level fusion	*Graft substitute* Achieves comparable fusion rates as autologous ICBG while obviating the need for autologous graft entirely

Source: Aghdasi B et al., *Surgeon;* 11(1):39–48, 2013. With permission.

5.3.1 Histology and DBM Composition

5.3.1.1 Histology of DBM

A histological comparison of healing revealed that demineralized freeze-dried bone allografts (DFDBAs) had a significantly higher percentage of vital bone and a significantly lower mean percentage of residual graft particles compared to freeze-dried bone allografts (FDBAs).[11] Bone particles between 250 and 710 microns were within the optimal size range, and an approximately 2% level of residual calcium was optimally osteoinductive, resulting in new bone formation in the DBM.[8] Histologically, most DBM preparations can be recognized as non-mineralized shavings of cortical bone, which appear to be necrotic. DBM is not thought to be significantly antigenic to the host and is thus not usually associated with inflammation. However, it is necessary to understand that (1) the demineralized spicules of DBM material should not be misinterpreted as a tumor osteoid when encountered at the site of a prior tumor, and (2) the lack of cells in the lacunae of the DBM material should not be misinterpreted as ischemic necrosis of host bone.[7]

5.3.1.2 DBM Composition

DBM is produced by removing calcium phosphate using acid extraction.[12] It contains type-1 collagen (93%), non-collagenous proteins, and glycoproteins, including osteoinductive growth factors, such as bone morphogenetic proteins (BMPs)-2, BMP-4, IGF-1, TGF-β1, approximately 5% of vascular endothelial growth factor (VEGF), and 2% residual mineralized matrix 2.[10,12-13] The TGF-β superfamily includes a number of factors that are known to stimulate the migration, differentiation, and activity of potential bone-forming mesenchymal cells in addition to BMPs.[4,5]

The factors that are known to be osteoinductive are BMPs, growth differentiation factors (GDFs), and potentially TGF-β1, TGF-β2, and TGF-β3.[4] BMP-2, BMP-4, and BMP-7 appear to be responsible for the formation of bone, where BMPs attract mesenchymal stem cells via chemotaxis and act as morphogens that differentiate these cells into an osteochondrogenic lineage.[14]

5.3.1.3 Carrier for DBM

DBM is difficult to handle, and its tendency to migrate from graft sites and its lack of stability after surgery can be clinical problems.[15] The carrier must be biocompatible with the surrounding tissue without interfering with the sequence of bone induction. Moreover, the carrier must be degradable or porous to enable the diffusion of BMPs.[15]

Currently, available DBM is produced using carrier vehicles. Different forms on the market include injectables, moldable paste, putty for void filling, strips, gel, pellets, freeze-dried powder, blocks, and granules.[6,16] Available DBM carriers include calcium sulfate, water-soluble polymers such as sodium hyaluronate or carboxymethylcellulose, anhydrous, starch, collagen, bovine gelatin, and water-miscible solvents such as glycerol to improve the handling properties.[17] Osteoinduction is affected by the carrier. The glycerol carrier is very acidic with a low pH, which may specifically have detrimental effects in large quantities especially.[18,19] Furthermore, DBM with a glycerol carrier should be used carefully in pediatric patients due to risk of renal disease.[20]

Advanced studies on carriers have been previously reported. Tian et al. presented the possibility of a thermogelling chitosan carrier via an in vitro study.[15] In addition, in studies using human acellular dermal matrix (AM), DBM/AM induced a significantly higher spinal fusion rate than autologous bone graft for posterolateral lumbar fusion,[17] and AM may increase the handling convenience when mixed with DBM, which does not inhibit the bone formation capacity of DBM.[21]

5.3.2 Screening Donors and Procuring Tissues

Evaluations of the medical, social history, environmental risks, physical assessment, specific medical conditions, and cause of death were performed for every donor (Table 5.4). The technique of procuring the tissues is dictated by the American Association of Tissue Banks (AATB) with guidance from the U.S. Food and Drug Administration (FDA).[22]

5.3.2.1 Serological and Microbiological Testing

Disease transmission, such as viral or bacterial infection, is extremely rare[23] with allobone, in which the last incidence of a fatality by disease transmission occurred in 2001.[22]

Infectious disease testing was performed by the FDA, and AATB requires an evaluation of donor eligibility, including human immunodeficiency virus (HIV), hepatitis B, hepatitis C, syphilis, etc. (Table 5.5). The FDA Center for Biologics Evaluation and Research (CBER) regulates human cells, tissues, and cellular-based products (HCT/Ps) under federal law.[24] DBM is not considered to be a medical device, but it is categorized under HCT/Ps.[20] Code of Federal Regulations (CFR) Title 21 created a unified registration and listing system for establishments that manufacture HCT/Ps, and also outlined the establishment of donor eligibility, good tissue practice, and other guidelines to prevent the introduction, transmission, and spread of communicable diseases, such as HIV, hepatitis B virus (HBV), hepatitis C virus (HCV), Treponema pallidum, and human T-lymphotropic virus (HTLV).[24]

5.3.2.2 Processing and Sterilization of DBM

The processing of DBM is needed to remove antigenicity without compromising the biomechanical and biochemical integrity. DBM is treated in two basic steps: aseptic processing and terminal sterilization.[26]

Aseptic processing includes the chemical agent and the physical cleaning of tissues to reduce bioburden and cellular antigens.[26] The processing methods vary depending on the type of final products. Steps in the processing of DBM are as follows: Initial processing involves stripping of the soft tissue and sectioning approximately 5 mm in diameter. The bone is cleaned and decontaminated using saline, acetone, ethanol, or hydrogen peroxide to remove residual bioburden and antigenicity. The microbiological treatment is performed using antimicrobial, antimycotics, and antifungal solutions. Next, processing involves freezing in liquid nitrogen, dehydration, and final sectioning. Demineralization with hydrochloric acid is performed to produce the DBM.[24] The sterility assurance level (SAL) measures of the Association for the Advancement of Medical Instrumentation indicates the probability of a single viable microorganism occurring on an item after sterilization. It is generally accepted that a sterility assurance level (SAL) of 10^{-6} is appropriate for items intended for contact with compromised tissue and can be labeled "sterile."[27]

TABLE 5.4

Risk Factors or Conditions for Donor Screening

1. Males who have had sex with another male in the preceding 5 years (risk factor for HIV and hepatitis B).
2. Persons who have injected drugs for a non-medical reason in the preceding 5 years (risk factor for HIV, hepatitis B and hepatitis C).
3. Persons with hemophilia or other related clotting disorders who have received human-derived clotting factor concentrates in the preceding 5 years (risk factor for HIV, hepatitis B and hepatitis C).
4. Persons who have engaged in sex in exchange for money or drugs in the preceding 5 years (risk factor for HIV, hepatitis B and hepatitis C).
5. Persons who have had sex in the preceding 12 months with any person described in criteria 1 through 4 of this section or with any person who has HIV infection, including a positive or reactive test for HIV virus, hepatitis B infection, or clinically active (symptomatic) hepatitis C infection.
6. Persons who have been exposed in the preceding 12 months to known or suspected HIV, HBV, and/or HCV-infected blood through percutaneous inoculation or through contact with an open wound, non-intact skin, or mucous membrane.
7. Children born to mothers with or at risk for HIV infection:
   • If 18 months of age or younger, or
   • If breast-fed within the preceding 12 months.
8. Persons who have been in juvenile detention, lock up, jail or prison for more than 72 consecutive hours in the preceding 12 months (risk factor for HIV, hepatitis B and hepatitis C).
9. Persons who have lived with (resided in the same dwelling) another person who has hepatitis B or clinically active (symptomatic) hepatitis C infection in the preceding 12 months.
10. Persons who have undergone tattooing, ear piercing or body piercing in the preceding 12 months, in which sterile procedures were not used, or shared instruments that had not been sterilized.
11. Persons who have had a past diagnosis of clinical, symptomatic viral hepatitis after their 11th birthday.
12. Persons who are deceased and have a documented medical diagnosis of sepsis or have documented clinical evidence consistent with a diagnosis of sepsis.
13. Persons who have had smallpox vaccination (vaccinia virus) in the preceding 8 weeks.
14. Persons who acquired a clinically recognizable vaccinia virus infection by contact with someone who received the smallpox vaccine.
15. Persons who have had a medical diagnosis or suspicion of WNV infection.
16. Persons who have tested positive or reactive for WNV infection using an FDA-licensed or investigational WNV NAT donor screening test in the preceding 120 days.
17. Persons who have been treated for or had syphilis within the preceding 12 months.
18. Reproductive HCT/P donors who have been treated for or had *Chlamydia trachomatis* or *Neisseria gonorrhea* infection in the preceding 12 months.
19. Persons who have been diagnosed with vCJD or any other form of CJD.
20. Persons who have been diagnosed with dementia or any degenerative or demyelinating disease of the central nervous system or other neurological disease of unknown etiology.
21. Persons who are at increased risk for CJD.
22. Persons who have a history of CJD in a blood relative.

Source: FDA Center for Biologics Evaluation and Research, Guidance for Industry: Eligibility Determination for Donors of Human Cells, Tissues, and Cellular and Tissue-Based Products (HCT/Ps), 2007. http://www.fda.gov/downloads/BiologicsBloodVaccines/GuidanceComplianceRegulatoryInformation/Guidances/Tissue/UCM091345.pdf.

TABLE 5.5

Donor Screening for Infectious Agents and HIV

Hepatitis B	*T. pallidum (Treponema pallidum [syphilis])*
Hepatitis C	*T. cruzi (Trypanosoma cruzi)*
Immunodeficiency virus type 1 and 2	WNV (West Nile virus)
Human T-lymphotropic virus types I and II	CMV (cytomegalovirus)

Source: FDA, Complete List of Donor Screening Assays for Infectious Agents and HIV Diagnostic Assays, 2013. http://www.fda.gov/biologicsbloodvaccines/bloodbloodproducts /approvedproducts/licensedproductsblas/blooddonorscreening/infectiousdisease /ucm080466 .htm.

Terminal sterilization includes gamma irradiation, gas sterilization, slow-freezing with glycerol, and equivalent chemical treatment.[28] Although gamma irradiation is appropriate for the terminal sterilization in clinical use due to its bactericidal characteristic,[29,30] it is less damaging to the osteoinductive index (OI).[20] However, damage to tissue by ionizing radiation occurs via two principal mechanisms. Photon depositing in the target results in the dislocation of outer electrons from molecules and the breakage of covalent bonds. Moreover, a chemical attack by free radicals and reactive oxygen species is typically generated by the interaction of radiation.[26,31]

An allograft is reduced by approximately 40% after irradiation compared with approximately 90% in non-irradiated bone allografts.[32] To prevent radiation damage, dry ice temperature during irradiation is important.[29,33]

Appropriate doses of terminal sterilization using gamma irradiation without inactivating DBM have been suggested. Low doses are insufficient for the inactivation of HIV, other radio-resistant viruses, and bacterial spores. However, high doses have adversely affected the osteoinductive properties and structural strength of the bone.[26] Alanay et al. described an aseptic procedure that required soaking 3% hydrogen peroxide for less than 1 hour; this and the 50-kGy terminal sterilization procedure are effective methods.[26] In addition, 30–50 kGy radiation doses are considered sufficient to sterilize and inactivate viruses, but do not degrade DBM.[20] The commercial levels of the bactericidal and fungicidal effects of radiation are given as 35 kGy.[29] Moreover, the International Atomic Energy Agency (IAEA) recommended 25 kGy as the standard dose for the sterilization of medical products.[34]

5.4 Bone Grafts with DBM

DBM is an advanced bone tissue product that is used by a number of orthopedic surgeons, oral and maxillofacial surgeons, neurosurgeons, periodontists, and dentists.[16,21,35] The field of clinical application includes:

1. Clinical dentistry, oral and maxillofacial surgery[36] and periodontal procedures such as sinus lifts,[37,38] alveolar augmentation, implant placement, and socket preservation and guided tissue regeneration

2. Orthopedic procedures such as revision total hip replacement, revision total knee replacement, nonunion repair, and ankle repair and replacements

3. Neurosurgical and other procedures such as cervical fusions and frontal sinus obliteration[39]

Most studies have demonstrated the clinical success of DBM. However, several studies have reported poor bone formation[40,41] or nonunion in large defects; thus, it is not recommended to use DBM alone in large defects.[42] DBM with autogenous bone has a synergistic osteogenic effect. However, bone healing using DBM is affected by characteristics of the recipient defect. There is variability among DBM products in the composition and osteoinductive index. As such, DBM is not recommended for the enhancement of facial or cranial contour deficits and in high compressive loads due to the tendency for resorption and graft collapse.

5.5 Limitations and Future DBM Studies

There is a significant variability in the osteoinductive capacity among different commercially available DBM (Table 5.6). Several factors, such as different amounts of DBM, donor age, metabolic characteristics, carrier, demineralization times, residual bone mineral content, particle size, and terminal sterilization method affect the osteoinductive properties of DBM.[14,43,44] In particular, the DBM content (17%–100%) among different commercial products is non-standardized and inconsistent and results in different osteoinductive capacities.[20] The ability of DBM to induce new bone formation is suggested to be age dependent, with DBM from older donors being less likely to have strong bone-inducing activity, although this hypothesis is controversial.[45,46]

In comparison to commercially available DBM for spinal fusion, all DBM products have significant osteoinductive capabilities. Moreover, there are significant differences among DBM products.[43,47] The authors demonstrated that the reliable use of DBM in spinal surgery is questionable due to the differences in osteoinduction of the products and the inconsistencies of the fusion rates between the different lots of the same products.[43]

While animal studies have documented the osteoinductive effects of DBM, the level-of-evidence ratings in the clinical care recommendation are C grade (poor quality evidence for or against recommending intervention).[3] Human studies on DBM are weak because DBM is used as a bone graft extender rather than DBM alone. Consequently, the efficacy for DBM has not been clearly elucidated.[20]

TABLE 5.6

Commercially Available DBM Products and Characteristics

Manufacturer/ Product name	Delivery	Morphology	Properties	Recommended use
Bonus II DBM	Paste	Non-load-bearing	OI + OC	Injectable. Use with bone marrow aspirate. Use in nonunions, revision arthroplasty, ankle fusion and tumor surgery
EquivaBone (DBM+ calciumphosphate)	Paste	Resorbable	OI + OC	Bone void filler in spinal and trauma surgery
Optium DBM	Gel/putty	DBM particle size 125 to 850 μm. Calcium content < 8%	OI + OC	Spinal fusion, bone voids, tumors, spine, pelvis, ankle and calcaneal fractures Non-load-bearing
Optecure	Putty	81% concentration of DBM by weight, non-load-bearing	OI + OC	Mix with blood or autograft
Opteform	Paste	Non-water-soluble, non-load-bearing	OI + OC	Multiple uses given on website but not load-bearing
Accell Connexus	Putty in syringe	Non-load-bearing	OI + OC	Spinal fusion, bone voids, revision hip and knee surgery
Accell 100	Putty in syringe	Non-load-bearing	OI + OC	Spinal fusion, bone voids
Dynagraft II	Putty/gel	Non-load-bearing, void filling	OI + OC	Bone graft extender for extremity, pelvis, or spine
Integra Accell Evo3	Putty/gel	Non-load-bearing, void filling	OI + OC	Bone graft extender for extremity, pelvis, or spine
Orthoblast	Putty, paste	50% macroporous, 50% microporous, non-load-bearing	OI + OC	Contained defects, ankle/foot fusions, nonunions
Grafton	Matrix, paste, putty, gel	Non-load-bearing	OI + OC	Multiple uses: Spinal fusion, void filler, trauma, arthrodesis

(Continued)

TABLE 5.6 (*Continued*)

Commercially Available DBM Products and Characteristics

Plexure (DBM+ polylactide-coglycolide)	Granules, wedge, blocksheet	Resorbable	OI + OC	Void filler, oncology bone surgery, tibial plateau fractures, and arthroplasty surgery
DBX	Putty	Non-load-bearing applications	OI + OC	Void filler in long bones and pelvis
Allomatrix (DBM+ calciumsulfate carrier: Osteoset)	Paste,chips	Non-load-bearing		Bone void filler in trauma surgery Lumbar spine surgery Tumor resection surgery and long bone nonunion Non-load-bearing applications
Osteoset II DBM (DBM+ calcium sulfate)	Pellets	53% vol DBM. Contains BMP-2, BMP-4, IGF-1, TGF-β1. Resorbable, rapid remodeling	OC	Spinal surgery, trauma, treatment of benign cysts and adult reconstruction To treat avascular necrosis of the femoral head when combined with autograft
Ignite (DBM+ calciumsulfate, bonemarrow aspirate)	Paste	Resorbable	OI + OC	Used in cases of suspected nonunion where no callus is seen at 6–8 weeks Cases of delayed union with well-fixed hardware Use in fresh fractures where there is high risk of nonunion, e.g., smokers or diabetics Contraindicated in infected cases or when bone gap > 3 mm, and when there are signs of hardware loosening

(*Continued*)

TABLE 5.6 (*Continued*)

Commercially Available DBM Products and Characteristics

ProStim (DBM+ PRO-DENSE)	Paste	Resorbable, 40 MPa initial compressive strength, 75% calcium sulfate, 25% calcium phosphate	OI + OC	Calcaneal, tibial plateau, distal radius, and proximal humerus fractures as bone void filler Used in treatment of benign bone cysts and in osteotomy and decompression surgery

Source: From Kurien T et al., *Bone Joint J* 2013 95-B (5):583–597.
Abbreviations: OI, osteoinductive; OC, osteoconductive.

Studies on bone protein extraction (BPE) as a new generation of DBM have been advanced.[48,49] BPE is obtained from animals, demineralized using HCl and EDTA, and lyophilized in the final step. It exhibits osteoconductivity, osteoinductivity, and osteogenicity, and it has utility as an alternative for DBM.[49]

Kasten et al. studied the seeding efficacy using human bone marrow stromal cells in various resorbable biomaterials, and demonstrated that DBM showed more homogeneous distribution throughout the matrix, with significantly high osteocalcin values and excellent seeding efficacy.[50] DBM quickly revascularizes and acts as a suitable matrix for bone marrow cells.[1]

Lin et al. reported that crosslinking heparin to DBM plus BMP-2 dramatically increases the mechanical intensity and specific BMP-2 binding ability and enhances osteogenesis.[51] Recently, studies of remineralization of DBM have continued to improve the mechanical properties and osteoconductivity of the collagenous matrix of DBM. The remineralization method has been applied in the clinic via many studies, such as the "mineralization by inhibitor exclusion" method,[52] the "polymer-induced liquid precursor" method,[53] and the "alternating solution immersion" method.[54] DBM is a potential vehicle for the delivery of endogenous and exogenous therapeutics. Drug delivery from DBM represents an attractive product synergy.[55]

Currently available DBM has limits such as low mechanical stability and variations in the efficacy of osteoinduction. However, if the scientific and therapeutic studies for clinical application are continued, it is certain that DBM will be one of the most effective bone materials in bone repair.

References

1. Ozer K, Kevin CC. The use of bone grafts and substitutes in the treatment of distal radius fractures. *Hand Clinics* 2012; 28(2):217–223.
2. Zimmermann G, Arash M. Allograft bone matrix versus synthetic bone graft substitutes. *Injury* 2011; 42(Suppl 2):S16–S21.
3. De Long WG Jr, Einhorn TA, Koval K, McKee M, Smith W, Sanders R, Watson T. Bone grafts and bone graft substitutes in orthopaedic trauma surgery. A critical analysis. *J Bone Joint Surg Am* 2007; 89(3):649–658.
4. Kolk A, Handschel J, Drescher W, Rothamel D, Kloss F, Blessmann M, Heiland M, Wolff K-D, Smeets R. Current trends and future perspectives of bone substitute materials—From space holders to innovative biomaterials. *J Craniomaxillofac Surg* 2012; 40(8):706–718.
5. Schimandle JH, Boden SD. Bone substitutes for lumbar fusion:present and future. *Oper Tech Orthop* 1997; 7(1):60–67
6. Bhatt RA, Rozental TD. Bone Graft Substitutes. *Hand Clinics* 2012; 28(4):457–468.
7. Bauer TW. An overview of the histology of skeletal substitute materials. *Arch Pathol Lab Med* 2007; 131(2):217–24.
8. Zhang M, Powers RM Jr, Wolfinbarger L Jr. Effect(s) of the demineralization process on the osteoinductivity of demineralized bone matrix. *J Periodontol* 1997; 68(11):1085–1092.
9. Khan SN, Tomin E, Lane JM. Clinical applications of bone graft substitutes. *Orthop Clin North Am* 2000; 31(3):389–398.
10. Aghdasi B, Montgomery SR, Daubs MD, Wang JC. A review of demineralized bone matrices for spinal fusion: The evidence for efficacy. *Surgeon* 2013; 11(1):39–48.
11. Wood RA, Mealey BL. Histologic comparison of healing after tooth extraction with ridge preservation using mineralized versus demineralized freeze-dried bone allograft. *J Periodontol* 2012; 83 (3):329–336.
12. Kurien T, Pearson RG, Scammell BE. Bone graft substitutes currently available in orthopaedic practice: The evidence for their use. *Bone Joint J* 2013 95-B (5):583–597.
13. Wildemann B, Kadow-Romacker A, Haas NP, Schmidmaier G. Quantification of various growth factors in different demineralized bone matrix preparations. *J Biomed Mater Res A* 2007; 81(2):437–442.
14. van Bergen CJ, Kerkhoffs GM, Ozdemir M, Korstjens CM et al. Demineralized bone matrix and platelet-rich plasma do not improve healing of osteochondral defects of the talus: An experimental goat study. *Osteoarthritis Cartilage* 2013; 21(11):1746–1754.
15. Tian M, Yang Z, Kuwahara K, Nimni ME, Wan C, Han B. Delivery of demineralized bone matrix powder using a thermogelling chitosan carrier. *Acta Biomater* 2012; 8(2):753–762.
16. Kanigan R. Market evaluation of demineralized bone matrix products in Canada: Research highlights. Canadian Council for Donation and Transplantation, 2006; http://www.organsandtissues.ca/s/wp-ontent/uploads/2011/11/Market_Evaluation.pdf

17. Qiu QQ, Shih MS, Stock K, Panzitta T, Murphy PA, Roesch SC, Connor J. Evaluation of DBM/AM composite as a graft substitute for posterolateral lumbar fusion. *J Biomed Mater Res B Appl Biomater* 2007; 82(1):239–245.

18. Lee KJH, Roper JG, Wang JC. Demineralized bone matrix and spinal arthrodesis. *Spine J* 2005; 5(6, Supplement):217S–223S.

19. Wang JC, Kanim LE, Nagakawa IS, Yamane BH, Vinters HV, Dawson EG. Dose-dependent toxicity of a commercially available demineralized bone matrix material. *Spine (Phila Pa 1976)* 2001; 26(13):1429–1435; discussion 1435–1436.

20. Gruskin E, Doll BA, Futrell FW, Schmitz JP, Hollinger JO. Demineralized bone matrix in bone repair: History and use. *Adv Drug Deliv Rev* 2012; 64(12):1063–1077.

21. Kim J, Lee KW, Ahn JH, Kim JY, Lee TY, Choi B. Osteoinductivity depends on the ratio of demineralized bone matrix to acellular dermal matrix in defects in rat skulls. *Tissue Eng Regen Med* 2013; 10(5):246–251.

22. Wilkins RM, Gitelis S, Hart RA, Gross AE. 2013. Human allograft bone processing and safety. *AAOS Now,* March 2013; http://www.aaos.org/news/aaosnow/mar13/research2.asp.

23. Michael JJ, Greenwald AS, Boden S, Brubaker S, Heim CS. 2008. Musculoskeletal allograft tissue safety. In *American Academy of Orthopaedic Surgeons, 75th Annual Meeting,* San Francisco, California, 2008.

24. Holtzclaw D, Toscano N, Eisenlohr L, Callan D. The safety of bone allografts used in dentistry: A review. *J Am Dent Assoc* 2008; 139 (9):1192–1199.

25. FDA. Complete List of Donor Screening Assays for Infectious Agents and HIV Diagnostic Assays. 2013. http://www.fda.gov/biologicsbloodvaccines/bloodbloodproducts/approvedproducts/licensedproductsblas/blooddonorscreening/infectiousdisease/ucm080466.htm.

26. Alanay A, Wang JC, Shamie AN, Napoli A, Chen C, Tsou P. A novel application of high-dose (50kGy) gamma irradiation for demineralized bone matrix: Effects on fusion rate in a rat spinal fusion model. *The Spine J* 2008; 8(5):789–795.

27. AAMI (Association for the Advancement of Medical Instrumentation). Comprehensive guide to steam sterilization and sterility assurance in health care facilities, Amendment 2. 2011.

28. Gross RH. The use of bone grafts and bone graft substitutes in pediatric orthopaedics: An overview. *J Pediatr Orthop* 2012; 32(1):100–105.

29. Glowacki J. A review of osteoinductive testing methods and sterilization processes for demineralized bone. *Cell Tissue Bank* 2005; 6(1):3–12.

30. Vangsness CT Jr, Garcia IA, Mills CR, Kainer MA, Roberts MR, Moore TM. Allograft transplantation in the knee: Tissue regulation, procurement, processing, and sterilization. *Am J Sports Med* 2003; 31(3):474–481.

31. Grieb TA, Forng R-Y, Stafford RE, Lin J et al. Effective use of optimized, high-dose (50kGy) gamma irradiation for pathogen inactivation of human bone allografts. *Biomater* 2005; 26(14):2033–2042.

32. Deakin DE, Bannister GC. Graft incorporation after acetabular and femoral impaction grafting with washed irradiated allograft and autologous marrow. *J Arthroplasty* 2007; 22(1):89–94.

33. Dziedzic-Goclawska A, Ostrowski K, Stachowicz W, Michalik J, Grzesik W. Effect of radiation sterilization on the osteoinductive properties and the rate of remodeling of bone implants preserved by lyophilization and deep-freezing. *Clin Orthop Relat Res* 1991; (272):30–37.

34. Nguyen H, Morgan DA, Forwood MR. Sterilization of allograft bone: Is 25 kGy the gold standard for gamma irradiation? *Cell Tissue Bank* 2007; 8(2):81–91.
35. Germain M, Mohr JW, Rogers C. Demineralized bone matrix market in Canada. *American Association of Tissue Banks 30th Annual Meeting*: American Association of Tissue Banks, 2006.
36. Lye KW, Deatherage JR, Waite PD. The use of demineralized bone matrix for grafting during Le Fort I and Chin osteotomies: Techniques and complications. *J Oral Maxillofac Surg* 2008; 66(8):1580–1585.
37. Schwartz Z, Goldstein M, Raviv E, Hirsch A, Ranly DM, Boyan BD. Clinical evaluation of demineralized bone allograft in a hyaluronic acid carrier for sinus lift augmentation in humans: A computed tomography and histomorphometric study. *Clin Oral Implants Res* 2007; 18(2):204–211.
38. Kim YK, Kim SG, Lim SC, Lee HJ, and Yun PY. A clinical study on bone formation using a demineralized bone matrix and resorbable membrane. *Oral Surg Oral Med Oral Pathol Oral Radiol Endod* 2010; 109(6):e6–e11.
39. Rodríguez IZ, Uceda MIF, Lobato RD, Aniceto GS. 2013. Postraumatic frontal sinus obliteration with calvarial bone dust and demineralized bone matrix: A long term prospective study and literature review. *Int J Oral Maxillofac Surg* 2013; 42(1):71–76.
40. Bielecki T, Cieslik-Bielecka A, Żelawski M, Mikusek W. A side-effect induced by the combination of a demineralized freeze-dried bone allograft and leucocyte and platelet-rich plasma during treatment for large bone cysts: A 4-year follow-up clinical study. *Transfus Apher Sci* 2012; 47(2):133–138.
41. Pflum, ZE, Palumbo SL, Li WJ. Adverse effect of demineralized bone powder on osteogenesis of human mesenchymal stem cells. *Exp Cell Res* 2013; 319(13):1942–1955.
42. Emad B, Sherif el-M, Basma GM, Wong RW, Bendeus M, Rabie AB. Vascular endothelial growth factor augments the healing of demineralized bone matrix grafts. *Int J Surg* 2006; 4(3):160–166.
43. Wang JC, Alanay A, Mark D, Kanim LE, Campbell PA, Dawson EG, Lieberman JR. A comparison of commercially available demineralized bone matrix for spinal fusion. *Eur Spine J* 2007; 16(8):1233–1240.
44. Kumaran ST, Arun KV, Sudarsan S, Talwar A, Srinivasan N. Osteoblast response to commercially available demineralized bone matrices—An in-vitro study. *Indian J Dent Res* 2010; 21(1):3–9.
45. Schwartz Z, Somers A, Mellonig JT, Carnes DL Jr, Dean DD, Cochran DL, Boyan BD. Ability of commercial demineralized freeze-dried bone allograft to induce new bone formation is dependent on donor age but not gender. *J Periodontol* 1998 69(4):470–478.
46. Traianedes, K, Russell JL, Edwards JT, Stubbs HA, Shanahan IR, Knaack D. Donor age and gender effects on osteoinductivity of demineralized bone matrix. *J Biomed Mater Res B Appl Biomater* 2004; 70(1):21–29.
47. Lee YP, Jo M, Luna M, Chien B, Lieberman JR, Wang JC. The efficacy of different commercially available demineralized bone matrix substances in an athymic rat model. *J Spinal Disord Tech* 2005; 18(5):439–44.
48. Li H, Zou X, Springer M, Briest A, Lind M, Bunger C. Instrumented anterior lumbar interbody fusion with equine bone protein extract. *Spine (Phila Pa 1976)* 2007; 32(4):E126–E129.

49. Zhou Z, Zou L, Li H, Bunger C, Zou X. An overview on bone protein extract as the new generation of demineralized bone matrix. *Sci China Life Sci* 2012; 55(12):1045–1056.
50. Kasten P, Luginbühl R, van Griensven M, Barkhausen T, Krettek C, Bohner M, Bosch U. Comparison of human bone marrow stromal cells seeded on calcium-deficient hydroxyapatite, β-tricalcium phosphate and demineralized bone matrix. *Biomater* 2003; 24(15):2593–2603.
51. Lin H, Zhao Y, Sun W, Chen B, Zhang J, Zhao W, Xiao Z, Dai J. The effect of crosslinking heparin to demineralized bone matrix on mechanical strength and specific binding to human bone. *Biomater* 2008; 29(9): 1189-97.

Part III

Biologic Delivery for Bone Grafts

6

Bone Morphogenetic Proteins BMP-2 and BMP-7

Junya Sonobe and Kazuhisa Bessho

CONTENTS

6.1 Introduction

Bone morphogenetic proteins (BMPs) belong to the transforming growth factor-β superfamily. BMPs play important roles in the migration of osteoblast progenitor cells, proliferation of mesenchymal cells, differentiation to chondrogenic or osteogenic cells, vascular invasion, and bone remodeling. BMPs may have a wide potential for clinical applications, including jaw reconstruction, orthognathic surgery, alveolar ridge augmentation, and the diagnosis of osteogenic lesions. We describe our studies and previous studies of BMP-2 and BMP-7 in this chapter.

6.2 BMP-2

6.2.1 Purified BMP-2 and Recombinant Human BMP-2

Difficulties are associated with the purification of bone morphogenetic protein (BMP) because it is present in markedly smaller amounts than those of other non-collagenous proteins in the bone matrix and is relatively insoluble. BMP was found to be soluble in 4M guanidine hydrochloride[1,2] and 6M urea[3] in the 1980s, and its isolation and purification have progressed rapidly. Several BMPs have become available through cloning and genetic engineering. However, some problems are still associated with the bone-inducing activity of recombinant human BMP (rhBMP), the most important of which is that the bone-inducing activity of rhBMP-2 is lower than that of phBMP. The results of bioassays revealed that the bone activity of rhBMP-2 was less than one-tenth that of phBMP. We examined the bone-inducing activity of rhBMP-2 and compared it to that of purified BMP derived from human BMP (phBMP).[4] Fifty micrograms of rhBMP-2 or phBMP was mixed with 3mg of atelopeptide type I collagen, and specimens were implanted in the calf muscles of Wister rats. New bone had formed in rhBMP-2 and phBMP-implanted muscles after 4 weeks and was visible radiographically and histologically (Figure 6.1 shows soft x-ray and histological findings with phBMP and rhBMP-2). Histological findings revealed that the

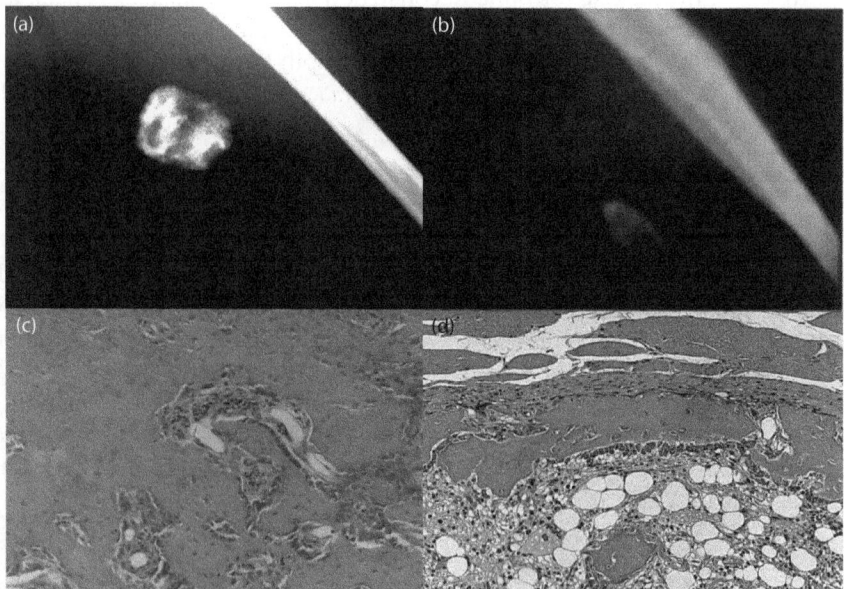

FIGURE 6.1
Soft x-ray and histological findings with phBMP (a, c) and rhBMP-2 (b, d).

maturity levels of rhBMP-2- and phBMP-induced bones were different after implantation: rhBMP-2-induced bone consisted of rich bone marrow containing angioid tissue and a poorer bone matrix. On the other hand, phBMP-induced bone had a small amount of bone marrow and a rich bone matrix. The bone-inducing activity of rhBMP-2 was found to be lower than that of phBMP. However, the clinical application of BMP is more favorable if rhBMP could be easily synthesized and obtained because phBMPs may have immunological problems and a prior risk of viral infections, and are limited in supply.

6.2.2 Suitable Carriers for rhBMP-2

Why rhBMP-2 has lower activity than phBMP needs to be determined, and methods that facilitate the clinical use of rhBMP-2 in conjunction with other suitable carriers to increase bone-inducing activity also need to be established. Recombinant human BMPs are soluble in vivo and disperse shortly after implantation; they do not induce bone formation in large quantities without a carrier. Therefore, in addition to recombinant BMPs, a carrier capable of acting as a slow-delivery system is required to allow sufficient bone induction in vivo. The evaluation of bone-inducing activities using a purer carrier is desirable. We previously reported that atelopeptide type I collagen could also be a useful delivery system for rhBMP-2.[5] Soft x-ray analysis revealed that bone induction was only observed in the part of the implanted material containing rhBMP-2, while histological analysis showed that bone induced by rhBMP-2 consisted of a small amount of bone marrow and a poor bone matrix. As the antigenicity of atelopeptide type I collagen is weak, it does not inhibit osteoinduction. However, problems with some unknown infections such as prions and strength have been reported when collagen has been used. Although the strength of porous hydroxyapatite and titanium is ideal for their application as scaffolds, they are not suitable for use as BMP-2 delivery systems because of their slow delivery rate. Weak biodegradable polymers are suitable as BMP-2 delivery systems, but are not strong enough to be used as scaffolds. Therefore, a synthetically stronger and slowly degradable carrier for BMP-2 is needed before BMP can be used more widely in a clinical setting. Recombinant human BMP-2, obtained by a bacterial expression system, was evaluated in rats due to the potential for large quantities of rhBMP-2 to be produced in this bacterial expression system at a low cost for its clinical application.[6] However, the rhBMP-2 produced by this bacterial expression system was not cheap enough for clinical use because of its low efficiency in humans and other issues.[7] An adenoviral vector system has certain advantages, including the production of a high titer of recombinant virus with ease and high transduction efficiency, especially in primates,[8] as well as its ability to transfer the target gene into nondividing cells. We constructed a BMP-2 gene-expressing recombinant adenoviral vector based on these findings.

6.2.3 Osteoinduction by BMP-2 Gene Therapy In Vivo via Adenoviral Vectors

Adenoviral vectors can more efficiently transfer and express a gene of interest into several kinds of cells. We previously demonstrated that the expression of BMP-2 via an adenoviral vector in C2C12 myoblasts induced differentiation into an osteoblastic lineage.[9] We recognized the ability of this vector to transduce and express a gene of interest into animals via a direct injection. However, adenoviruses are known to induce an immune response that obstructs the duration of gene expression in vivo. Because infected host cells are eliminated by the T-cell mediated immune response, transgene expression cannot be sustained. We evaluated osteoinduction at intramuscular sites under transient immunosuppression. The results obtained revealed that gene therapy with an adenovirus carrying the BMP-2 gene under immunosuppression could induce a larger amount of bone than that with a slow delivery system with rhBMP-2 (Figure 6.2 shows soft x-ray and histological findings with or without immunosuppression). However, the vector could not induce bone formation in immunocompetent rats because of the host immune response. Therefore, we attempted to identify solutions to control or avoid the host immune response against the vector. We showed that osteoinduction could be achieved by the vector

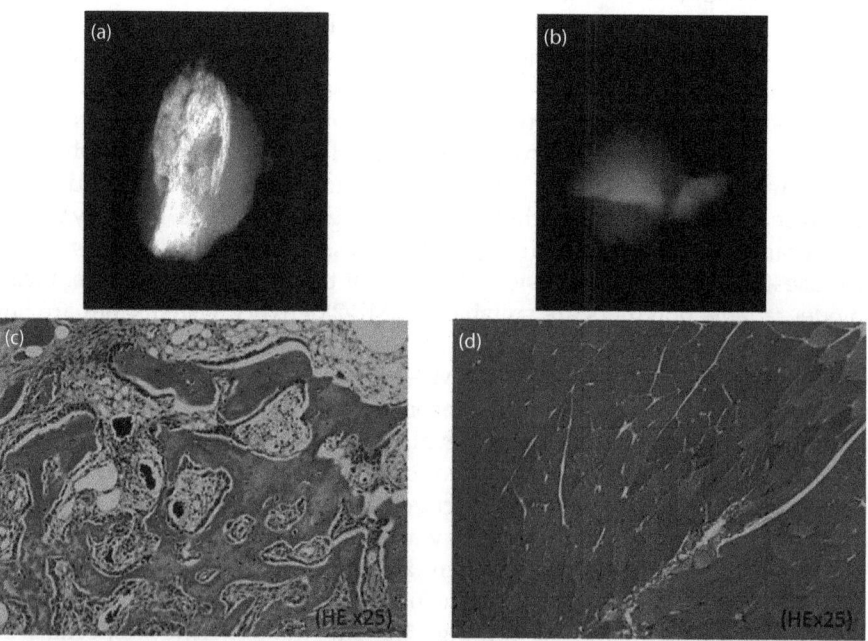

FIGURE 6.2
Soft x-ray and histological findings with adenoviral vector with (a, c) or without (b, d) immunosuppression.

after immunosuppression with cyclophosphamide or FK506.[10,11] We also observed osteoinduction when collagen was used as a masking material to block the host immune system.[12] Although gene therapy with a viral vector is very efficient, potential cytotoxicity and immunogenicity may limit its clinical use.

6.2.4 Osteoinduction by BMP-2 Gene Therapy with Plasmid Vector In Vivo

Gene-based delivery methods for BMP-2 are generally divided into two categories: those using viral vectors and those using nonviral vectors. Nonviral delivery methods do not require immunosuppression for successful gene delivery. We previously reported the successful transfer of the human BMP-2 gene to skeletal muscle in vivo by transcutaneous electroporation[13] (Figure 6.3 shows in vivo electroporation with the plasmid BMP-2 gene to rat skeletal muscles), and showed that it induced ectopic bone formation in the target muscle. A histological examination of ectopic bone specimens in the target muscle revealed well-mineralized trabecular bone with mature bone marrow, including the presence of active osteoblasts and osteoclasts. The expression of human BMP-2 mRNA and secretion of BMP-2 after in vivo transcutaneous electroporation have been reported. This method is simple and inexpensive because it does not require surgery.

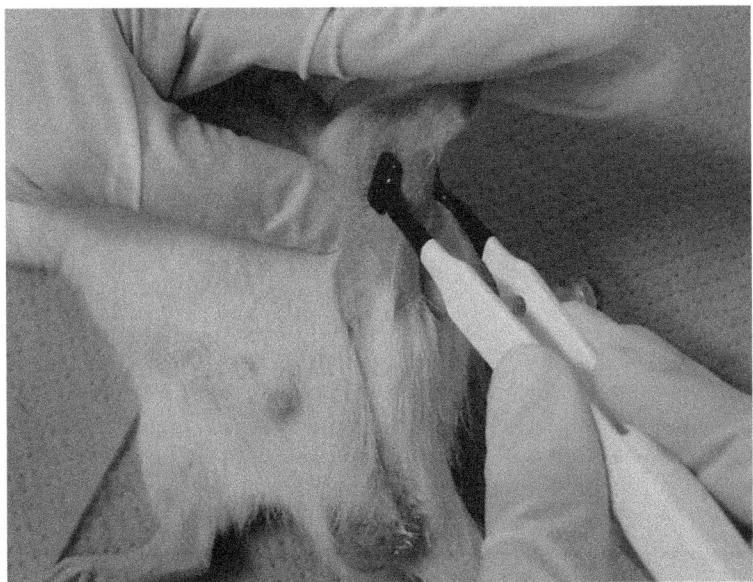

FIGURE 6.3
In vivo electroporation with plasmid BMP-2 gene to rat skeletal muscles.

Although this method has the potential to be used for clinical applications, concerns regarding tissue damage induced by electric pulses need to be addressed. Electroporation also requires special equipment, and the optimization of parameters is necessary. We previously reported osteoinduction by the microbubble-enhanced transcutaneous sonoporation of BMP-2 plasmid DNA.[14] This method also appears to be safer than electroporation, but requires special equipment and the optimization of ultrasound parameters. A direct transcutaneous injection can be repeated as necessary and does not require other special equipment. A very simple approach to promote the osteoinduction of human BMP-2 plasmid DNA needs to be developed. We evaluated the repeated injection of human BMP-2 plasmid DNA, and showed that osteoinduction in mouse skeletal muscle was caused by a direct transcutaneous injection of the human BMP-2 gene.[15]

The results of our previous study showed that the implantation of rhBMP-2 with a carrier matrix, adenovirus-mediated gene transfer, transcutaneous electroporation, or sonoporation achieved osteoinduction. However, practical limitations reduce the probability that these procedures will be used extensively. The purification of rhBMP-2 requires considerable labor and expense, and problems with antigenicity, biocompatibility, biodegradability, and infection have been reported with carrier matrices. Surgical procedures are also required to implant a carrier matrix. The delivery of human BMP-2 genes with adenoviral vectors causes an immune response that needs to be systemically or locally suppressed. Naked plasmid DNA delivery is associated with weak toxicity or immunogenicity. A plasmid encoding the BMP-2 (pCAGGS-BMP-2) gene was injected into the skeletal muscles of mice, and mature bone was observed in mice injected repeatedly with pCAGGS-BMP-2. Human BMP-2 gene therapy by a direct injection was demonstrated with the possibility of effective clinical use.

6.2.5 Clinical Use with BMP-2

Recent clinical studies demonstrated that an absorbable collagen sponge (ACS) with recombinant human bone morphogenetic protein-2 (rhBMP-2) could induce bone formation. A concentration of 1.5 mg/mL rhBMP-2/ACS (INFUSE® Bone Graft, Medtronic Spinal and Biologics, Memphis, TN) was approved by the U.S. Food and Drug Administration (FDA) as an autograft replacement for certain interbody spinal fusion procedures in 2002.[16] The European Commission also approved the Marketing Authorization Application (MAA) for rhBMP-2/ACS for use in the treatment of acute tibia fractures in adults in the European Union (EU) in 2002.

INFUSE® Bone Graft was approved for open tibial factures with intermedullary nail fixation in 2004.[16] INFUSE® Bone Graft was approved as an alternative to autogenous bone grafts for sinus augmentations in defects associated with extraction sockets in March 2007 (Table 6.1 shows rhBMP-2 and rhBMP-7 clinical products).[16]

TABLE 6.1

Recombinant Human BMP-2 and rhBMP-7 Clinical Products

INFUSE® BONE Graft Kits (Medtronic, Inc)	xx Small Kit	x Small Kit	Small Kit	Medium Kit	Large Kit	Large II Kit
rhBMP-2 (mg)	1.05	2.1	4.2	8.4	12	12
BMP-2 concentration (mg/mL)	1.5	1.5	1.5	1.5	1.5	1.5
Total graft volume (mL)	0.7	1.4	2.8	5.6	5.6	8
Absorbable collagen sponge (cm)	1.27×5.08	2.54×5.08	2.54×5.08	2.54×5.08	2.54×5.08	7.62×10.16
OP-1™ IMPLANT (OLYMPUS®)						20 mL vial
rhBMP-7 (mg)						3.3
Purified Type I bovine collagen (g)						1
OP-1™ PUTTY (OLYMPUS®)						
OP-1 IMPLANT (20 mL vial)						
rhBMP-7 (mg)						3.3
Purified Type I bovine collagen (g)						1
Putty Additive (10 mL vial)						
Carboxymethylcellulose (CMC) (mg)						230

6.3 BMP-7

BMP-7, which is also known as OP-1 (osteogenic protein 1), is a growth factor specific to bone growth and formation. The protein encoded by the BMP-7 gene is a member of the TGF-β superfamily. It plays a role in the transformation of mesenchymal cells into bone and cartilage. BMP-7 is inhibited by noggin and chordin, which are expressed in the Spemann–Mangold organizer. It may be involved in bone homeostasis and is expressed in the brain, kidneys, and bladder.[17] BMP-7 has the potential to be used in the treatment of chronic kidney disease.[18,19] BMPs interact with specific receptors on cell surfaces, referred to as bone morphogenetic protein receptors. Signal transduction through these receptors results in the mobilization of members of the SMAD family of proteins. BMP-7 was shown to induce the phosphorylation of SMAD 1 and SMAD 5, which induce the transcription of numerous osteogenic genes.[20] Treatment with BMP-7 was reported to be sufficient to induce all of the genetic markers of osteoblast differentiation in many cell types.[17]

6.3.1 Clinical Use for Bone Reconstruction

Human recombinant BMP-7 has surgical applications and is marketed under the brand name OP-1™ (sold by Olympus, who bought it from Stryker). It can be used to aid in the fusion of vertebral bodies in order to prevent neurological trauma,[21] and in the treatment of tibial non union, which has frequently been observed in cases in which a bone graft has failed.[22] Recombinant human BMP-2 is more widely used clinically because bone growth is better with it than with rhBMP-7 or other BMPs.[23] Stryker reported that OP-1™ Putty and OP-1™ Implant are currently approved in the United States under Humanitarian Device Exemptions (HDE) for revision posterolateral lumbar spine fusion and the treatment of long bone nonunion fractures, respectively.[24] OP-1™ Implant has been approved in 28 additional countries, including Australia, Canada, and the European Union. Approximately 40,000 patients have been treated globally with OP-1 products (Table 6.1 shows rhBMP-2 and rhBMP-7 clinical products).[24]

OP-1™ has also been utilized in cases of jaw reconstruction. Ten patients with mandibular defects following resection of ameloblastoma or osteomyelitis were treated with a combination of BMP-7 and demineralized bone matrix.[25] The postoperative course was uneventful and bone formation was identified radiographically. No complications were observed in jaw function or aesthetic appearance one year after surgery. The HA/OP-1 composite implant applied to a vascularized pedicled bone flap was demonstrated to be useful in reconstructing half of the human mandible. An MRSA infection of the graft led to its failure five months after surgery. However, this case successful demonstrated osteoinduction using the HA/OP-1 composite implant in the human skeletal muscle.[26]

6.3.2 Clinical Use for Kidney Disease

Pre-clinical research reported the potential of BMP-7 to cure most kidney diseases in humans, with the possibility of relieving the suffering of hundreds of thousands of people now on dialysis and millions of others with pre-dialysis kidney diseases.[27] The expression of BMP-7 in adults is selectively limited to bone and the kidneys. High levels of BMP-7 have been reported in the distal convoluted tubules of the renal cortex. BMP-7 was previously shown to be localized to the outer medullary collecting ducts.[28,29] TGF-β and its downstream Smad cascade are known to be key mediators in the pathogenesis of renal fibrosis both in experimental models and human kidney diseases.[30-32] The up-regulation of TGF-β and its downstream Smad cascade is prevalent in many types of kidney diseases. TGF-β mediates progressive renal fibrosis by stimulating the production of the extracellular matrix, while inhibiting its degradation. TGF-β is also considered to induce the tubular epithelial–mesenchymal transition of injured tubule epithelial cells,[33] whereas the in vivo relevance of the epithelial–mesenchymal transition remains controversial. TGF-β was also shown to mediate the accumulation of the mesangial matrix in diabetic nephropathy.[34,35] Several strategies to inhibit the TGF-β signaling pathway have been proposed, including the administration of neutralizing antibodies against TGF-β. BMP-7 exerts several functions in various types of kidney cells. It antagonizes TGF-β-dependent fibrosis[36] and reduces the amount of apoptosis in tubular epithelial cells and podocytes.[37,38] In contrast to anti-TGF-β strategies that may augment inflammation, BMP-7 has been shown to attenuate the renal expression of inflammatory cytokines[39,40] and reduce the infiltration of inflammatory cells. Collectively, BMP-7 promotes various aspects of the repair process during kidney diseases.

Evidence to support the important roles of BMP antagonists in developing and diseased kidneys is increasing.[41,42] Among the many BMP antagonists examined, uterine sensitization-associated gene-1 (USAG-1) and gremlin are the most intensively studied. USAG-1 is a 28-kDa secretory protein that acts as a BMP antagonist.[43] USAG-1 null mice exhibited prolonged survival, preserved renal function, and reduced renal fibrosis in animal models of acute and chronic kidney injuries.[44,45] Renal BMP signaling was significantly enhanced in USAG-1 null mice during renal injury, whereas the administration of a neutralizing antibody against BMP-7 abolished renoprotection, indicating that USAG-1 plays a role in modulating the renoprotective action of BMP-7.[44]

6.3.3 Clinical Use for Supernumerary Tooth Formation

USAG-1 is a BMP antagonist and modulates Wnt signaling. We previously reported that USAG-1 deficient mice have supernumerary teeth.[46] The supernumerary maxillary incisor appears to form as a result of the successive development of the rudimentary upper incisor. USAG-1 abrogation rescued the apoptotic elimination of odontogenic mesenchymal cells. We confirmed that BMPs were expressed in both the epithelium and mesenchyme of the rudimentary incisor at E14 and E15. BMP signaling in the rudimentary maxillary incisor, assessed by the expression of Msx and Dlx2 and the phosphorylation of Smad protein, was significantly enhanced. The inhibition of BMP signaling was shown to rescue supernumerary tooth formation in an E15 incisor explant culture (Figure 6.4 shows supernumerary tooth formation in a USAG-1 knockout mouse).

Based on these results, we concluded that enhanced BMP signaling results in supernumerary teeth and BMP signaling was modulated by Wnt signaling in the USAG-1 deficient mouse model.[47]

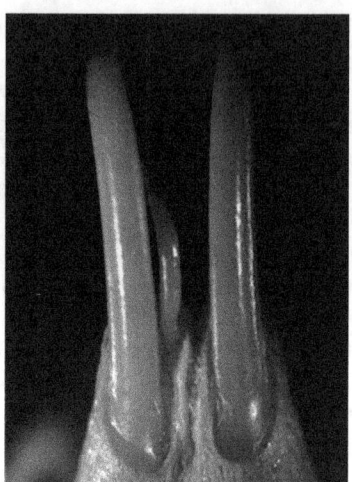

FIGURE 6.4
Supernumerary tooth formation of USAG-1 knockout mouse.

References

1. Takaoka K., Ono K., Amitani K. et al. 1980. Solubilization and concentration of a bone-inducing substance from a murine osteoma. *Clin Orthop* 148: 274–280.
2. Hanamura H., Higuchi Y., Nakagawa M. et al. 1980. Solubilized bone morphogenetic protein (BMP) from mouse osteosarcoma and rat demineralized bone matrix. *Clin Orthop* 148: 281–290.
3. Urist M.R., Leitze A., Mizutani H. et al. 1982. A bovine low molecular weight bone morphogenetic protein (BMP) fraction. *Clin Orthop* 162: 219–232.
4. Bessho K., Kusumoto K., Fujimura K. et al. 1999. Comparison of recombinant and purified human bone morphogenetic protein. *Br J Oral Maxillofac Surg* 37: 2–5.
5. Fujimura K., Bessho K., Kusumoto K. et al. 1995. Experimental studies on bone inducing activity of composites of atelopeptide type I collagen as a carrier for ectopic osteoinduction by rhBMP-2. *Biochem Biophys Res Commun* 208: 316–22.
6. Bessho K., Konishi Y., Kaihara S. et al. 2000. Bone induction by Escherichia coli-derived recombinant human bone morphogenetic protein-2 compared with Chinese hamster ovary cell-derived recombinant human bone morphogenetic protein-2. *Br J Oral Maxillofac Surg* 38: 645–649.
7. Boyne P.J. 2001. Application of bone morphogenetic proteins in the treatment of clinical oral and maxillofacial osseous defects. *J Bone Joint Surg Am* 83-A Suppl 1: S146–150.
8. Saito I. 1994. Adenovirus vector. *Uirusu* 44: 100–104.
9. Okubo Y., Bessho K., Fujimura K. et al. 1999. Expressing of bone morphogenetic protein-2 via adenoviral vector in C2C12 myoblasts induces differentiation into the osteoblast lineage. *Biochem Biophys Res Commun* 262: 730–743.
10. Okubo Y., Bessho K., Fujimura K. et al. 2000. Osteoinduction by bone morphogenetic protein-2 via adenoviral vector under transient immunosuppression. *Biochem Biophys Res Commun* 267: 382–387.

11. Sonobe J., Bessho K., Kaihara S. et al. 2002. Bone induction by BMP-2 expressing adenoviral vector in rats under treatment with FK506. *J Musculoskeletal Res* 6: 23–29.

12. Sonobe J., Okubo Y., Kaihara S. et al. 2004. Osteoinduction by bone morphogenetic protein 2-expressing adenoviral vector: Application of biomaterial to mask the host immune response. *Hum Gene Ther* 15: 659–668.

13. Kawai M., Bessho K. Kaihara S. et al. 2003. Ectopic bone formation by human morphogenetic protein-2 gene transfer to skeletal muscle using transcutaneous electroporation. *Hum Gene Ther* 14: 1547–1556.

14. Osawa K., Okubo Y., Nakao K. et al. 2009. Osteoinduction by micro bubble-enhanced transcutaneous sonoporation of human bone morphogenetic protein-2. *J Gene Med* 11: 633–641.

15. Osawa K., Okubo Y., Nakao K. et al. 2010. Osteoinduction by repeat plasmid injection of human bone morphogenetic protein-2. *J Gene Med* 12: 937–944.

16. Mckay W.M., Peckham S.M, and Badura J.M. 2007. A comprehensive clinical review of recombinant human bone morphogenetic protein-2 (INFUSE® Bone Graft). *Int Orthop.* 31: 729–734.

17. Chen D., Zhao M., and Mundy G.R. 2004. Bone morphogenetic proteins. *Growth Factors* 22: 233–41.

18. Gould S.E., Day M., Jones S.S. et al. 2002. BMP-7 regulates chemokine, cytokine, and hemodynamic gene expression in proximal tubule cells. *Kidney Int.* 61: 51–60.

19. Gonzalez E.A., Lund R.J. Martin K.J. et al. 2002. Treatment of a murine model of high-turnover renal osteodystrophy by exogenous BMP-7. *Kidney Int.* 61: 1322–1331.

20. Itoh F., Asao H., Sugamura K. et al. 2001. Promoting bone morphogenetic protein signaling through negative regulation of inhibitory Smads. *EMBO J.* 20: 4132–4142.

21. Vaccaro A.R., Whang P.G., Patel T. et al. 2008. The safety and efficacy of OP-1 (rhBMP-7) as a replacement for iliac crest autograft for posterolateral lumbar arthrodesis: Minimum 4-year follow-up of a pilot study. *Spine* J8: 457–465.

22. Zimmermann G., Muller U., Loffer C. et al. 2007. Therapeutic outcome in tibia pseudarthrosis: Bone morphogenetic protein 7 (BMP-7) versus autologous bone grafting for tibial fractures. *Unfallchirurg* 110: 931–938.

23. Even J., Eskander M., and Kang J. 2012. Bone morphogenetic protein in spine surgery: Current and future uses. *J Am Acad Orthop Surg* 20: 547–552.

24. Stryker Inc. Osteoinductive-OP-1/BMP-7. An overview of OP-1 products. http://www.stryker.com/cn/products/Orthobiologicals/Osteoinductive/OP-1/index/htm (accessed October 28, 2013).

25. Cameron M.L. and George K.B. 2008. Reconstruction of 10 major mandibular defects using bioimplants containing BMP-7. *JCDA* 74, no.1 (February): 67–72. http://www.cda-adc.ca/jcda/vol-74/issue-1/67.html (accessed October 28, 2013).

26. Heliotis M., Lavery U., Ripamonti U. et al. 2006. Transformation of a prefabricated hydroxyapatite/osteogenic protein-1 implant into a vascularised pedicled bone flap in the human chest. *Int J Oral Maxillofac Surg* 35: 265–269.

27. Frank Baker. BMP-7: Human trials now to end kidney disease. http://www.ipetitions.com/petition/bmp7/ (accessed October 28, 2013).

28. Wang S., Lapage J., and Hirschberg R. 2001. Loss of tubular bone morphogenetic protein-7 (BMP7) in diabetic nephropathy. *J Am Soc Nephrol* 12: 2392–2399.

29. Wetzel P., Haag J., Campean V. et al. 2006. Bone morphogenetic protein-7 expression and activity in the human adult normal kidney is predominantly localized to the distal nephron. *Kidney Int* 70: 717–723.

30. Lan H.Y. 2008. Diverse roles of TGF-beta/Smads in renal fibrosis and inflammation. *Int J Biol Sci* 7: 1056–1067.

31. Decleves A.E. and Sharma K. 2010. New pharmacological treatments for improving renal outcomes in diabetes. *Nat Rev Nephrol* 6: 371–380.

32. Bottinger E.P. 2007. TGF-beta in renal injury and disease. *Semin Nephrol* 27: 309–320.

33. Lan H.Y. 2003. Tubular epithelial-myofibroblast trans differentiation mechanisms in proximal tubule cells. *Curr Opin Nephrol Hypertens* 12: 25–29.

34. Sharma K. and Ziyadeh F.N. 1995. Hyperglycemia and diabetic kidney disease. The case for transforming growth factor-beta as a key mediator. *Diabetes* 44: 1139–1146.

35. Sharma K. and McGowan T.A. 2000. TGF-beta in diabetic kidney disease: Role of novel signaling pathways. *Cytokine Growth Factor Rev* 11: 115–123.

36. Wang S., Chen Q., Simon T.C. et al. 2006. Bone morphogenetic protein-7 (BMP-7), a novel therapy for diabetic nephropathy. *Kidney Int* 63: 2037–2049.

37. Mitu G.M., Wang S., and Hirschberg R. 2007. BMP7 is a podocyte survival factor and rescues podocytes from diabetic injury. *Am J Physiol* 293: F1641–F1648.

38. De Petris L., Hruska K.A., Chiechio S. et al. 2007. Bone morphogenetic proteon-7 delays podocytes injury due to high glucose. *Nephrol Dial Transplant* 22: 3442–3450.

39. Gould S.E., Day M., Jones S.S. et al. 2001. BMP-7 regulates chemokine, cytokine, and hemodynamic gene expression in proximal tubule cells. *Kidney Int* 61: 51–60.

40. Zhang X.L., Selbi W., de la Motte C. et al. 2005. Bone morphogenetic protein-7 inhibits monocyte-stimulated TGF-beta 1 generation in renal proximal tubular epithelial cells. *J Am Soc Nephrol* 16: 79–89.

41. Nakamura J. and Yanagita M. 2012. BMP modulators in kidney disease. *Discov Med* 13: 57–63.

42. Yanagita M. 2010. Antagonists of bone morphogenetic proteins in kidney disease. *Curr Opin Investig Drugs* 11: 315–322.

43. Yanagita M., Oka M., Watanabe T. et al. 2004. USAG-1: A bone morphogenetic protein antagonist abundantly expressed in the kidney. *Biochem Biophys Res Commun* 316: 490–500.

44. Yanagita M., Okuda T., Endo S. et al. 2006. Uterine sensitization-associated gene-1(USAG-1), a novel BMP antagonist expressed in the kidney, accelerates tubular injury. *J Clin Invest* 116: 70–79.

45. Tanaka M., Asada M., Higashi A.Y. et al. 2010. Loss of the BMP antagonist USAG-1 ameliorates disease in a mouse model of the progressive hereditary kidney disease Alport syndrome. *J Clin Invest* 120: 768–777.

46. Murashima-Suginami A., Takahashi K., Kawabata T. et al. 2007. Rudiment incisors survive and erupt as supernumerary teeth as a result of USAG-1 abrogation. *Biochem Biophys Res Commun* 359: 549–555.

47. Murashima-Suginami A., Takahashi K., Sakata T. et al. 2008. Enhanced BMP signaling results in supernumerary tooth formation in USAG-1 deficient mouse. *Biochem Biophys Res Commun* 369: 1012–1016.

7

Biologics for Bone Regeneration and Local Delivery Mechanisms

Scott A. Guelcher

CONTENTS

7.1 Introduction

Local delivery of rhBMP-2 is a clinically proven strategy for bone regeneration [1–4]. Collagen, which is the primary protein component of bone, is an effective carrier for rhBMP-2 due to its biocompatibility and ability to bind rhBMP-2 [5]. The U.S. Food and Drug Administration (FDA) has approved the use of rhBMP-2 delivered on an absorbable collagen sponge (sold commercially as INFUSE® Bone Graft by Medtronic Sofamor Danek) for posterolateral lumbar fusion, grafting fractures of the tibial mid-diaphysis, sinus lift procedures, and alveolar ridge augmentations [6]. Considering recent reports that rhBMP-2 promotes bone healing as well as autograft [7], it has become a common standard of care for treating severe fractures. The bolus release of rhBMP-2 from collagen [1,8] recruits local osteoprogenitor cells and initiates osteogenesis [9]. However, the majority of the rhBMP-2 is released in the first few days [10], which has been associated with the need to deliver supra-physiological doses of rhBMP-2 to induce a robust osteogenic effect. Rapidly released rhBMP-2 may diffuse from the fracture site prior to significant infiltration of osteoprogenitor cells into the scaffold [1]. Furthermore, rapid release of the drug may result in complications such as inflammation and ectopic bone formation [11,12].

While rhBMP-2 is considered a standard of care for treating many types of bone defects, a number of other osteobiologics are currently under study as alternatives for bone regeneration. Considering that bone healing is dependent on vascularization [13–16] and that the processes of vasculogenesis and bone repair are highly coupled, local delivery of recombinant angio-osteogenic factors such as platelet-derived growth factor (rhPDGF), vascular endothelial growth factor (VEGF), and fibroblast growth factor (FGF) has been investigated as a potential strategy for bone restoration and repair. These factors have been reported to have angiogenic properties and have been investigated for their potential to heal bone defects. They have also been investigated for their potential to enhance the osteoinductive properties of rhBMP-2. In addition to these recombinant human proteins, small molecule drugs have also been investigated for treatment of bone fractures. Statins, a family of natural compounds that inhibit 3-hydroxy-3-methylglutaryl-coenzyme A (HMG-CoA) reductase and reduce serum cholesterol, are known to increase BMP2 expression and stimulate bone formation in vivo and in vitro [17–21].

In this chapter, alternative osteobiologics to rhBMP-2 are reviewed, including their mechanism of action and efficacy in preclinical and clinical studies. Consideration is also given to the release kinetics that support optimum bone healing, as well as combination of these drugs with rhBMP-2 to enhance healing.

7.2 Recombinant Human Growth Factors

Bone regeneration is a complex event that requires the interaction of numerous growth factors. In addition to BMP-2, a number of factors play an active role in fracture repair, including FGF, VEGF, and PDGF. These properties have prompted researchers to investigate the potential of these factors for inducing new bone formation, both alone and in combination with each other and/or rhBMP-2. In this section, the effects of local delivery of rhFGF, rhVEGF, and rhPDGF from bone grafts on healing of bone defects is reviewed.

7.2.1 Recombinant Human Fibroblast Growth Factor (rhFGF)

FGF and FGF receptor (FGFR) signaling is an important pathway involved in skeletal development and fracture healing [22]. Twenty-two FGFs have been identified, and FGF-1, 2, 5, 6, 8, 16, and 18 are up-regulated during fracture healing [22]. In a recent study, the role of FGF-9 in long bone repair was investigated in mice. Treatment with FGF-9 promoted angiogenesis and rescued the healing capacity of mice lacking the FGF-9 gene [23]. Furthermore, although other angio-osteogenic factors, including FGF-2, FGF-18, BMP-2, were expressed in FGF-9-deficient mice, bone healing was still impaired, which underscores the important role of FGF-9 in long bone repair.

Considering the importance of FGF in bone regeneration, a number of studies have investigated the effects of local delivery of rhFGF on healing of craniofacial bone defects. Several studies have reported that rhFGF delivered from injectable and implantable scaffolds enhances periodontal regeneration. Delivery of rhFGF-2 from an injectable macroporous calcium phosphate cement (CaP) enhanced healing of bone and the periodontal ligament (PDL) in intra-bony periodontal defects in Wistar rats compared to CaP alone and CaP augmented with rhBMP-2 [24]. In canine buccal gingival recession [25] and intra-bony [26] defects, rhFGF-2 delivered from β-tricalcium phosphate (β-TCP) enhanced new bone and cementum formation compared to β-TCP alone. rhFGF-2 has also been reported to enhance healing of critical-size calvarial defects in preclinical models. When combined with DNA/protamine complex paste (D/P), rhFGF-2 increased both new bone formation as well as osteogenic gene expression in rat calvarial defects at 3 months post-implantation [27]. In another rat calvarial defect study, delivery of rhFGF-2 from an absorbable collagen sponge (ACS) increased blood vessel and new bone formation at 28 days in a dose-responsive manner [28].

Scaffolds augmented with rhFGF have been also investigated for their potential to heal orthopedic bone defects. Slow release of rhb-FGF from crosslinked gelatin hydrogels was more effective at healing mouse femoral defects compared to fast release [29]. Delivery of rhFGF-2 from a β-TCP/collagen paste increased new bone formation and flexural strength in rabbit tibial shaft segmental defects at 12 weeks [30]. In another femoral segmental defect study in rats, local delivery of rhbFGF from porous carbonate apatite scaffolds increased new bone formation at 2 and 12 weeks compared to the scaffold alone [31]. rhFGF has also been shown to be effective approach for healing osteochondral defects. Delivery of 100 μg/ml rhFGF-2 from a porous hydroxyapatite/collagen scaffold enhanced both bone and cartilage regeneration in a rabbit osteochondral defect model [32]. Despite the success of local delivery of rhFGF in regenerating new bone in rodent models, its utility in larger animals and in patients has not been extensively investigated.

7.2.2 Platelet-Derived Growth Factor (rhPDGF)

Recombinant human PDGF BB homodimer (rhPDGF-BB) is a potent recruiter of mesenchymal stem cells (MSCs) and tenocytes, which are crucial for musculoskeletal tissue repair [33]. As shown in Figure 7.1, rhPDGF-BB also up-regulates chemotaxis, angiogenesis, macrophage activation, and

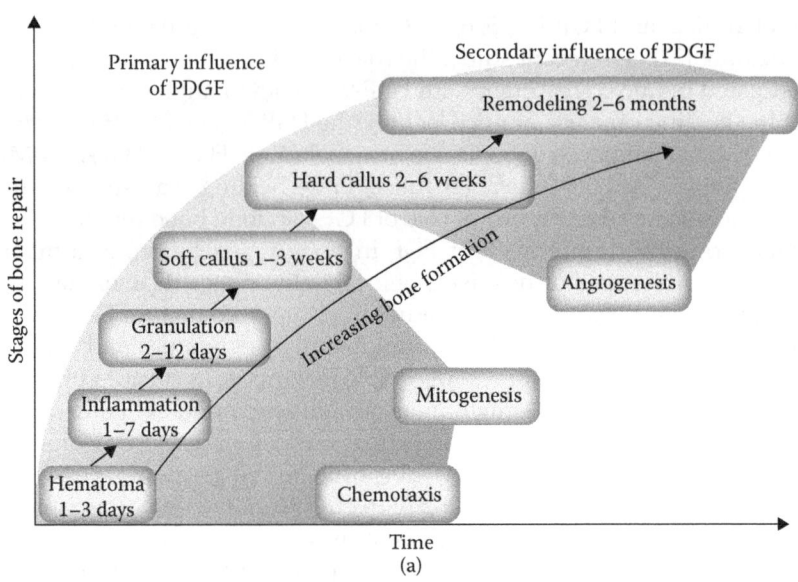

FIGURE 7.1
RhPDGF in bone repair. (a) Role of rhPDGF on the stages of bone repair. (b) Comparison of growth factors in bone healing. (Adapted from Chang PC et al. *Biomaterials*; 34:9990–7, 2013. With permission.)

mitogenesis, which enable it to trigger the cascade of bone and adjoining soft tissue repair and regeneration [33–35]. Recent studies further suggest that PDGF recruits pericytes from their abluminal location and stimulates their mitotic expansion [36]. Thus, PDGF contributes to the stabilization of newly formed vessels that drive new bone formation. Consequently, rhPDGF-BB has been investigated extensively for enhancing bone healing, with the result that several products are under commercial development. Based on clinical studies demonstrating its safety and efficacy, the FDA has approved products for regeneration of alveolar bone lost to periodontal disease and for healing of chronic foot ulcers [33]. A third product comprising rhPDGF-BB delivered from an osteoconductive bone matrix is the in late stages of development for foot and ankle fusion.

The safety and efficacy of local delivery of rhPDGF-BB for regeneration of craniofacial bone has been highlighted in a number of preclinical and clinical studies, and has been recently reviewed [37]. Delivery of rhPDGF from a β-TCP carrier reduced probing pocket depth, increased clinical attachment level, and increased bone growth in 18 patients with infrabony defects at 12 months compared to the hydroxyapatite control [38]. Another clinical study of 135 patients with one localized periodontal osseous defect has reported treatment with 0.3 or 1.0 mg/mL rhPDGF-BB delivered from a β-TCP carrier significantly increased clinical attachment level and linear bone growth compared to the carrier alone [39]. In a recent study, sequential delivery of rhPDGF-BB followed by lovastatin from double-walled PLGA microspheres accelerated periodontal regeneration compared to either molecule alone in a rat model [40]. While rhPDGF-BB has been investigated most extensively for craniofacial bone defects, it has also been found to be a safe and effective alternative to autograft bone for foot and ankle fusion procedures [35]. Due to its angiogenic properties, it is being investigated in preclinical models of diabetes-impaired fracture healing [41] and distraction osteogenesis [42]. The properties of rhPDGF-BB are compared to those of rhBMP-2 in Figure 7.1b. While the mechanism of action of rhBMP-2 is induction, the mechanisms of action for rhPDGF are chemotaxis, mitogenesis, and angiogenesis. Consequently, there is no risk of ectopic bone formation, in contrast to rhBMP-2. rhPDGF is also administered at a lower dose (0.3 mg/mL) compared to rhBMP-2 (1.5 mg/mL).

7.2.3 Vascular Endothelial Growth Factor (rhVEGF)

VEGF increases bone formation by promoting vascularization and osteoblast differentiation, which are essential for bone healing [43]. The osteoinductivity of rhVEGFA has been compared to that of rhBMP-2 and rhFGF-2. In a rat calvarial defect model, rhVEGFA and rhBMP-2 showed similar angiogenic and bone healing capacities, which exceeded those of rhFGF-2 [44]. Another critical-size calvarial defect study in mice has reported that the release kinetics of rhVEGF regulates bone healing [45]. Sustained release of rhVEGF from a biphasic calcium phosphate scaffold for up to 28 days promoted vascularization and new bone formation, while a burst release of the drug did not promote bone healing. Local delivery of rhVEGF from biodegradable microspheres has also been investigated as a strategy for vascularization of cortical bone allografts [46]. While rhFGF-2 had minimal effect on allograft vascularization, rhVEGF increased cortical bone blood as well as new bone formation in frozen allografts implanted with an arteriovenous bundle in rat femoral diaphyseal defects. In another segmental defect study in the rabbit radius, rhVEGF delivered from a β-TCP scaffold enhanced bone healing, as assessed by histology and biomechanical testing, compared to the scaffold alone at 12 weeks [47]. Co-delivery of rhVEGF with MSCs has also been investigated as a strategy for healing bone defects in elderly patients. Delivery of MSCs and a bolus release of rhVEGF from collagen scaffolds enhanced healing of segmental femoral defects in mice compared to MSCs or rhVEGF alone [48]. While these studies in rodent models highlight the osteoinductive potential of rhVEGF, its utility in large-animal models merits further studies.

7.2.4 Combinations with rhBMP-2

Vasculogenesis and bone repair are highly coupled, as exemplified by the stimulation of angiogenesis through osteoblast-derived VEGF [49]. Consequently, enhancement of either process is beneficial to the other, which has prompted many studies investigating the effects of dual delivery of rhVEGF or rhPDGF and the osteogenic factor rhBMP-2 on bone healing. However, there are conflicting reports about the efficacy of dual delivery of rhVEGF and rhBMP-2. Mechanistic studies have suggested that dual delivery of rhVEGF and rhBMP-2 enhances new bone formation compared to either drug alone. In one study, human periosteium-derived cells were transfected with BMP-2, VEGF, or VEGF+BMP-2 and implanted in the muscle of nude mice [50]. VEGF+BMP-2-transfected cells formed significantly more ectopic bone at 4 weeks. Furthermore, VEGF increased the number of blood vessels compared to treatments without VEGF. Another recent study has reported that VEGF and BMP-2 promote new bone formation by mobilizing endogenous stem cells and directing their endothelial and osteogenic differentiation [51]. Preclinical studies in models of bone regeneration have found that the release kinetics of rhVEGF and rhBMP-2 have an important effect on bone regeneration. One study has reported that a burst release of rhVEGF and sustained release of rhBMP-2 from a poly(propylene fumarate) scaffold did not increase vasculogenesis or new bone formation relative to rhBMP-2 alone in a segmental defect model (Figure 7.2) [52]. A similar study in a rat calvarial defect model also found that a burst release of both rhVEGF and rhBMP-2 did not increase new bone formation compared to rhBMP-2 alone at 12 weeks [53]. In contrast, a sustained release of both rhBMP-2 and rhVEGF has been reported to have a synergistic effect on bone healing. As shown in Figure 7.3a, silk hydrogels supported a sustained release of rhBMP-2 and rhVEGF at similar rates, in contrast to the sequential delivery approach shown in Figure 7.2a. Sustained delivery of both factors increased new bone formation at 12 weeks in a rabbit sinus floor model (Figure 7.3c–h), presumably due to increased angiogenesis supported by rhVEGF (Figure 7.3b) [54]. Another study found that sustained release of

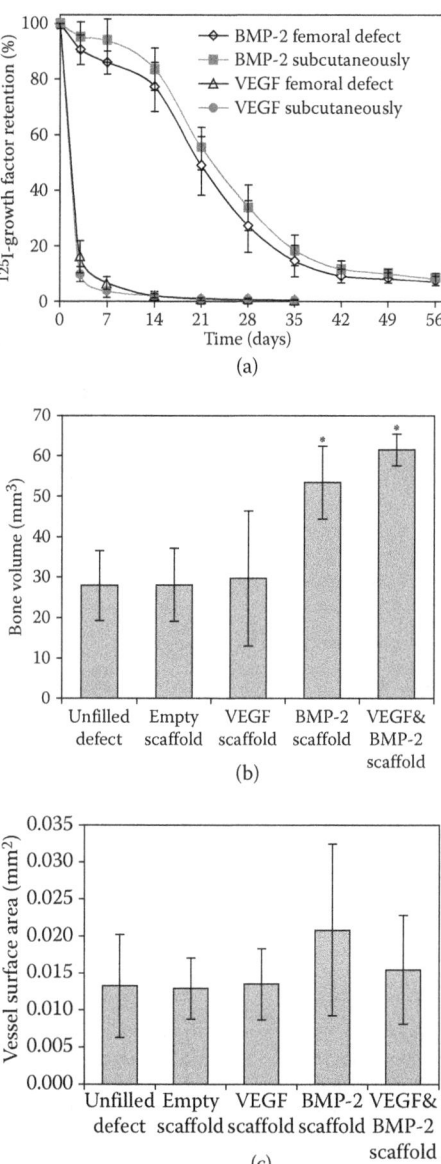

FIGURE 7.2

Sequential delivery of rhVEGF and rhBMP-2 in a 5-mm rat segmental defect model. (a) rhVEGF and rhBMP-2 were radio-labeled with ^{125}I and their retention in the scaffold determined by measurements of γ-irradiation. Release of rhVEGF is complete on day 14, while the rhBMP-2 release is sustained for >56 days. (b) Quantification of new bone volume in the defect by μCT showed significant differences between rhBMP-2- and non-rhBMP-2-treated groups. Sequential delivery of rhVEGF and rhBMP-2 did not significantly increase new bone formation. (c) Surface area of new blood vessels at 8 weeks showed no significant differences between rhVEGF, rhBMP-2, and rhVEGF + rhBMP-2.

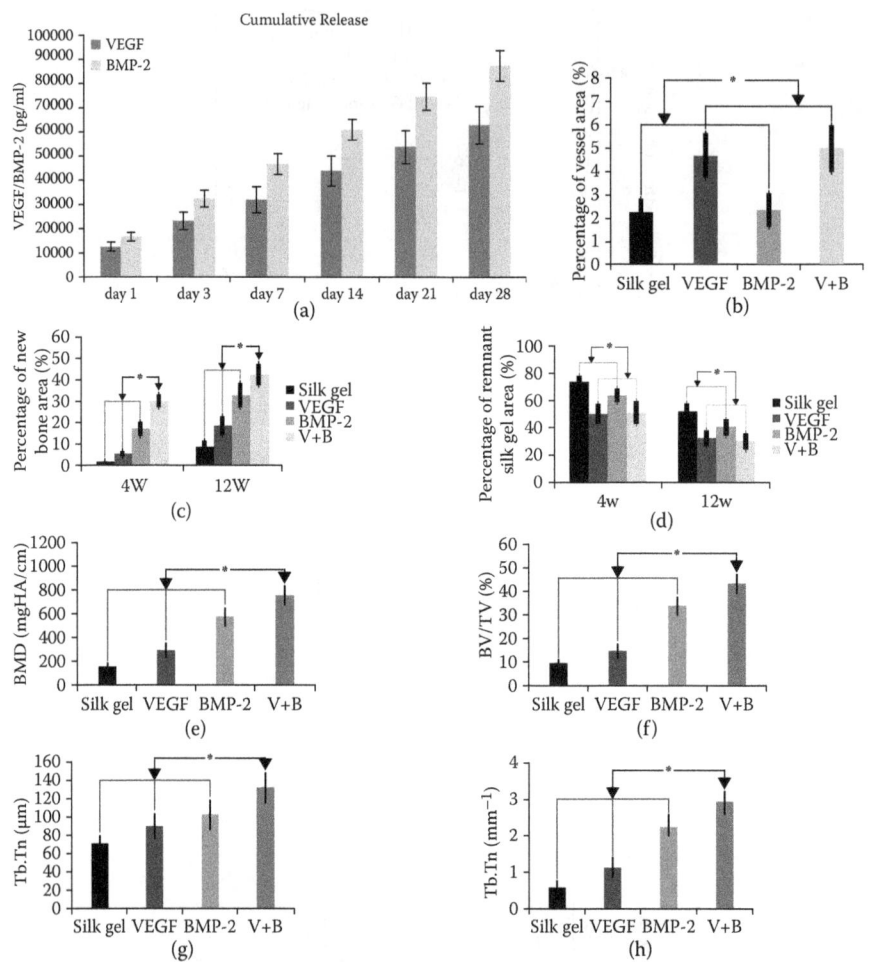

FIGURE 7.3
Co-delivery of rhVEGF and rhBMP-2 from silk scaffolds for elevation of the maxillary sinus floor [54]. (a) Release kinetics shows that rhVEGF and rhBMP-2 are released at approximately the same rate. (b) Delivery of rhVEGF alone or rhVEGF and rhBMP-2 enhances formation of new blood vessels at 12 weeks. (c,d) Histomorphometric analysis of bone healing. (c) New bone formation and (d) residual silk gel for four groups at 4 and 12 weeks post-operation (* indicates significant differences, $p < 0.05$). (e–h) Quantitative analysis of μCT scans of (e) bone mineral density (BMD), (f) the ratio of bone volume to total volume (BV/TV), (g) trabecular thickness (Tb.Th), and (h) trabecular number (Tb.N) were calculated to assess the quality of newly formed bone in the different groups. (Adapted from Zhang W et al., *Biomaterials*; 32:9415–24, 2011. With permission.)

rhVEGF and rhBMP-2 increased new bone formation at 4 weeks, but not at 12 weeks, compared to rhBMP-2 alone in a rat femoral defect model [55]. Taken together, these studies suggest that both the dose of rhVEGF and rhBMP-2 as well as the release kinetics must be optimized to enhance bone healing compared to either factor alone.

The effects of dual delivery of rhPDGF-BB and rhBMP-2 on new bone formation have also been investigated. Bone marrow–derived MSCs were transfected to expression BMP-2 using an adenoviral vector and co-delivered with rhPDGF-BB in critical-size rat defects [56]. Dual delivery of rhPDGF-BB and BMP-2 increased new bone formation and bone mineral density compared to either factor alone, which was attributed to the modulation of rhPDGF-BB on BMP-2-induced new bone formation. In a similar study, MSCs were transfected (using an adenovirus) to express PDGF and BMP-7 and seeded on silk scaffolds followed by implantation in femoral defects in ovariectomized rats [57]. Dual-delivery of PDGF and BMP-7 enhanced new bone formation at 4 weeks compared to either factor alone. However, the effects of the release kinetics of rhPDGF and rhBMP-2 on bone healing have not been extensively explored.

7.2.5 Summary

Preclinical studies in rodent models of bone regeneration have highlighted the osteoinductive potential of rhVEGF, rhFDF, and rhPDGF. Local delivery of rhPDGF-BB from a β-TCP carrier supports new bone formation and healing of periodontal and foot and ankle bone defects in human patients. However, the potential of rhPDGF-BB for healing other types of bone defects is not well known and warrants further investigation. Studies investigating the co-delivery of rhVEGF, rhFGF, or rhPDGF and rhBMP-2 have been motivated by the potential for enhancing the osteogenic potential of rhBMP-2 by enhancing angiogenesis at early time points. However, these co-delivery studies have given mixed results due to the challenges associated with delivering two different growth factors at biologically relevant release rates. Furthermore, the data suggest that sustained release of both factors appears to be a more effective strategy for regenerating new bone than sequential delivery of rhVEGF followed by rhBMP-2.

7.3 Statins

In a seminal 1999 study, Mundy et al. reported that statins induced osteogenic differentiation in vitro and new bone formation in vivo [17]. This family of natural compounds are mediators of the mevalonate pathway by inhibiting HMG-CoA reductase. Statins are promising candidates for bone regeneration due to their lower cost of synthesis compared to recombinant human growth factors [17] and favorable safety record in treatment of hypercholesterolemia [58,59]. Therefore, the benefits of statins for treating of bone injuries have increasingly generated interest among researchers and clinicians [60–63].

7.3.1 Drug Delivery Strategies

A barrier to the clinical application of statins for bone regeneration is an effective delivery system. Statins are limited in their ability to stimulate bone formation when administered orally by their susceptibility to first-pass metabolism in the liver, and therefore they do not reach sufficient concentrations at distant bone sites [58]. While local delivery of statins may be preferable for effective bone regeneration, there are a number of challenges that must be overcome. Statins disperse quickly and have short half-lives [17] when injected locally. Excessively fast release of statins in the bone environment may lead to accumulation of high local concentrations, resulting in undesirable side effects, such as cytotoxicity or an adverse inflammatory response [64,65]. Therefore, a suitable delivery system is required to optimize the dose and release kinetics that promote bone regeneration without inducing inflammation.

Several studies have investigated carriers for sustained release of statins. Ceramic delivery systems have generated considerable interest. Marine exoskeletons were hydrothermally converted to β-TCP and investigated as a carrier for simvastatin [66]. Coating with a layer of hydroxyapatite (HA) was found to reduce the burst release by 25%. Poly(D,L-lactic-co-glycolide) (PLGA) has also been investigated as a delivery system for simvastatin [67]. PLGA microspheres were prepared by electrospraying from a dichloromethane solution, with a simvastatin encapsulation efficiency of >90%. The resulting microspheres supported cell attachment and proliferation and sustained release of simvastatin for up to 3 weeks. Sustained release of simvastatin in vitro has also been accomplished by grafting the statin to hydrolytically degradable PLGA microspheres [64]. In other studies, sustained local delivery of lovastatin from poly(DL-lactide) (PLA) nanoparticles (~200 nm) for up to 21 days enhanced fracture repair [66]. Hydrogels have also been investigated as carriers for statins. Sustained release of fluvastatin from a poly(ethylene glycol) (PEG) hydrogel delivery system induced osteogenic differentiation in vitro [65]. Another study has investigated gelatin-poly(ethylene glycol)-tyramine (GPT) hydrogels as carriers for simvastatin [68]. GPT hydrogels exhibited a burst followed by a sustained release of simvastatin, and the burst release increased with decreasing crosslinking and stiffness of the gels. Furthermore, osteoblast differentiation increased in a simvastatin dose-responsive manner, thereby highlighting their potential for use in bone tissue engineering.

7.3.2 Regeneration of Craniomaxillofacial Bone Defects

A number of studies have investigated the effects of local delivery of statins on healing of craniofacial bone defects. In a preclinical study in critical-size rat calvarial defects, calcium sulfate augmented with 1 mg simvastatin showed less bone and soft tissue inflammation compared to calcium sulfate alone at 2 and 4 weeks. However, at 8 weeks the simvastatin showed dramatically new bone formation [65]. Thus, while this early study showed the potential of simvastatin for regenerating craniofacial bone, it also demonstrated that the dose and release kinetics must be optimized to minimize inflammation. Electrospun poly(epsilon-caprolactone) (PCL) nonwoven membranes have also been investigated as carriers for simvastatin [69]. Simvastatin was added either during electrospinning or was loaded into the membranes after they had been formed. New bone formation was greatest when the drug was incorporated into the scaffolds during electrospinning. In mechanistic studies in rat cavarial defects, simvastatin released from α-TCP was found to increase proliferation and migration of osteoprogenitor cells from the dura from day 3 to 10 [70]. Furthermore, BMP-2 expression was higher in the simvastatin group on days 3 and 14, and new bone formation was consequently increased on days 14 and 21. Thus, these observations suggest that simvastatin enhanced new bone formation through recruitment of osteoprogenitor cells and increased expression of BMP-2 and TGF-β1. Other calcium phosphates, such as α-TCP, β-TCP, and HA, have been investigated as carriers for simvastatin in a 5-mm rat calvarial defect model [71]. The α-TCP and β-TCP groups augmented with 0.1 mg simvastatin generated more new bone compared to HA at 6 and 8 weeks. The faster degradation of the TCP groups compared to HA was conjectured to result in more new bone formation when the calcium phosphates were combined with simvastatin. In a recent study, local delivery of fluvastatin from gelatin scaffolds on new bone formation in rat calvarial defects was found to increase new bone formation at 7, 14, and 28 days compared to gelatin alone [72].

Statins have been investigated extensively for regeneration of mandibular and periodontal bone defects. In an early study, local delivery of simvastatin from a gelatin sponge resulted in significantly more new bone than the gelatin sponge control in 3-mm rat mandibular defects at 14 days [73], which highlighted the potential of statins for healing mandibular bone. A more recent study in a dog dehiscence bilateral defect model has reported that local delivery of 10 mg of simvastatin from HA-collagen grafts induced modest amounts of new bone formation in closed injection sites over a periosteal surface [74]. However, minimal new bone formation was observed in dehiscence defects lacking periosteum. Similarly, a pilot study in infra-bony and fenestration defects in dogs showed a reduction in ridge height at 2 months when 3 weekly injections of 0.5 or 2.0 mg simvastatin were administered [75]. Consequently, this study cautioned against multiple injections of simvastatin. While simvastatin has been shown to generate new bone in mandibular defects, higher doses of simvastatin have been associated with bone resorption and inflammation. Consequently, the effect of dual-delivery of the anti-resorption agent alendronate and simvastatin on bone regeneration has been investigated in rat periodontal defects [76]. Rat fenestration defects were treated with simvastatin alone, alendronate alone, or simvastatin and alendronate and followed for 21 or 48 days. In addition, some rats injected with simvastatin alone were also treated with systemic alendronate. While all groups showed nearly complete bone healing at 21 days, at 42 days local delivery of simvastatin and systemic delivery of alendronate resulted in 2–3 times more bone width compared to simvastatin or alendronate alone. These observations suggest that short-term systemic alendronate treatment could reduce bone resorption. Finally, a randomized clinical trial in 72 patients has shown that 1.2 mg simvastatin delivered sub-gingivally was effective at healing patients with class II furcation defects [77]. Compared to those receiving scaling and root planing (SRP) alone, patients receiving SRP and 1.2 mg simvastatin achieved significantly more bone fill and relative and horizontal attachment levels. Thus, local delivery of simvastatin was found to both enhance new bone formation and also improve clinical outcomes.

7.3.3 Regeneration of Orthopedic Bone Defects

Statins have also been investigated for their potential to heal bony defects in orthopedic preclinical models. Recent studies have evaluated the ability of simvastatin-loaded coatings on orthopedic implants to improve implant osseointegration. Simvastatin was adsorbed onto roughened implants and implanted in the tibiae of ovariectomized rats [78]. Adsorption of simvastatin showed faster growth of new bone and bone-to-implant contact on the implant surface compared to untreated implants. In another study, titanium implants were coated with PLA incorporating three doses of simvastatin [79]. At 56 days, 20% of the rats with the high dose of simvastatin showed resorption near the implant surface at 8 weeks, and the pull-out strength was significantly lower than that of implants with no simvastatin. Thus, this study showed impaired osseointegration of simvastatin-coat implants.

The effects of local delivery of statins on new bone formation have also been investigated in bony defects. Apatite cements augmented with simvastatin supported the formation of denser bone compared to the cement control in osteoporotic rats [80]. Sustained release of lovastatin from lysine-derived polyurethane scaffolds enhanced new bone formation in rat femoral condyle plug defects at 4 weeks [81]. Sustained release of lovastatin was observed for up to 4 weeks. In a follow-up study, lovastatin microspheres with a release period of 14 days (Figure 7.4a) were injected into polyurethane scaffolds implanted in rat segmental defects [82]. While injection of lovastatin microspheres at 0 or 2 weeks did not improve bone healing at 8 weeks, delayed injection of lovastatin at 4 weeks enhanced new bone formation at 8 weeks (Figure 7.4b–e). Since the period of lovastatin release from the microspheres was only 2 weeks, these observations point to either (a) delaying injection of lovastatin until time points at which cells have infiltrated the scaffold, or (b) designing a carrier that can release lovastatin for up to 8 weeks as an effective strategy for healing open fractures. In another study, delivery of simvastatin (3 or 5 mg) from PLGA/HA composite microspheres enhanced

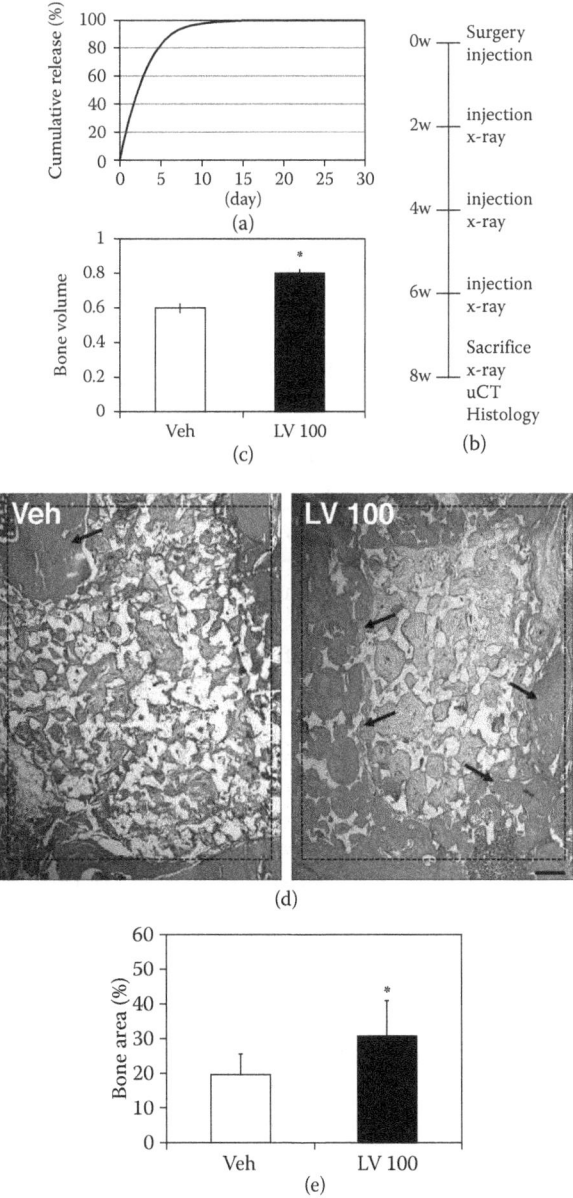

FIGURE 7.4

Local delivery of lovastatin from lysine-derived poly(ester urethane) scaffolds in segmental femoral defects. (a) Lovastatin was released from the particles for a period of two weeks. (b) Schematic showing the timing of injections (every 2 weeks). Animals were injected with the vehicle (saline) or 100 μg lovastatin (LV 100). (c) μCT quantitative analysis shows significantly more new bone formation at 8 weeks in the LV 100 group. (d) Images of histological sections of Veh- and LV 100–treated defects show more new bone in the LV 100–treated group (e). (Adapted from Yoshii T et al., *J Tissue Eng Regen Med*, 2012. With permission.)

healing of segmental bone defects in mice at 4 weeks [83]. B-TCP carriers have also been shown to effective carriers for local delivery of simvastatin in ovariectomized mice [84].

A few studies have investigated the effects of statin dose and release kinetics on bone healing. Hyaluronic acid (HyA) hydrogels loaded with 0.1–1.0 mg simvastatin showed comparable cytotoxicity to the hydrogel with the drug, and 1 mg drug loading enhanced osteogenic differentiation in vitro and new bone formation in vivo [85]. In another study, PLGA nanoparticles prepared by an oil-in-water emulsion technique showed 97% release of lovastatin at 7 days [86]. While alkaline phosphatase (ALP) activity in human osteoblasts was stimulated by PLGA nanoparticles augmented with simvastatin, concentrations exceeding 4 µg/ml inhibited ALP activity. This observation is consistent with previous studies showing that bone healing was inhibited at higher doses of statins. Another study investigated the effect of lovastatin injections into bony defects on new bone formation and gene expression [87]. Injection of simvastatin increased new bone formation, as well as expression of ALP and BMP-2. Interestingly, simvastatin also reduced the number of tartrate-resistant acid phosphatase-positive (TRAP) multi-nucleated cells and expression of cathepsin K. Furthermore, new bone formation was not sustained when the injections were stopped. Thus, these findings point to the importance of sustained release of statins for new bone formation.

7.3.4 Summary

Numerous studies in craniomaxillofacial and orthopedic models of bone regeneration highlight the potential of statins for bone regeneration and repair. However, these studies also point to the need to optimize the dose and release kinetics of the drug. Relatively high local concentrations of statins have been associated with bone resorption and inflammation. Furthermore, unlike rhBMP-2, statins have limited angiogenic properties. Further studies are needed to assess the utility of statins for healing bone defects in the clinic.

7.4 Conclusions

While rhBMP-2 is the most extensively investigated drug for enhanced bone formation, several other angio-osteogenic factors have been investigated for their potential to heal craniofacial and orthopedic bone defects. Recombinant human PDGF, VEGF, and FGF have been evaluated both alone and in combination with other factors, including rhBMP-2. The most commercially successful factor is rhPDGF delivered from a calcium phosphate carrier, which has been approved for treatment of regeneration of alveolar bone lost to periodontal disease. Combination of these angio-osteogenic factors with rhBMP-2 has shown some potential for enhancing bone healing, but also presents numerous challenges due to the need to control the dose and release kinetics for multiple growth factors. Statins, a class of synthetic drugs for treatment of hypercholesterolemia, have also been investigated for their potential to treat bone defects. Preclinical studies are promising, but more testing is required to resolve questions of optimal dose and release kinetics.

References

1. Seeherman H, Wozney JM. Delivery of bone morphogenetic proteins for orthopedic tissue regeneration. *Cytokine Growth Factor Rev* 2005;16:329–45.
2. Haidar ZS, Hamdy RC, Tabrizian M. Delivery of recombinant bone morphogenetic proteins for bone regeneration and repair. Part B: Delivery systems for BMPs in orthopaedic and craniofacial tissue engineering. *Biotechnol Lett* 2009;31:1825–35.
3. Haidar ZS, Hamdy RC, Tabrizian M. Delivery of recombinant bone morphogenetic proteins for bone regeneration and repair. Part A: Current challenges in BMP delivery. *Biotechnol Lett* 2009;31:1817–24.
4. Li RH, Wozney JM. Delivering on the promise of bone morphogenetic proteins. *Trends Biotechnol* 2001;19:255–65.
5. Kirker-Head C. Potential applications and delivery strategies for bone morphogenetic proteins. *Advanced Drug Deliv Reviews* 2000;43:65–92.
6. Wenke JC, Guelcher SA. Dual delivery of an antibiotic and a growth factor addresses both the microbiological and biological challenges of contaminated bone fractures. *Expert Opinion on Drug Delivery* 2011:1–15.
7. Jones AL, Bucholz RW, Bosse MJ, Mirza SK, Lyon TR, Webb LX, et al. Recombinant human BMP-2 and allograft compared with autogenous bone graft for reconstruction of diaphyseal tibial fractures with cortical defects. A randomized, controlled trial. *J Bone Joint Surg Am* 2006;88:1431–41.
8. Uludag H, Gao T, Porter T, Friess W, Wozney J. Delivery systems for BMPS: Factors contributing to the protein retention at an application site. *J Bone Joint Surg* 2001;83–A:S128–S35.
9. Cho TJ, Gerstenfeld LC, Einhorn TA. Differential temporal expression of members of the transforming growth factor beta superfamily during murine fracture healing. *J Bone Miner Res* 2002;17:513–20.
10. Brown KV, Li B, Guda T, Perrien DS, Guelcher SA, Wenke JC. Improving bone formation in a rat femur segmental defect by controlling bone morphogenetic protein-2 release. *Tissue Eng Part A* 2011.
11. Swiontkowski MF, Aro HT, Donell S, Esterhai JL, Goulet J, Jones A, et al. Recombinant human bone morphogenetic protein-2 in open tibial fractures. A subgroup analysis of data combined from two prospective randomized studies. *J Bone Joint Surg Am* 2006;88:1258–65.

12. Govender S, Csimma C, Genant HK, Valentin-Opran A, Amit Y, Arbel R, et al. Recombinant human bone morphogenetic protein-2 for treatment of open tibial fractures: A prospective, controlled, randomized study of four hundred and fifty patients. *J Bone Joint Surg Am* 2002;84-A:2123–34.

13. Gung YW, Cheng CK, Su CY. A stereomorphologic study of bone matrix apposition in HA-implanted cavities observed with SEM, being prepared by a microvascular cast and freeze-fracture method. *Med Eng Phys* 2003;25:565–71.

14. Lienau J, Schmidt-Bleek K, Peters A, Haschke F, Duda GN, Perka C, et al. Differential regulation of blood vessel formation between standard and delayed bone healing. *J Orthop Res* 2009;27:1133–40.

15. Li R, Stewart DJ, von Schroeder HP, Mackinnon ES, Schemitsch EH. Effect of cell-based VEGF gene therapy on healing of a segmental bone defect. *J Orthop Res* 2009;27:8–14.

16. Geiger F, Bertram H, Berger I, Lorenz H, Wall O, Eckhardt C, et al. Vascular endothelial growth factor gene-activated matrix (VEGF165-GAM) enhances osteogenesis and angiogenesis in large segmental bone defects. *J Bone Miner Res* 2005;20:2028–35.

17. Mundy G, Garrett R, Harris S, Chan J, Chen D, Rossini G, et al. Stimulation of bone formation in vitro and in rodents by statins. *Science* 1999;286:1946–9.

18. Garrett IR, Gutierrez G, Mundy GR. Statins and bone formation. *Curr Pharm Des* 2001;7:715–36.

19. Maeda T, Matsunuma A, Kawane T, Horiuchi N. Simvastatin promotes osteoblast differentiation and mineralization in MC3T3-E1 cells. *Biochem Biophys Res Commun* 2001;280:874–7.

20. Maeda T, Matsunuma A, Kurahashi I, Yanagawa T, Yoshida H, Horiuchi N. Induction of osteoblast differentiation indices by statins in MC3T3-E1 cells. *J Cell Biochem* 2004;92:458–71.

21. Baek KH, Lee WY, Oh KW, Tae HJ, Lee JM, Lee EJ, et al. The effect of simvastatin on the proliferation and differentiation of human bone marrow stromal cells. *J Korean Med Sci* 2005;20:438–44.

22. Du X, Xie Y, Xian CJ, Chen L. Role of FGFs/FGFRs in skeletal development and bone regeneration. *J Cell Physiol* 2012;227:3731–43.

23. Behr B, Sorkin M, Manu A, Lehnhardt M, Longaker MT, Quarto N. Fgf-18 is required for osteogenesis but not angiogenesis during long bone repair. *Tissue Eng Part A* 2011;17:2061–9.

24. Oortgiesen DA, Walboomers XF, Bronckers AL, Meijer GJ, Jansen JA. Periodontal regeneration using an injectable bone cement combined with BMP-2 or FGF-2. *J Tissue Eng Regen Med* 2014;8:202–9.

25. Ishii Y, Fujita T, Okubo N, Ota M, Yamada S, Saito A. Effect of basic fibroblast growth factor (FGF-2) in combination with beta tricalcium phosphate on root coverage in dog. *Acta Odontologica Scandinavica* 2013;71:325–32.

26. Oi Y, Ota M, Yamamoto S, Shibukawa Y, Yamada S. Beta-tricalcium phosphate and basic fibroblast growth factor combination enhances periodontal regeneration in intrabony defects in dogs. *Dental Materials Journal* 2009;28:162–9.

27. Shinozaki Y, Toda M, Ohno J, Kawaguchi M, Kido H, Fukushima T. Evaluation of bone formation guided by DNA/protamine complex with FGF-2 in an adult rat calvarial defect model. *J Biomed Mater Res B Appl Biomater* 2014;102(8):1669–76.

28. Kigami R, Sato S, Tsuchiya N, Yoshimakai T, Arai Y, Ito K. FGF-2 angiogenesis in bone regeneration within critical-sized bone defects in rat calvaria. *Implant Dentistry* 2013;22:422–7.

29. Furuya H, Tabata Y, Kaneko K. Bone regeneration for murine femur fracture by gelatin hydrogels incorporating basic fibroblast growth factor with different release profiles. *Tissue Eng Part A* 2014;20:1531–41.

30. Komaki H, Tanaka T, Chazono M, Kikuchi T. Repair of segmental bone defects in rabbit tibiae using a complex of beta-tricalcium phosphate, type I collagen, and fibroblast growth factor-2. *Biomaterials* 2006;27:5118–26.

31. Keiichi K, Mitsunobu K, Masafumi S, Yutaka D, Toshiaki S. Induction of new bone by basic FGF-loaded porous carbonate apatite implants in femur defects in rats. *Clin Oral Implants Res* 2009;20:560–5.

32. Maehara H, Sotome S, Yoshii T, Torigoe I, Kawasaki Y, Sugata Y, et al. Repair of large osteochondral defects in rabbits using porous hydroxyapatite/collagen (HAp/Col) and fibroblast growth factor-2 (FGF-2). *J Orthop Res* 2010;28:677–86.

33. Friedlaender GE, Lin S, Solchaga LA, Snel LB, Lynch SE. The role of recombinant human platelet-derived growth factor-BB (rhPDGF-BB) in orthopaedic bone repair and regeneration. *Current Pharmaceutical Design* 2013;19:3384–90.

34. Shah P, Keppler L, Rutkowski J. A review of Platelet Derived Growth Factor playing pivotal role in bone regeneration. *The Journal of Oral Implantology* 2012;40(3):330–40.

35. DiGiovanni CW, Lin S, Pinzur M. Recombinant human PDGF-BB in foot and ankle fusion. *Expert Review of Medical Devices* 2012;9:111–22.

36. Caplan AI, Correa D. PDGF in bone formation and regeneration: New insights into a novel mechanism involving MSCs. *J Orthop Res* 2011;29:1795–803.

37. Kaigler D, Avila G, Wisner-Lynch L, Nevins ML, Nevins M, Rasperini G, et al. Platelet-derived growth factor applications in periodontal and peri-implant bone regeneration. *Expert Opinion on Biological Therapy* 2011;11:375–85.

38. Thakare K, Deo V. Randomized controlled clinical study of rhPDGF-BB + beta-TCP versus HA + beta-TCP for the treatment of infrabony periodontal defects: Clinical and radiographic results. *Int J Periodontics Restorative Dent* 2012;32:689–96.

39. Nevins M, Kao RT, McGuire MK, McClain PK, Hinrichs JE, McAllister BS, et al. Platelet-derived growth factor promotes periodontal regeneration in localized osseous defects: 36-month extension results from a randomized, controlled, double-masked clinical trial. *J Periodontol* 2013;84:456–64.

40. Chang PC, Dovban AS, Lim LP, Chong LY, Kuo MY, Wang CH. Dual delivery of PDGF and simvastatin to accelerate periodontal regeneration in vivo. *Biomaterials* 2013;34:9990–7.

41. Al-Zube L, Breitbart EA, O'Connor JP, Parsons JR, Bradica G, Hart CE, et al. Recombinant human platelet-derived growth factor BB (rhPDGF-BB) and beta-tricalcium phosphate/collagen matrix enhance fracture healing in a diabetic rat model. *J Orthop Res* 2009;27:1074–81.

42. Moore DC, Ehrlich MG, McAllister SC, Machan JT, Hart CE, Voigt C, et al. Recombinant human platelet-derived growth factor-BB augmentation of new-bone formation in a rat model of distraction osteogenesis. *J Bone Joint Surg Am* 2009;91:1973–84.

43. Leedy MR, Jennings JA, Haggard WO, Bumgardner JD. Effects of VEGF-loaded chitosan coatings. *J Biomed Mater Res A* 2014;102:752–9.

44. Behr B, Sorkin M, Lehnhardt M, Renda A, Longaker MT, Quarto N. A comparative analysis of the osteogenic effects of BMP-2, FGF-2, and VEGFA in a calvarial defect model. *Tissue Eng Part A* 2012;18:1079–86.

45. Wernike E, Montjovent MO, Liu Y, Wismeijer D, Hunziker EB, Siebenrock KA, et al. VEGF incorporated into calcium phosphate ceramics promotes vascularisation and bone formation in vivo. *Eur Cell Mater* 2010;19:30–40.

46. Willems WF, Larsen M, Giusti G, Friedrich PF, Bishop AT. Revascularization and bone remodeling of frozen allografts stimulated by intramedullary sustained delivery of FGF-2 and VEGF. *J Orthop Res* 2011;29:1431–6.

47. Yang P, Wang C, Shi Z, Huang X, Dang X, Li X, et al. rhVEGF 165 delivered in a porous beta-tricalcium phosphate scaffold accelerates bridging of critical-sized defects in rabbit radii. *J Biomed Mater Res A* 2010;92:626–40.

48. Gao C, Harvey EJ, Chua M, Chen BP, Jiang F, Liu Y, et al. MSC-seeded dense collagen scaffolds with a bolus dose of VEGF promote healing of large bone defects. *Eur Cell Mater* 2013;26:195–207; discussion.

49. Deckers MM, van Bezooijen RL, van der Horst G, Hoogendam J, van Der Bent C, Papapoulos SE, et al. Bone morphogenetic proteins stimulate angiogenesis through osteoblast-derived vascular endothelial growth factor A. *Endocrinology* 2002;143:1545–53.

50. Samee M, Kasugai S, Kondo H, Ohya K, Shimokawa H, Kuroda S. Bone morphogenetic protein-2 (BMP-2) and vascular endothelial growth factor (VEGF) transfection to human periosteal cells enhances osteoblast differentiation and bone formation. *J Pharmacol Sci* 2008;108:18–31.

51. Zhang W, Zhu C, Wu Y, Ye D, Wang S, Zou D, et al. VEGF and BMP-2 promote bone regeneration by facilitating bone marrow stem cell homing and differentiation. *Eur Cell Mater* 2014;27:1–11; discussion 11–2.

52. Kempen DH, Lu L, Heijink A, Hefferan TE, Creemers LB, Maran A, et al. Effect of local sequential VEGF and BMP-2 delivery on ectopic and orthotopic bone regeneration. *Biomaterials* 2009;30:2816–25.

53. Young S, Patel ZS, Kretlow JD, Murphy MB, Mountziaris PM, Baggett LS, et al. Dose effect of dual delivery of vascular endothelial growth factor and bone morphogenetic protein-2 on bone regeneration in a rat critical-size defect model. *Tissue Eng Part A* 2009;15:2347–62.

54. Zhang W, Wang X, Wang S, Zhao J, Xu L, Zhu C, et al. The use of injectable sonication-induced silk hydrogel for VEGF(165) and BMP-2 delivery for elevation of the maxillary sinus floor. *Biomaterials* 2011;32:9415–24.

55. Hernandez A, Reyes R, Sanchez E, Rodriguez-Evora M, Delgado A, Evora C. In vivo osteogenic response to different ratios of BMP-2 and VEGF released from a biodegradable porous system. *J Biomed Mater Res A* 2012;100:2382–91.

56. Park SY, Kim KH, Shin SY, Koo KT, Lee YM, Seol YJ. Dual delivery of rhPDGF-BB and bone marrow mesenchymal stromal cells expressing the BMP2 gene enhance bone formation in a critical-sized defect model. *Tissue Eng Part A* 2013;19:2495–505.

57. Zhang Y, Cheng N, Miron R, Shi B, Cheng X. Delivery of PDGF-B and BMP-7 by mesoporous bioglass/silk fibrin scaffolds for the repair of osteoporotic defects. *Biomaterials* 2012;33:6698–708.

58. Schachter M. Chemical, pharmacokinetic and pharmacodynamic properties of statins: An update. *Fundam Clin Pharmacol* 2005;19:117–25.

59. Armitage J. The safety of statins in clinical practice. *Lancet* 2007;370:1781–90.

60. Mundy GR. Statins and their potential for osteoporosis. *Bone* 2001;29:495–7.
61. Gonyeau MJ. Statins and osteoporosis: A clinical review. *Pharmacotherapy* 2005;25:228–43.
62. Gutierrez GE, Lalka D, Garrett IR, Rossini G, Mundy GR. Transdermal application of lovastatin to rats causes profound increases in bone formation and plasma concentrations. *Osteoporos Int* 2006;17:1033–42.
63. Toh S, Hernandez-Diaz S. Statins and fracture risk. A systematic review. *Pharmacoepidemiol Drug Saf* 2007;16:627–40.
64. Stein D, Lee Y, Schmid MJ, Killpack B, Genrich MA, Narayana N, et al. Local simvastatin effects on mandibular bone growth and inflammation. *J Periodontol* 2005;76:1861–70.
65. Nyan M, Sato D, Oda M, Machida T, Kobayashi H, Nakamura T, et al. Bone formation with the combination of simvastatin and calcium sulfate in critical-sized rat calvarial defect. *J Pharmacol Sci* 2007;104:384–6.
66. Chou J, Ito T, Bishop D, Otsuka M, Ben-Nissan B, Milthorpe B. Controlled release of simvastatin from biomimetic beta-TCP drug delivery system. *PLoS One* 2013;8:e54676.
67. Nath SD, Son S, Sadiasa A, Min YK, Lee BT. Preparation and characterization of PLGA microspheres by the electrospraying method for delivering simvastatin for bone regeneration. *Int J Pharm* 2013;443:87–94.
68. Park YS, David AE, Park KM, Lin CY, Than KD, Lee K, et al. Controlled release of simvastatin from in situ forming hydrogel triggers bone formation in MC3T3-E1 cells. *The AAPS Journal* 2013;15:367–76.
69. Piskin E, Isoglu IA, Bolgen N, Vargel I, Griffiths S, Cavusoglu T, et al. In vivo performance of simvastatin-loaded electrospun spiral-wound polycaprolactone scaffolds in reconstruction of cranial bone defects in the rat model. *J Biomed Mater Res A* 2009;90:1137–51.
70. Nyan M, Miyahara T, Noritake K, Hao J, Rodriguez R, Kuroda S, et al. Molecular and tissue responses in the healing of rat calvarial defects after local application of simvastatin combined with alpha tricalcium phosphate. *J Biomed Mater Res B Appl Biomater* 2010;93:65–73.
71. Rojbani H, Nyan M, Ohya K, Kasugai S. Evaluation of the osteoconductivity of alpha-tricalcium phosphate, beta-tricalcium phosphate, and hydroxyapatite combined with or without simvastatin in rat calvarial defect. *J Biomed Mater Res A* 2011;98:488–98.
72. Tanabe K, Nomoto H, Okumori N, Miura T, Yoshinari M. Osteogenic effect of fluvastatin combined with biodegradable gelatin-hydrogel. *Dental Materials Journal* 2012;31:489–93.
73. Ozec I, Kilic E, Gumus C, Goze F. Effect of local simvastatin application on mandibular defects. *J Craniofac Surg* 2007;18:546–50.
74. Rutledge J, Schieber MD, Chamberlain JM, Byarlay M, Killeen AC, Giannini PJ, et al. Simvastatin application to augment facial jaw bone in a dog model: Pilot study. *J Periodontol* 2011;82:597–605.
75. Morris MS, Lee Y, Lavin MT, Giannini PJ, Schmid MJ, Marx DB, et al. Injectable simvastatin in periodontal defects and alveolar ridges: Pilot studies. *J Periodontol* 2008;79:1465–73.
76. Killeen AC, Rakes PA, Schmid MJ, Zhang Y, Narayana N, Marx DB, et al. Impact of local and systemic alendronate on simvastatin-induced new bone around periodontal defects. *J Periodontol* 2012;83:1463–71.

77. Pradeep AR, Priyanka N, Kalra N, Naik SB, Singh SP, Martande S. Clinical efficacy of subgingivally delivered 1.2-mg simvastatin in the treatment of individuals with Class II furcation defects: A randomized controlled clinical trial. *J Periodontol* 2012;83:1472–9.
78. Yang G, Song L, Guo C, Zhao S, Liu L, He F. Bone responses to simvastatin-loaded porous implant surfaces in an ovariectomized model. *Int J Oral Maxillofac Implants* 2012;27:369–74.
79. Pauly S, Back DA, Kaeppler K, Haas NP, Schmidmaier G, Wildemann B. Influence of statins locally applied from orthopedic implants on osseous integration. *BMC Musculoskeletal Disorders* 2012;13:208.
80. Hamada H, Ohshima H, Otsuka M. Dissolution medium responsive simvastatin release from biodegradable apatite cements and the therapeutic effect in osteoporosis rats. *Journal of Applied Biomaterials & Functional Materials* 2012;10:22–8.
81. Yoshii T, Hafeman AE, Nyman JS, Esparza JM, Shinomiya K, Spengler DM, et al. A sustained release of lovastatin from biodegradable, elastomeric polyurethane scaffolds for enhanced bone regeneration. *Tissue Engineering Part A* 2010;16:2369–79.
82. Yoshii T, Hafeman AE, Esparza JM, Okawa A, Gutierrez G, Guelcher SA. Local injection of lovastatin in biodegradable polyurethane scaffolds enhances bone regeneration in a critical-sized segmental defect in rat femora. *J Tissue Eng Regen Med* 2012;8(8):589–95.
83. Tai IC, Fu YC, Wang CK, Chang JK, Ho ML. Local delivery of controlled-release simvastatin/PLGA/HAp microspheres enhances bone repair. *International Journal of Nanomedicine* 2013;8:3895–904.
84. Chou J, Ito T, Otsuka M, Ben-Nissan B, Milthorpe B. Simvastatin-loaded beta-TCP drug delivery system induces bone formation and prevents rhabdomyolysis in OVX mice. *Advanced Healthcare Materials* 2013;2:678–81.
85. Bae MS, Yang DH, Lee JB, Heo DN, Kwon YD, Youn IC, et al. Photo-cured hyaluronic acid-based hydrogels containing simvastatin as a bone tissue regeneration scaffold. *Biomaterials* 2011;32:8161–71.
86. Ho MH, Chiang CP, Liu YF, Kuo MY, Lin SK, Lai JY, et al. Highly efficient release of lovastatin from poly(lactic-co-glycolic acid) nanoparticles enhances bone repair in rats. *J Orthop Res* 2011;29:1504–10.
87. Ayukawa Y, Yasukawa E, Moriyama Y, Ogino Y, Wada H, Atsuta I, et al. Local application of statin promotes bone repair through the suppression of osteoclasts and the enhancement of osteoblasts at bone-healing sites in rats. *Oral Surg Oral Med Oral Pathol Oral Radiol Endod* 2009;107:336–42.

8

Infection-Related Considerations for Bone Grafts

Joseph J. Pearson, Joo Ong, and Teja Guda

CONTENTS

8.1 Introduction

Bone grafts are important for healing various bone-related defects. Grafts can be created from the patient (autograft), another person (allograft), or other synthetic materials. In the United States alone, nearly 500,000 people undergo treatment for bone defects with a cost of $2.5 billion annually. This number are expected to double by 2020 due to a variety of population trends including a large aged population, and increased life expectancy and obesity.[1] These numbers express the importance of an effective treatment that provides the long-term solution. Otherwise, secondary treatment costs alone can steeply increase costs.

The gold standard for bone grafts is an autograft from the iliac crest. However, there are concerns with this procedure, including donor site morbidity that can lead to infection and other complications. In addition to donor site morbidity, the harvesting tissues from a secondary site of a same donor usually does not provide sufficient bone grafting materials for large nonunion defects.[2] The second option for bone is the use of cadaver tissues or allografts. The risks of allografts include infection, immune response, the loss of functional bone properties, and still an insufficient supply for the demand,[1] which explains the need for other synthetic alternatives. Not only is the availability of adequate graft material a concern, but many bone graft procedures lead to infections which can cause graft failure.

In a military study, Burns et al. detailed bone graft failures in open traumatic tibia injuries.[3] They found that 22% of the injuries led to amputation due to infections,[3] whereas the infection rate in civilian extreme lower
extremity trauma is 23.2%.[4] In a retrospective study on open traumatic tibia
injuries sustained by military personnel and comparing the various factors
influencing the personnel's ability to return to duty, 92% of these personnel that developed complications from osteomyelitis (bone infection) were
unable to return to duty.[5] Focusing on the complex nature of open traumatic
tibia fractures along with the added complications of large soft tissue deficits that are often found in conjunction with bone fractures, another study
reported that 33% of injuries led to chronic osteomyelitis.[6] As such, these
complex injuries require much consideration on multiple treatment variables
in order to provide a one-time treatment solution to combat infection. One
such treatment variable that is debated is the timing to close an open wound.

Eardley et al. discuss how the solution to treat infections is not necessar-
ily clear, but is in fact a balance between eliminating infection and scarring.[7]
Although initial cleaning of necrotic tissues and removal of any foreign objects
with early closing of the wound reduces scarring, it has been reported that
early closure of the wound site can lead to infection, especially for battlefield
injuries because of the difficulty in completely cleansing the wound.[7] Morshed
et al. utilized U.S. data from 2000 to 2004 to discern the effect of femoral fracture fixation time post-injury when the injury involved multiple systems and
concluded that delaying fracture fixation to after the first 12 hours actually
reduced the mortality rate by 50%, thereby allowing the stabilization of the
patient and other systems.[8] Another reason for the need of a one-time treatment solution to combat infection is that in normal total joint operations with
bone graft usage, there is a 1% or less risk for infection in primary surgeries and
a greater than 20% risk for infection when revisions are needed.[9] A 2011 study
discussed the different outcomes of early and late amputation and infections,
with the late amputation group having greater complications with infection
thereby affecting the ability to salvage the remaining limb.[10]

When developing strategies to eliminate infection in critical traumatic
wounds, it is thus essential to know which infections are prominent in order
to tailor the graft material used. A military study conveyed that the initial and
secondary infections in the majority of patients were from different bacterial
strands, with the initial infection found to be primarily gram negative and
subsequent infections found to be gram positive and primarily *Staphylococcus*.[10]
These findings suggested that even though early infection cultures do not
show gram positive bacteria, preemptive treatment against these bacteria may
reduce subsequent infection. Such preemptive treatment was reported in a
2014 case study whereby tobramycin and vancomycin beads were employed
to treat gram negative and gram positive infections in a calcaneal defect.[10]

Another complication in military traumatic injuries is the location of the
occurrence. Although a 2011 review of battle wounds with infectious complications were suggested to be equivalent to that of civilian rates, the authors

decidedly admitted that the infection rate is likely higher due to lack of long-term registries of treatment.[11] 47.6% of the infectious cases reported were mostly gram negative and these were indicative of initial infections.[11] Another study on damage control by orthopedic surgeons using external fixation followed by intramedullary fixation led to a 40% infection rate and a 17% rate of osteomyelitis. Table 8.1 summarizes the infection information discussed within this introduction with examples from both the military and civilian communities.

The previous studies mentioned so far in this chapter beg for the need of not only an osteoinductive graft material[2] but also for a combination of synthetic materials that combat infection.[12] These strategies incorporate a local delivery of antibiotics or drugs to treat the infection, thereby effectively limiting the dosage required as well as eliminating any systemic side effects that are associated with systemic toxicity as a result of supraphysiologic dosages.[13] Since it is essential to know the infections prior to treatment, subsequent paragraphs below will first explore the types of osteomyelitis and

TABLE 8.1

Bone Infection Data Reported in the Literature

Journal	Author	Year	Patients	Environment	Data
J of Trauma	Burns et al.	2012	192	Combat	27% Infection, 22% Amputation[3]
J of Ortho Trauma	Cross et al.	2012	115	Combat	18% Return to Duty (RTD), 8% RTD with osteomyelitis[5]
Euro J of Plast Surg	Franken et al.	2010	17	Civilian	18% of chronic osteomyelitis cases had recurrence after surgery[6]
J of Ortho Trauma	Harris et al.	2009	545	Civilian	28.3% of patients developed osteomyelitis[4]
J Trauma Inj, Inf, CC	Huh et al.	2011	213	Combat	13.9%, 16.7%, and 54.5% osteomyelitis for salvage, early amputation, and late amputation, respectively[105]
Infection Combat-Rel Fractures	Johnson et al.	2007	62	Combat	Gram negative and positive for early and recurrent infections, respectively[106]
J Trauma Inj, Inf, CC	Murray et al.	2011	18,463	Combat	5.5% infection with 47.6% gram negative (26.7% skin/wound and 14.6% lung infection)[11]
J Trauma Inj, Inf, CC	Mody et al.	2009	58	Combat	17% osteomyelitis[107]

more in-depth information on current debridement and treatment technologies prior to discussing the synthetic approaches.

8.2 Types of Osteomyelitis

There are multiple types of osteomyelitis, some of which have been mentioned briefly in the introduction. Since the treatment used relates directly to the type of osteomyelitis, it is critical to establish guidelines prior to continuing the care for the patients. There are multiple clinical scales used to classify osteomyelitis.[14] Cierny et al. developed one scale separating osteomyelitis into four distinct categories with three physiologic classifications for the patient, the combination of which forms the overall clinical stage of the patient.[15]

Based on where the infection is occurring, the Cierny–Mader system distinguishes osteomyelitis into four types (Table 8.2,). Type 1 osteomyelitis relates to infection located within the bone or in the medullary, whereas type 2 osteomyelitis occurs superficially on the bone surface, which may involve the surrounding soft tissues. Type 3 osteomyelitis is considered localized and is a combination of type 1 and type 2 osteomyelitis, and this is usually the result of a traumatic injury in which osteomyelitis occurs throughout the entire thickness of a specific bone segment. Type 4 osteomyelitis is referred to as a diffused infection and is considered "through and through,"

TABLE 8.2

An Overview of the Cierny–Mader System of Categorizing Injury Type and Physiological Status of the Patient in Order to Select the Most Appropriate Treatment Strategy

Cierny–Mader System			
	Type		**Physiologic Considerations**
1	Medullary	**A**	Normal
2	Superficial	**B**	Systemic, Local or both compromised
3	Localized	**C**	Treatment worse than disease
4	Diffuse		

Class B Examples	
Localized	**Systemic**
Venous stasis	Malnutrition
Arteritis	Immune deficiency
Extensive scarring	Diabetes mellitus
Major vessel compromise	Malignancy
Radiation fibrosis	Extremes of age

Source: Adapted from Cierny III G et al., *Clinical Orthopaedics and Related Research*; 414:7–24, 2003.

meaning it encompasses both soft and hard tissue. An example of a diffuse-type osteomyelitis is an infected critical-sized (nonunion) defect.[15]

In addition to the types of infection, the Cierny–Mader system also takes into consideration the physiological or immunological status of the patient, and such status has a large effect on the management of patients. The first physiological consideration is an otherwise normal patient which is designated Class A. A patient with compromised physiological considerations is designated Class "B," which is further split into systemic and local conditions. Table 8.2 gives examples of systemic and local conditions, and these conditions are denoted as either Class B or Bl, respectively. Lastly, a patient is classified Class C if the treatment required would make the status worse than the current disease and the patient is not recommended for surgery.[15] In combination with the type of osteomyelitis, these physiological considerations form a "clinical stage" of a patient which, in turn, helps the surgeon to determine an appropriate treatment. As an example, consider a patient who has osteomyelitis that covers the surface of the bone and has malnutrition. This patient will be considered to have type 2 osteomyelitis and Class B (systemic) for malnutrition. Together the overall clinical stage of the patient would be 2-Bs.

Taking into account the lack of blood supply to infected regions, Waldevogel et al. further distinguish osteomyelitis by how long the disease lasts (acute or chronic) and where the infection originates, that is whether infection begins in the bone or in a surrounding tissue.[16] The chronic osteomyelitis in Waldevogel's system involves antibiotics and surgical intervention because the bone is necrotic and requires treatment, whereas acute osteomyelitis is associated with just antibiotics.[17]

8.3 Treatment Options and Strategies

Knowing the overall clinical stage of the patient, management for the different types of osteomyelitis differ as well, but all treatment options involve antibiotic therapy for a period of time. The normal length of treatment for types 1 and 2 osteomyelitis lasts for 4 weeks and 2 weeks, respectively, whereas the normal length of treatment for types 3 and 4 osteomyelitis ranges from 4 to 6 weeks. The success of antibiotic treatment is dependent largely on debridement treatment. If the treatment is unsuccessful, the treatment cycle is repeated and this can lead to chronic wounds.[18] Thomas et al. discuss the important relationship between infection, inflammation, and successful bone healing,[22] with inflammation being necessary for successful healing; however, it can lead to chronic issues if not promptly resolved.[19] Another important part of treatment is the temporary use of external fixation in lower extremity trauma. The stabilization of traumatic injuries is vital, especially in military and civilian environments that require time to transport patients to a facility in which adequate treatment can be acquired.[20]

Debridement is an essential part of successful treatments of bone-related injuries. This process removes debris and necrotic bone tissues from the wound site in order to allow the underlying viable tissue to heal properly. There are multiple techniques used for debridement, with the gold standard being to debride through surgical removal of the tissues and debris. Although not always practical, the gold standard is an effective technique since it requires an experienced surgeon to ensure adequate removal.[21] Another technique is the use of maggots to cleanse the wound. Termed "biodebridement," a 2012 study revealed that this technique is inconclusive due to inadequate follow-up procedures.[22] Autolytic debridement is a natural technique that uses the body's own enzymatic autolytic processes for debridement.[21] Although it can take time, autolytic debridement is enhanced through incorporation of enzymes such as collagenase and papain within wound dressings. Additionally, enzymatic debridement is often accompanied by drugs that encourage removal of necrotic tissues.[23] Mechanical debridement is also a common technique that is used, but it can damage healthy tissue due to a dry environment.[21] Other techniques include the development of a debrider that is made of monofilaments.[24] This tool showed adequate durability and no chemical reactions or fragmentations of the debrider into the wound site.

Besides the debrider made from monofilament, other debridement tools used include the use of ultrasound,[25] hydrosurgery,[26] and plasma-mediated bipolar radiofrequency ablation (PBRA).[21] Used in maxillofacial and ear surgery as well as in chronic wound healing, the PBRA technique uses a current that is generated between two electrodes with radiofrequencies in saline to remove the necrotic tissue.[21] By comparing the different debridement techniques to no debridement in a porcine model, Nusbaum et al. reported significantly less methicillin-resistant *Staphylococcus aureus* (MRSA) counts with debridement using the PBRA technique.[27] With the use of low frequency with high- or low-intensity ultrasound, either in contact with the wound site or as a non-contact therapy for debridement, it was inconclusive that the use of ultrasound enhances overall wound healing, although reports have indicated signs of decreased wound size.[25] Using a high-pressure jet of water and removing foreign particles and necrotic tissues through suction, a 2011 report indicated lower bacterial content in 50% of the patient population studied when using a hydrosurgery system such as the VERSAJET debridement system.[26]

Negative pressure therapy[28–30] or a vacuum-assisted[31,32] closure system creates a negative pressure that aids in the removal of excess tissue, fluid, and foreign objects. In a clinical study comparing vacuum-assisted closure to conventional treatment of osteomyelitis, Tan et al. reported negative bacterial readings occurring in 90.6% of the patients and one case of recurrence 1 month post discharge with vacuum-assisted treatment, whereas only 50% of the patients had negative bacterial readings and there were seven recurrences in the conventional group.[31] In a meeting of an international group of professionals to discuss and to vote on the consensus use of negative pressure treatment in various wound situations, the following three recommendations were made: (1) negative pressure must be considered for use for success of grafting; (2) negative pressure should be continuously used for at least the initial 3–7 days after graft placement; and (3) negative pressure should be used between debridements or when immediate closure is not likely in open fractures.[28] When the vacuum-assisted closure technique was combined with drainage systems to aid in healing of traumatic civilian and military injuries, Rispoli reported reduced edema and that the combined systems provided a means to avoid cordoning off of the deeper cavity tissues.[32]

Until now, this chapter has provided an idea on the clinical outlook on osteomyelitis, and discussed how the classifications and treatments for bone injuries vary greatly depending on the patient's physiological status, the wound location, and the involvement of surrounding tissues and systems. The following section will discuss possible synthetic graft materials that not only heal the defect, but can also provide solutions to complications associated with infections.

8.4 Synthetic Bone Graft Materials

As stated previously, autologous grafts are the gold standard for repairing bone defects. These grafts leave much to be desired with complications of donor site morbidity, infection, and the inability to fill large defects due to limited supply. Allografts are another option but they come with risks of immune response and loss of functionality in the transplantation process. The ability to develop synthetic graft materials to replace these options has been studied over the past few decades with the emergence of biomaterial design.

Before considering a material for synthetic grafts, it is important to briefly review the structure and composition of bone. Structurally, bone is made up of both cortical and trabecular (spongy) components. The structure of bone depends on the location of the body where bone is found. As an example, in long bones, the shaft is composed of cortical bone and the ends are made up of a cortical shell covering the trabecular bone on the inside. With the marrow contained within the bone shaft and trabeculae, the cortical portion of the bone is only 10% porous, whereas the trabecular bone has up to 95% porosity. Bone is composed of both an inorganic mineral component and a non-mineral component which pay a role in the remodeling and structural integrity of bone.[33] The inorganic mineral component is primarily a biological apatite and the non-mineral component is made up of mostly collagen (primarily Type 1), proteoglycans (biglycan and decorin), and non-collagenous proteins (osteocalcin).

Since one of the components of bone is a biological apatite, hydroxyapatite (HA), with the chemical formula $Ca_{10}(PO_4)_6(OH)_2$, can be synthetically produced and used as a graft material for bone applications. Since HA is one phase of the calcium phosphate (CaP) material, other well-known phases to the biomedical community include tricalcium phosphate (TCP), which has the chemical formula $Ca_3(PO_4)_2$. Known for its biocompatibility, HA is well-known to be osteoconductive. HA is also capable of being fabricated into a three-dimensional scaffold or construct for bone grafting applications. One form of fabrication technique is the template coating method, which typically is performed by coating a porous polymeric sponge with HA slurry, followed by high-temperature sintering to remove the polymeric sponge and leaving behind a porous HA scaffold.[2,34–36] In addition to HA, biphasic composite scaffolds composed of HA and TCP can also be fabricated in order to tailor the overall properties of the scaffolds. These ceramics are also known to possess similar mechanical compressive properties to bone.[37–39] In addition to incorporating antibiotics[40–43] to HA scaffolds for osteomyelitis treatment, the use of calcium sulfate as a bone graft substitute has also been extensively studied.[44]

Bioactive glass has been suggested for use as a bone graft substitute material.[45,46] Although the composition of bioactive glass can vary depending on the manufacturer, these materials are biocompatible and possess bone regenerative capabilities. Researchers have shown that these materials can also provide antibacterial properties that are beneficial for prevention of infection.[47,48] Although Lindfors et al. had observed encouraging results using a type of bioactive glass as a bone substitute alternative and for treating infection, the lack of angiogenesis was also reported.[49] This is yet another complication in the bone regenerative enigma and to remedy this problem, some researchers investigated the angiogenetic capacity of bioactive glass[46] and also encouraged angiogenesis through the incorporation and release of vascular endothelial growth factor.[50] In addition to the incorporation of growth factors, other investigators have included the incorporation of antibiotics such a vancomycin to bioactive glass.[51]

Natural and synthetic polymers have also been a popular choice of materials for bone regeneration.[52] While the most frequently used natural polymer is collagen type I, which is naturally found in bone,[38] other natural polymers such as silk[53,54] have also been explored. Some popular synthetic polymers used for bone regeneration include poly(lactic acid),[55,56] poly(glycolic acid),[56] poly(caprolactone),[57] and poly(methylmethacrylate).[55,58] These polymers have been chosen because they can achieve properties similar to bone and are biocompatible. Also, depending on the polymer chosen, varying modes of biodegradation can occur over predictable timeframes.[59–62]

Metals have also been used as bone grafting materials, in bone fixation, and for total joint replacements. Depending on the grade, titanium,[63,64] cobalt chromium,[65] and magnesium[66] are just a few examples of such metals that have been FDA-approved. Metals are often coated with osteoinductive or osteoconductive materials to encourage rapid osseointegration. Coatings of synthetic bone grafts are also utilized to decrease the chances of infection.[67,68] One example includes coating of titanium with vancomycin-incorporated chitosan that eventually releases and delivers vancomycin at localized sites.[67]

Figure 8.1 represents the bone regenerative strategies for the successful treatment of bone graft patients, and these strategies include the consideration of bone grafting materials, growth factors, and cells, and the

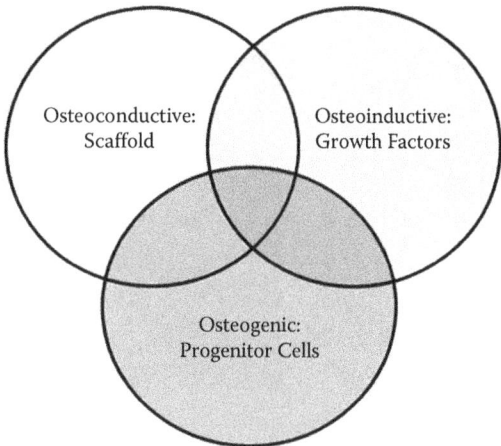

FIGURE 8.1
Schematic showing combinational strategies for bone graft patients. The components include osteoconductive scaffolds, osteoinductive growth factors, osteogenic cells, and the incorporation of antibiotics.

incorporation of antibiotics to combat infection. Various pieces of this puzzle will continue to be discussed throughout this chapter.

8.5 Antibiotics and Drug Delivery Systems

Drug delivery systems have been developed for the treatment of osteomyelitis for multiple reasons, including optimization of the required dosages for efficacy and the systemic side effects associated with antibiotics. Earlier in this chapter we discussed the differences between gram positive and negative infection in early and late infections. As such, knowledge on the types of antibiotics used for treating osteomyelitis will provide an understanding on the current drug delivery systems as well as allow investigators to strategize and develop more optimal systems in the future.

Some antibiotics that have been reportedly used in studies for the treatment of osteomyelitis are vancomycin,[13,51,69–74] tobramycin,[13] gentimicin,[75,76] teicoplanin,[77] and amikacin.[13,69,70] Of these antibiotics, vancomycin seems to be the most widely utilized for treatment of MRSA. Figure 8.2 provides histological images of *Staphylococcus aureus* (*S. aureus*) infection in a rabbit condyle model to show how infection can affect the success of HA bone grafts that are not incorporated with antibiotics. The autograft control group (Figures 8.2a and 8.2b) revealed a lot of void space with little regeneration, whereas the implanted HA scaffolds revealed less void space. Overall, Figure 8.2 provides a view of the effect of infection on bone regeneration.

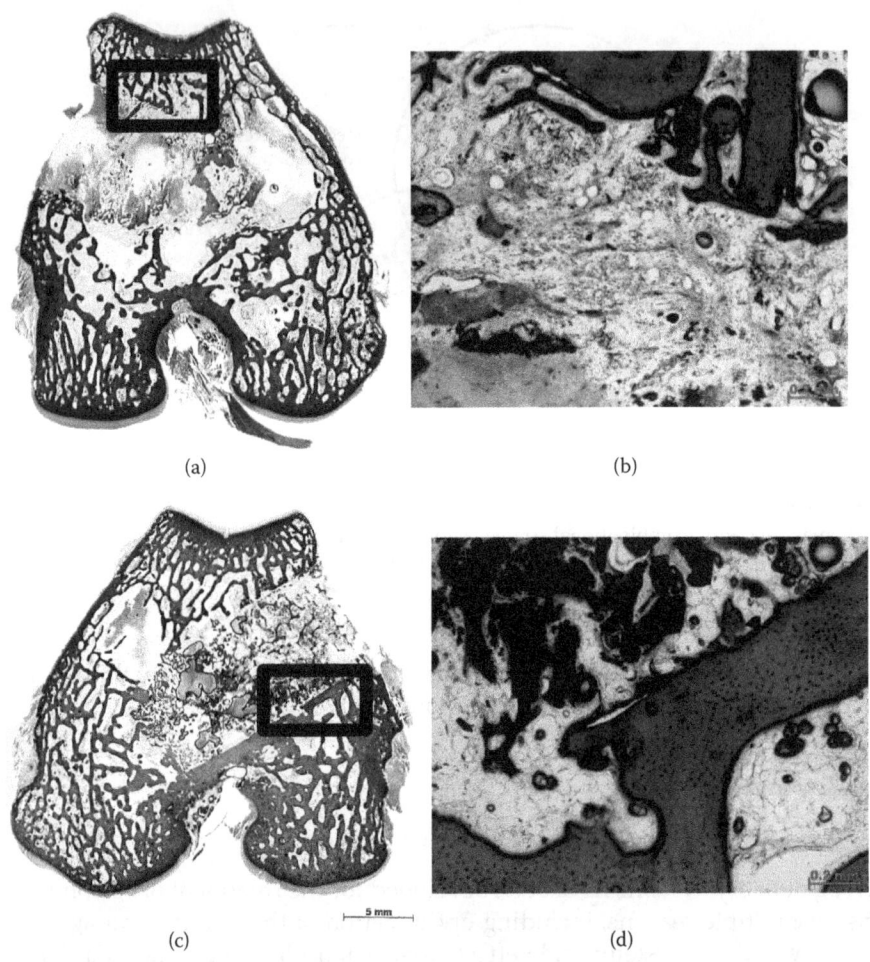

(a)   (b)

(c)   (d)

FIGURE 8.2
Histological images (von Kossa staining) of rabbit femoral condylar critical-sized defects with S. aureus infections after 8-week in vivo study. (a) and (b) show a defect filled with an autograft. (c) and (d) display the defect filled with a hydroxyapatite scaffold. (b) and (d) are enhanced views of the boxed region in (a) and (c), respectively.

In a 2011 study by Rathbone et al. on the effect of 21 different antibiotics at the cellular level in bone, it was reported that vancomycin, amikacin, and tobramycin had the least effect on osteogenic activities, whereas penicillin, gentamicin, ciprofloxacin, and minocycline showed decreased osteogenic activities.[13] In addition to the types of antibiotics, having an optimal drug release system is also critical for combating infection. Anytime a drug release system is being developed, it is important to understand the release profile needed for the application at hand. Release profiles can be burst, sustained, dual, or any combinations of the three profiles. A burst release provides a complete dumping of the drug into the environment, whereas a sustained release is used for continuous drug release over a period of time and at an optimal concentration that is directly related to the degradation of the biomaterial. The dual release system is typically used to release multiple drugs or growth factors using different materials and release patterns. An example is the release of recombinant human bone morphogenetic protein-2 (rhBMP-2) and vascular endothelial growth factor (VEGF) for osteogenesis[78,79] and angiogenesis,[50,80] respectively. Other examples include a drug release system that was developed by Shah et al. using a layer-by-layer approach with polyelectrolyte films to release growth factors at different times.[81]

An example of biomaterials containing antibiotics to treat infection is the impregnation of poly(methyl methacrylate) (PMMA) beads or cement[82,83] with tobramycin and colistin in order to treat *Pseudomonas aeruginosa* infection.[84] Although PMMA beads are the most common form of drug delivery with a combination of antibiotics including vancomycin and tobramycin, PMMA is not biodegradable.[85] However, a combination of different antibiotics is often prescribed to provide a defense against gramnegative (tobramycin) and grampositive (vancomycin) bacteria. Gentamicin along with tobramycin is in the aminoglycoside family for treating gram negative infections.[86]

Creating a phospholipid gel with vancomycin and gentamicin that was biodegradable and was able to be applied throughout the wound because of its pliability, Penn-Barwell et al. reported that the gel produced greater reduction of infection in a rat femoral critical-sized defect model.[87] A coating of a lipid and polymeric carrier system on titanium would also alleviate infection.[88] Other strategies such as the use of bioactive borate glass as a degradable carrier have been attempted to release vancomycin[51] and teicoplanin[77] for chronic osteomyelitis. By combining phosphate glass with poly(ε-caprolactone), vancomycin was released from the system.[89] With advances in technology towards the use of nanomaterials, sustained release of vancomycin for up to 35 days and releasing 95% of the drug was reported from a silica and calcium phosphate nanocomposite, with the average daily release at therapeutic levels.[74]

Chitosan[69,70,90], calcium phosphates,[71] polyurethane,[72] and composites have all been used as drug carriers. With biphasic calcium phosphate cement loaded with gentamicin, an initial burst release of the antibiotics was observed followed by a sustained release, with the antibiotics retaining their antibacterial activity after 30 days with *Staphylococcus aureus* and *Pseudomonas aeruginosa*.[91] Through understanding of the material's properties, Uskokovic et al. tuned the composition of calcium phosphates to control the biodegradable timescale, thereby creating a sustained release of the drugs over the time period of choice, which is typically around 6 weeks for osteomyelitis treatments.[92] In addition to modifying calcium phosphate composition, the combination of nano-HA particles and chitosan have also been studied for sustained release.[93]

An example of a system with a porous biodegradation polyurethane material is a sustained release of vancomycin throughout the treatment of osteomyelitis, alleviating the need for removing PMMA beads impregnated with antibiotics during recovery.[72] In another study comparing the standard PMMA beads to calcium sulfate, the authors found that the calcium sulfate provided similar or better reduction in infection than PMMA.[94] Similarly, when Beenken et al. coated calcium sulfate scaffolds with chitosan to release daptomycin, it was observed that these coatings significantly reduced the amount of infection present.[95]

In addition to the reliance on biomaterials and its properties for delivering antibiotics, another approach to drug release is to utilize physiologic changes caused by osteomyelitis. Since normal, average physiological pH for humans is 7.4 for humans,[96,97] the pH drops to an acidic level in a septic condition.[98] Understanding this concept, researchers have sought to harness this change by tailoring release of drugs using pH-sensitive materials, and this allows for release of the antibiotics at the time of infection. Chung et al. developed such a system by encapsulating vancomycin within poly(DL-lactic-co-glycolic acid) (PLGA) particles and placing these particles in an injectable calcium phosphate paste.[99] PLGA and its copolymers have also been used for drug release[100] because of their ability to have variable release characteristics based on polymer composition ratios, molecular weight, and crystallinity.[101] In a review of polymeric nanoparticles, Cheng et al. go further to suggest that in addition to the pH triggering the release of the drug, the nanoparticles themselves also have the ability to use temperature, redox reactions, and magnetic fields to trigger drug release.[102] These capabilities make polymeric particles an enticing solution for designing delivery systems tuned to a specific application and strategy. As such, when developing polymeric drug delivery systems for antibiotics, one must also consider the interactions of the material and any combinations of antibiotics that are to be used to ensure efficacy and that the materials have no effect on bone regeneration.[103]

From the above discussions, many techniques have been examined, including current research strategies and ideas on utilizing local delivery of antibiotics for osteomyelitis. Some strategies focus on the incorporation of antibiotics within materials that are already currently used for bone regeneration while others use a combination of different materials for antibiotics delivery. One example of a combined approach is the use of a fibrin gel embedded with vancomycin containing alginate beads and seeded with bone marrow-derived mesenchymal stem cells.[73] Other investigators made use of ethyl cellulose microparticles as a drug carrier that was incorporated in an HA-polyurethane scaffold for osteogenesis.[104] These approaches incorporate the strategies to combat infection together with bone regenerative capabilities.

As researchers continue to develop strategies to maintain bone regenerative capabilities while inserting infectious deterrents through local antibiotic delivery, it is important to consider the drug release profile and how the wound environment will affect that profile. By understanding the infectious environment, natural cues such as changes in pH can be harnessed for drug release. Table 8.3 summarizes some of the local antibiotic release studies for the treatment of osteomyelitis.

TABLE 8.3

Examples of Antibiotics That Have Been Used in Local Release Studies for the Treatment of Osteomyelitis

Journal	Author	Year	Antibiotic	Bacteria	Scaffold
Biomaterials	Zhang et al.	2010	Teicoplanin	MRSA	Borate bioactive glass[77]
J Cont Release	Xie et al.	2009	Vancomycin	MRSA	Borate glass, calcium sulfate[51]
J Biomed Mat Res Part B	Teller et al.	2006	Gentamicin	*S. aureus*	BONIT matrix®, Synthacer®[75]
J Ortho Trauma	Stinner et al.	2010	Vancomycin, amikacin	*S. aureus, P. aeruginosa*	Chitosan[69]
Clin Ortho Rel Res	Noel et al.	2010	Vancomycin, amikacin	*S. aureus, P. eruginosa*	Chitosan sponges[70]
J of Mat Sci	Makarov et al.	2010	Vancomycin	N/A release study	Calcium phosphate/polymer[71]
J Controlled Release	Li et al.	2010	Vancomycin	Target MRSA	Polyurethane[72]
J Ortho Trauma	Penn-Barwell et al.	2014	Vancomycin, gentamicin	*S. aureus*	Phospholipid gel[87]
Intl J Antimicro Agents	Krajewski et al.	2014	Colistin, tobramycin	*P. aeruginosa*	PMMA spacer[84]
J Biomed Mat Res B	McConoughey et al.	2015	Vancomycin	*S. aureus, S. epidermidis, P. aeruginosa*	Calcium sulfate[94]

8.6 Conclusion

The focus of this chapter is to understand the nature of infection in bone graft surgery, and to provide a basis for developing strategies to provide one-time treatment solutions to injuries requiring bone graft implementation. These solutions must consider the status of the patient on a case-by-case basis. The focus should be to provide the best overall combination of surgical strategy and graft type for that individual patient. In this chapter, the Cierny–Mader system provides a way to classify patients according to the types of infection and the patient's physiological condition. Unlike the classification of the patient with osteomyelitis, there is currently no classification for graft options due to inadequate synthetic solutions. However, currently developed strategies using synthetic grafts must still be investigated and optimized through continuous research. In addition to combating infection, the ultimate goal of the graft is to also provide functional regeneration of bone tissues. As such, the ability for angiogenesis as well for a continuous supply of nutrition must also be considered. Additionally, with the growing advancements in graft synthesis, 3D printing, and co-culture techniques, a bone graft of this quality may soon be a reality to mitigate infection and minimize the need for amputation.

References

1. Amini AR, Laurencin CT, Nukavarapu SP. Bone tissue engineering: Recent advances and challenges. *Critical Reviews™ in Biomedical Engineering.* 2012;40(5):363–408.
2. Guda T, Walker JA, Pollot BE, Appleford MR, Oh S, Ong JL, et al. In vivo performance of bilayer hydroxyapatite scaffolds for bone tissue regeneration in the rabbit radius. *Journal of Materials Science: Materials in Medicine.* 2011;22(3):647–56.
3. Burns TC, Stinner DJ, Mack AW, Potter BK, Beer R, Eckel TT, et al. Microbiology and injury characteristics in severe open tibia fractures from combat. *Journal of Trauma and Acute Care Surgery.* 2012;72(4):1062–7.
4. Harris AM, Althausen PL, Kellam J, Bosse MJ, Castillo R, Group LEAPS. Complications following limb-threatening lower extremity trauma. *Journal of Orthopaedic Trauma.* 2009;23(1):1–6.
5. Cross JD, Stinner DJ, Burns TC, Wenke JC, Hsu JR, Consortium STR. Return to duty after type III open tibia fracture. *Journal of Orthopaedic Trauma.* 2012;26(1):43–7.
6. Franken J, Hupkens P, Spauwen P. The treatment of soft-tissue defects of the lower leg after a traumatic open tibial fracture. *European Journal of Plastic Surgery.* 2010;33(3):129–33.
7. Eardley W, Brown K, Bonner T, Green A, Clasper J. Infection in conflict wounded. *Philosophical Transactions of the Royal Society of London B: Biological Sciences.* 2011;366(1562):204–18.
8. Morshed S, Miclau T, Bembom O, Cohen M, Knudson MM, Colford JM. Delayed internal fixation of femoral shaft fracture reduces mortality among patients with multisystem trauma. *The Journal of Bone & Joint Surgery.* 2009;91(1):3–13.
9. Geurts J, Arts JC, Walenkamp G. Bone graft substitutes in active or suspected infection. Contra-indicated or not? *Injury.* 2011;42:S82–S6.
10. Loder BG, Dunn KW. Functional reconstruction of a calcaneal deficit due to osteomyelitis with femoral head allograft and tendon rebalance. *The Foot.* 2014;24(3):149–52.
11. Murray CK, Wilkins K, Molter NC, Li F, Yu L, Spott MA, et al. Infections complicating the care of combat casualties during operations Iraqi Freedom and Enduring Freedom. *Journal of Trauma and Acute Care Surgery.* 2011;71(1):S62–S73.
12. Liu X, Xie Z, Zhang C, Pan H, Rahaman M, Zhang X, et al. Bioactive borate glass scaffolds: In vitro and in vivo evaluation for use as a drug delivery system in the treatment of bone infection. *Journal of Materials Science: Materials in Medicine.* 2010;21(2):575–82.

13. Rathbone CR, Cross JD, Brown KV, Murray CK, Wenke JC. Effect of various concentrations of antibiotics on osteogenic cell viability and activity. *Journal of Orthopaedic Research*. 2011;29(7):1070–4.

14. Calhoun JH, Manring M, Shirtliff M, editors. Osteomyelitis of the long bones. *Seminars in Plastic Surgery*; 2009: Thieme Medical Publishers.

15. Cierny III G, Mader JT, Penninck JJ. The Classic: A clinical staging system for adult osteomyelitis. *Clinical Orthopaedics and Related Research*. 2003;414:7–24.

16. Waldvogel FA, Medoff G, Swartz MN. Osteomyelitis: A review of clinical features, therapeutic considerations and unusual aspects. *New England Journal of Medicine*. 1970(282):198–206.

17. Lew DP, Waldvogel FA. Osteomyelitis. *The Lancet*. 2004;364(9431):369–79.

18. Lazzarini L, Mader JT, Calhoun JH. Osteomyelitis in long bones. *The Journal of Bone & Joint Surgery*. 2004;86(10):2305–18.

19. Thomas M, Puleo D. Infection, inflammation, and bone regeneration: A paradoxical relationship. *Journal of Dental Research*. 2011;90(9):1052–61.

20. Carroll EA, Andrew Koman L. External fixation and temporary stabilization of femoral and tibial trauma. *Journal of Surgical Orthopaedic Advances*. 2011;20(1):74.

21. Madhok BM, Vowden K, Vowden P. New techniques for wound debridement. *International Wound Journal*. 2013;10(3):247–51.

22. Zarchi K, Jemec GB. The efficacy of maggot debridement therapy—A review of comparative clinical trials. *International Wound Journal*. 2012;9(5):469–77.

23. Shi L, Ermis R, Kiedaisch B, Carson D. The effect of various wound dressings on the activity of debriding enzymes. *Advances in Skin & Wound Care*. 2010;23(10):456–62.

24. Haemmerle G, Duelli H, Abel M, Strohal R. The wound debrider: A new monofilament fibre technology. *British Journal of Nursing*. 2011;20(6):35.

25. Voigt J, Wendelken M, Driver V, Alvarez OM. xLow-frequency ultrasound (20-40 kHz) as an adjunctive therapy for chronic wound healing: A systematic review of the literature and meta-analysis of eight randomized controlled trials. *The International Journal of Lower Extremity Wounds*. 2011;10(4):190–9.

26. Fraccalvieri M, Serra R, Ruka E, Zingarelli E, Antoniotti U, Robbiano F, et al. Surgical debridement with VERSAJET: An analysis of bacteria load of the wound bed pre- and post-treatment and skin graft taken. A preliminary pilot study. *International Wound Journal*. 2011;8(2):155–61.

27. Nusbaum AG, Gil J, Rippy MK, Warne B, Valdes J, Claro A, et al. Effective method to remove wound bacteria: Comparison of various debridement modalities in an in vivo porcine model. *Journal of Surgical Research*. 2012;176(2):701–7.

28. Krug E, Berg L, Lee C, Hudson D, Birke-Sorensen H, Depoorter M, et al. Evidence-based recommendations for the use of Negative Pressure Wound Therapy in traumatic wounds and reconstructive surgery: Steps towards an international consensus. *Injury*. 2011;42:S1–S12.

29. Lehner B, Fleischmann W, Becker R, Jukema GN. First experiences with negative pressure wound therapy and instillation in the treatment of infected orthopaedic implants: A clinical observational study. *International Orthopaedics*. 2011;35(9):1415–20.

30. Bollero D, Driver V, Glat P, Gupta S, Lazaro-Martinez JL, Lyder C, et al. The role of negative pressure wound therapy in the spectrum of wound healing. *Ostomy Wound Manage*. 2010;56(5 Suppl):1–18.

31. Tan Y, Wang X, Li H, Zheng Q, Li J, Feng G, et al. The clinical efficacy of the vacuum-assisted closure therapy in the management of adult osteomyelitis. *Archives of Orthopaedic and Trauma Surgery*. 2011;131(2):255–9.

32. Rispoli DM, Horne BR, Kryzak TJ, Richardson MW. Description of a technique for vacuum-assisted deep drains in the management of cavitary defects and deep infections in devastating military and civilian trauma. *Journal of Trauma and Acute Care Surgery*. 2010;68(5):1247–52.

33. Martin RB, Burr DB, Sharkey NA. *Skeletal tissue mechanics*. Springer; 1998.

34. Guda T, Walker J, Singleton B, Hernandez J, Son J, Kim S, et al. Guided bone regeneration in long-bone defects with a structural hydroxyapatite graft and collagen membrane. *Tissue Engineering Part A*. 2013;19(17–18):1879.

35. Guda T, Walker JA, Singleton B, Hernandez J, Oh DS, Appleford MR, et al. Hydroxyapatite scaffold pore architecture effects in large bone defects in vivo. *Journal of Biomaterials Applications*. 2014;28(7):1016–27.

36. Rathbone C, Guda T, Singleton B, Oh D, Appleford M, Ong J, et al. Effect of cell-seeded hydroxyapatite scaffolds on rabbit radius bone regeneration. *Journal of Biomedical Materials Research Part A*. 2014;102(5):1458–66.

37. Agrawal CM, Ong J, Appleford MR, Mani G. *Introduction to Biomaterials: Basic Theory with Engineering Applications*. Cambridge, UK: Cambridge University Press; 2014.

38. Burdick JA, Mauck RL. *Biomaterials for Tissue Engineering Applications: A Review of the Past and Future Trends*. New York, NY: Springer Science & Business Media; 2010.

39. Blokhuis T, Arts JC. Bioactive and osteoinductive bone graft substitutes: Definitions, facts and myths. *Injury*. 2011;42:S26–S9.

40. Joosten U, Joist A, Gosheger G, Liljenqvist U, Brandt B, von Eiff C. Effectiveness of hydroxyapatite-vancomycin bone cement in the treatment of Staphylococcus aureus induced chronic osteomyelitis. *Biomaterials*. 2005;26(25):5251–8.

41. Saito T, Takeuchi R, Hirakawa K, Nagata N, Yoshida T, Koshino T, et al. Slow-releasing potential of vancomycin-loaded porous hydroxyapatite blocks implanted into MRSA osteomyelitis. *Journal of Biomedical Materials Research*. 2002;63(3):245–51.

42. Jiang J-L, Li Y-F, Fang T-L, Zhou J, Li X-L, Wang Y-C, et al. Vancomycin-loaded nano-hydroxyapatite pellets to treat MRSA-induced chronic osteomyelitis with bone defect in rabbits. *Inflammation Research*. 2012;61(3):207–15.

43. Shirtliff ME, Calhoun JH, Mader JT. Experimental osteomyelitis treatment with antibiotic-impregnated hydroxyapatite. *Clinical Orthopaedics and Related Research*. 2002;401:239–47.

44. Yashavantha Kumar C, Nalini K, Jagdish Menon DKP, Banerji B. Calcium sulfate as bone graft substitute in the treatment of osseous bone defects, a prospective study. *Journal of Clinical and Diagnostic Research* 2013;7(12):2926.

45. Fu Q, Huang W, Jia W, Rahaman MN, Liu X, Tomsia AP. Three-dimensional visualization of bioactive glass-bone integration in a rabbit tibia model using synchrotron x-ray microcomputed tomography. *Tissue Engineering Part A*. 2011;17(23–24):3077–84.

46. Leu A, Leach JK. Proangiogenic potential of a collagen/bioactive glass substrate. *Pharmaceutical Research*. 2008;25(5):1222–9.

47. Munukka E, Leppäranta O, Korkeamäki M, Vaahtio M, Peltola T, Zhang D, et al. Bactericidal effects of bioactive glasses on clinically important aerobic bacteria. *Journal of Materials Science: Materials in Medicine*. 2008;19(1):27–32.

48. Leppäranta O, Vaahtio M, Peltola T, Zhang D, Hupa L, Hupa M, et al. Antibacterial effect of bioactive glasses on clinically important anaerobic bacteria in vitro. *Journal of Materials Science: Materials in Medicine.* 2008;19(2):547–51.

49. Lindfors N, Hyvönen P, Nyyssönen M, Kirjavainen M, Kankare J, Gullichsen E, et al. Bioactive glass S53P4 as bone graft substitute in treatment of osteomyelitis. *Bone.* 2010;47(2):212–8.

50. Leach JK, Kaigler D, Wang Z, Krebsbach PH, Mooney DJ. Coating of VEGF-releasing scaffolds with bioactive glass for angiogenesis and bone regeneration. *Biomaterials.* 2006;27(17):3249–55.

51. Xie Z, Liu X, Jia W, Zhang C, Huang W, Wang J. Treatment of osteomyelitis and repair of bone defect by degradable bioactive borate glass releasing vancomycin. *Journal of Controlled Release.* 2009;139(2):118–26.

52. Sionkowska A. Current research on the blends of natural and synthetic polymers as new biomaterials: Review. *Progress in Polymer Science.* 2011;36(9):1254–76.

53. Kim HJ, Kim UJ, Leisk GG, Bayan C, Georgakoudi I, Kaplan DL. Bone regeneration on macroporous aqueous-derived silk 3-D scaffolds. *Macromolecular Bioscience.* 2007;7(5):643–55.

54. Kim HJ, Kim U-J, Kim HS, Li C, Wada M, Leisk GG, et al. Bone tissue engineering with premineralized silk scaffolds. *Bone.* 2008;42(6):1226–34.

55. Kretlow JD, Mikos AG. Bones to biomaterials and back again—20 years of taking cues from nature to engineer synthetic polymer scaffolds. *Journal of Biomedical Materials Research Part A.* 2011;98(3):323.

56. Rimondini L, Nicoli-Aldini N, Fini M, Guzzardella G, Tschon M, Giardino R. In vivo experimental study on bone regeneration in critical bone defects using an injectable biodegradable PLA/PGA copolymer. *Oral Surgery, Oral Medicine, Oral Pathology, Oral Radiology, and Endodontology.* 2005;99(2):148–54.

57. Son S-R, Linh N-TB, Yang H-M, Lee B-T. In vitro and in vivo evaluation of electrospun PCL/PMMA fibrous scaffolds for bone regeneration. *Science and Technology of Advanced Materials.* 2013;14(1):015009.

58. Poi MJ, Pisimisis G, Barshes NR, Darouiche RO, Lin PH, Kougias P, et al. Evaluating effectiveness of antibiotic polymethylmethacrylate beads in achieving wound sterilization and graft preservation in patients with early and late vascular graft infections. *Surgery.* 2013;153(5):673–82.

59. Anderson JM, Shive MS. Biodegradation and biocompatibility of PLA and PLGA microspheres. *Advanced Drug Delivery Reviews.* 2012;64:72–82.

60. Scott G. *Degradable Polymers: Principles and Applications.* New York, NY: Springer Science & Business Media; 2013.

61. LeBlon CE, Pai R, Fodor CR, Golding AS, Coulter JP, Jedlicka SS. In vitro comparative biodegradation analysis of salt-leached porous polymer scaffolds. *Journal of Applied Polymer Science.* 2013;128(5):2701–12.

62. Wang Y, Rudym DD, Walsh A, Abrahamsen L, Kim H-J, Kim HS, et al. In vivo degradation of three-dimensional silk fibroin scaffolds. *Biomaterials* 2008;29(24):3415–28.

63. Albrektsson T, Brånemark P-I, Hansson H-A, Lindström J. Osseointegrated titanium implants: Requirements for ensuring a long-lasting, direct bone-to-implant anchorage in man. *Acta Orthopaedica.* 1981;52(2):155–70.

64. Kujala S, Ryhänen J, Danilov A, Tuukkanen J. Effect of porosity on the osteointegration and bone ingrowth of a weight-bearing nickel–titanium bone graft substitute. *Biomaterials.* 2003;24(25):4691–7.

65. Brydone A, Meek D, Maclaine S. Bone grafting, orthopaedic biomaterials, and the clinical need for bone engineering. *Proceedings of the Institution of Mechanical Engineers, Part H: Journal of Engineering in Medicine.* 2010;224(12):1329–43.

66. Bohner M. Resorbable biomaterials as bone graft substitutes. *Materials Today.* 2010;13(1):24–30.

67. Swanson TE, Cheng X, Friedrich C. Development of chitosan–vancomycin antimicrobial coatings on titanium implants. *Journal of Biomedical Materials Research Part A.* 2011;97A(2):167–76.

68. Simchi A, Tamjid E, Pishbin F, Boccaccini AR. Recent progress in inorganic and composite coatings with bactericidal capability for orthopaedic applications. *Nanomedicine: Nanotechnology, Biology and Medicine.* 2011;7(1):22–39.

69. Stinner DJ, Noel SP, Haggard WO, Watson JT, Wenke JC. Local antibiotic delivery using tailorable chitosan sponges: The future of infection control? *Journal of Orthopaedic Trauma.* 2010;24(9):592–7.

70. Noel S, Courtney H, Bumgardner J, Haggard W. Chitosan sponges to locally deliver amikacin and vancomycin: A pilot in vitro evaluation. *Clinical Orthopaedics and Related Research.* 2010;468(8):2074–80.

71. Makarov C, Gotman I, Radin S, Ducheyne P, Gutmanas E. Vancomycin release from bioresorbable calcium phosphate–polymer composites with high ceramic volume fractions. *Journal of Materials Science.* 2010;45(23):6320–4.

72. Li B, Brown KV, Wenke JC, Guelcher SA. Sustained release of vancomycin from polyurethane scaffolds inhibits infection of bone wounds in a rat femoral segmental defect model. *Journal of Controlled Release.* 2010;145(3):221–30.

73. Hou T, Xu J, Li Q, Feng J, Zen L. In vitro evaluation of a fibrin gel antibiotic delivery system containing mesenchymal stem cells and vancomycin alginate beads for treating bone infections and facilitating bone formation. *Tissue Engineering Part A.* 2008;14(7):1173–82.

74. El-Ghannam A, Jahed K, Govindaswami M. Resorbable bioactive ceramic for treatment of bone infection. *Journal of Biomedical Materials Research Part A.* 2010;94(1):308–16.

75. Teller M, Gopp U, Neumann HG, Kühn KD. Release of gentamicin from bone regenerative materials: An in vitro study. *Journal of Biomedical Materials Research Part B: Applied Biomaterials.* 2007;81B(1):23–9.

76. Fleiter N, Walter G, Bösebeck H, Vogt S, Büchner H, Hirschberger W, et al. Clinical use and safety of a novel gentamicin-releasing resorbable bone graft substitute in the treatment of osteomyelitis/osteitis. *Bone and Joint Research.* 2014;3(7):223–9.

77. Zhang X, Jia W, Gu Y, Xiao W, Liu X, Wang D, et al. Teicoplanin-loaded borate bioactive glass implants for treating chronic bone infection in a rabbit tibia osteomyelitis model. *Biomaterials.* 2010;31(22):5865–74.

78. Shiels S, Oh S, Bae C, Guda T, Singleton B, Dean DD, et al. Evaluation of BMP-2 tethered polyelectrolyte coatings on hydroxyapatite scaffolds in vivo. *Journal of Biomedical Materials Research Part B: Applied Biomaterials.* 2012;100(7):1782–91.

79. Guda T, Darr A, Silliman DT, Magno MH, Wenke JC, Kohn J, et al. Methods to analyze bone regenerative response to different rhBMP-2 doses in rabbit craniofacial defects. *Tissue Engineering Part C: Methods.* 2014;20(9):749–60.

80. Young S, Patel ZS, Kretlow JD, Murphy MB, Mountziaris PM, Baggett LS, et al. Dose effect of dual delivery of vascular endothelial growth factor and bone

morphogenetic protein-2 on bone regeneration in a rat critical-size defect model. *Tissue Engineering Part A*. 2009;15(9):2347–62.

81. Shah NJ, Macdonald ML, Beben YM, Padera RF, Samuel RE, Hammond PT. Tunable dual growth factor delivery from polyelectrolyte multilayer films. *Biomaterials*. 2011;32(26):6183–93.

82. Wu P, Grainger DW. Drug/device combinations for local drug therapies and infection prophylaxis. *Biomaterials*. 2006;27(11):2450–67.

83. Barth RE, Vogely HC, Hoepelman AI, Peters EJ. 'To bead or not to bead?' Treatment of osteomyelitis and prosthetic joint-associated infections with gentamicin bead chains. *International Journal of Antimicrobial Agents*. 2011;38(5):371–5.

84. Krajewski J, Bode-Böger SM, Tröger U, Martens-Lobenhoffer J, Mulrooney T, Mittelstädt H, et al. Successful treatment of extensively drug-resistant Pseudomonas aeruginosa osteomyelitis using a colistin-and tobramycin-impregnated PMMA spacer. *International Journal of Antimicrobial Agents*. 2014;44(4):363–6.

85. Schlickewei CW, Yarar S, Rueger JM. Eluting antibiotic bone graft substitutes for the treatment of osteomyelitis in long bones. A review: Evidence for their use? *Orthopedic Research & Reviews*. 2014;6:71–79.

86. Hake ME, Young H, Hak DJ, Stahel PF, Hammerberg EM, Mauffrey C. Local antibiotic therapy strategies in orthopaedic trauma: Practical tips and tricks and review of the literature. *Injury*. 2015;46(8):1447–56.

87. Penn-Barwell JG, Murray CK, Wenke JC. Local antibiotic delivery by a bioabsorbable gel is superior to PMMA bead depot in reducing infection in an open fracture model. *Journal of Orthopaedic Trauma*. 2014;28(6):370–5.

88. Metsemakers W-J, Emanuel N, Cohen O, Reichart M, Potapova I, Schmid T, et al. A doxycycline-loaded polymer-lipid encapsulation matrix coating for the prevention of implant-related osteomyelitis due to doxycycline-resistant methicillin-resistant Staphylococcus aureus. *Journal of Controlled Release*. 2015;209:47–56.

89. Kim H-W, Lee E-J, Jun I-K, Kim H-E, Knowles JC. Degradation and drug release of phosphate glass/polycaprolactone biological composites for hard-tissue regeneration. *Journal of Biomedical Materials Research Part B: Applied Biomaterials*. 2005;75B(1):34–41.

90. Tan H-L, Ao H-Y, Ma R, Lin W-T, Tang T-T. In vivo effect of quaternized chitosan-loaded polymethylmethacrylate bone cement on methicillin-resistant staphylococcus epidermidis infection of the tibial metaphysis in a rabbit model. *Antimicrobial Agents and Chemotherapy*. 2014;58(10):6016–23.

91. Su W-Y, Chen Y-C, Lin F-H. A new type of biphasic calcium phosphate cement as a gentamicin carrier for osteomyelitis. *Evidence-Based Complementary and Alternative Medicine*. 2013;2013.

92. Uskoković V, Desai TA. Phase composition control of calcium phosphate nanoparticles for tunable drug delivery kinetics and treatment of osteomyelitis. I. Preparation and drug release. *Journal of Biomedical Materials Research Part A*. 2013;101(5):1416–26.

93. Uskoković V, Desai TA. In vitro analysis of nanoparticulate hydroxyapatite/chitosan composites as potential drug delivery platforms for the sustained release of antibiotics in the treatment of osteomyelitis. *Journal of Pharmaceutical Sciences*. 2014;103(2):567–79.

94. McConoughey SJ, Howlin RP, Wiseman J, Stoodley P, Calhoun JH. Comparing PMMA and calcium sulfate as carriers for the local delivery of antibiotics to infected surgical sites. *Journal of Biomedical Materials Research Part B: Applied Biomaterials.* 2015;103(4):870–7.

95. Beenken KE, Smith JK, Skinner RA, Mclaren SG, Bellamy W, Gruenwald MJ, et al. Chitosan coating to enhance the therapeutic efficacy of calcium sulfate-based antibiotic therapy in the treatment of chronic osteomyelitis. *Journal of Biomaterials Applications.* 2014;29(4):514–23.

96. Fox SI. *Human Physiology.* Boston, MA: McGraw-Hill; 2006.

97. Feher JJ. *Quantitative Human Physiology: An Introduction.* Waltham, MA: Elsevier/ Academic Press; 2012.

98. Lee J-H, Gu Y, Wang H, Lee WY. Microfluidic 3D bone tissue model for high-throughput evaluation of wound-healing and infection-preventing biomaterials. *Biomaterials.* 2012;33(4):999–1006.

99. Chung MF, Chia WT, Liu HY, Hsiao CW, Hsiao HC, Yang CM, et al. Inflammation-induced drug release by using a pH-responsive gas-generating hollow-microsphere system for the treatment of osteomyelitis. *Advanced Healthcare Materials.* 2014;3(11):1854–61.

100. Zhang Y, Chan HF, Leong KW. Advanced materials and processing for drug delivery: The past and the future. *Advanced Drug Delivery Reviews.* 2013;65(1):104–20.

101. Makadia HK, Siegel SJ. Poly lactic-co-glycolic acid (PLGA) as biodegradable controlled drug delivery carrier. *Polymers.* 2011;3(3):1377–97.

102. Cheng R, Meng F, Deng C, Klok H-A, Zhong Z. Dual and multi-stimuli responsive polymeric nanoparticles for programmed site-specific drug delivery. *Biomaterials.* 2013;34(14):3647–57.

103. Low SA, Kopeček J. Targeting polymer therapeutics to bone. *Advanced Drug Delivery Reviews.* 2012;64(12):1189–204.

104. Liu H-H, Zhang J-H, Xu Q-L, Zhang L, Li Y-B. Studies on hydroxyapatite/polyurethane scaffold containing drug-loaded microspheres for bone tissue engineering. *Wuji Cailiao Xuebao (Journal of Inorganic Materials).* 2011;26(10):1073–7.

105. Huh J, Stinner DJ, Burns TC, Hsu JR, Team LAS. Infectious complications and soft tissue injury contribute to late amputation after severe lower extremity trauma. *Journal of Trauma-Injury, Infection, and Critical Care.* 2011;71(1):S47–S51.

106. Johnson EN, Burns TC, Hayda RA, Hospenthal DR, Murray CK. Infectious complications of open type III tibial fractures among combat casualties. *Clinical Infectious Diseases.* 2007;45(4):409–15.

107. Mody RM, Zapor M, Hartzell JD, Robben PM, Waterman P, Wood-Morris R, et al. Infectious complications of damage control orthopedics in war trauma. *Journal of Trauma and Acute Care Surgery.* 2009;67(4):758–61.

9

Cell Sources for Orthopedic Defects

Christopher R. Rathbone, Marcello Pilia, and Jennifer S. McDaniel

CONTENTS

9.1 Introduction

The research directed toward gaining a better understanding of the role of stem cells in tissue injury has burgeoned in the past few decades. Accordingly, the development of methodologies to use stem cells has also increased. An improved understanding of the regenerative potential of adult (as opposed to embryonic) stem cells has resulted in a better acceptance of the study and use of stem cells by the general public. Importantly, patients with orthopedic injuries have benefitted directly from the remarkable advances in adult stem cell research. In addition to gaining a better comprehension of the mechanisms through which stem cells exert their effects, the discovery and isolation of stem cells from a large number of tissues has been an important advancement. This chapter will attempt to give the reader a better understanding of the sources of cells that are currently available for the clinician to apply and reliable sources for a basic scientist entering into the realm of stem cell biology to explore. The reader may notice there is an emphasis on mesenchymal stem cells (MSCs) derived from different tissues;

the majority of information and therapies concerning orthopedic injuries is focused on MSCs. However, this is not to say that cells with characteristics and capabilities equivalent or even superior to MSCs that are viable therapeutic options for orthopedic defects do not exist. The available sources of stem cells, especially MSCs,[1] and the discovery of several subtypes of stem cells within a given source, has grown dramatically. However, for the purposes of this chapter the discussion will be limited to sources that have been studied more thoroughly for bone repair. The use of bone marrow and adipose tissue as sources of stem cells, followed by other tissues (e.g., skeletal muscle) will be addressed, and specific topics covered include the isolation methods used to extract the stem cells, the delivery considerations, and the mechanisms of action.

9.2 Bone Marrow

Bone marrow is perhaps the most obvious and thoroughly studied source of stem cells when considering therapies for enhancing bone regeneration. The ability of bone marrow cells to produce mature bone when implanted subcutaneously provided strong evidence that stem cells resident within it would be a useful tool for future therapeutic applications for orthopedic injuries.[2] Subsequent discoveries of a plastic adherent stem cell within the bone marrow that was distinct from the hematopoietic stem cell revolutionized the field of stem cell biology, and, unbeknownst to the discoverers at the time, the field of regenerative medicine.[3-4] These unique cells were originally thought to primarily perform the function of supporting the hematopoietic niche; however, although their role in maintaining hematopoietic function is still appreciated,[5] it has also been recognized that they possess the capacity for multipotent differentiation to cells contributing to mesenchymal lineages including bone, cartilage, muscle, and adipose, hence the name mesenchymal stem cells (MSCs).[6-9] The difficulty in identifying their niche and fully understanding their potential has contributed to the difficulty in determining the most appropriate name, i.e., mesenchymal stem cell, multipotent mesenchymal stromal cells, marrow stromal cells, and marrow stromal cells, to name a few.[3,10-12] It is beyond the scope of this chapter to discuss the ambiguity in the nomenclature referring to these cells. For consistency for the remainder of the chapter they will be referred to as mesenchymal stem cells (MSCs).

MSCs are a relatively small fraction of cells within the bone marrow mononuclear cell fraction.[13,14] The discovery and thorough use of MSCs should not completely overshadow the therapeutic capacity of a bone marrow mononuclear (BM-MNC) cell fraction. In addition to MSCs there are several other types of stem/progenitor cells within the BM-MNC fraction, including hematopoietic stem cells (HSCs) and endothelial progenitor cells (EPCs).[15] Although BM-MNCs contain a heterogeneous mixture of stem cells, they should not be overlooked as a therapeutic cell source. Since they are a heterogeneous mixture of cells it is difficult to ascribe a specific experimental outcome to a specific cell type. However, the processing required to procure BM-MNCs is minimal, making them a viable clinical option.[16–19]

9.2.1 Isolation

The extraction of BM-MNCs, and by extension MSCs, is accomplished using bone marrow aspirate as the starting material. In humans the retrieval of bone marrow aspirates is accomplished by inserting an aspiration needle into the marrow cavity, removing the trochar and replacing it with a syringe, and establishing negative pressure until the desired amount of aspirate is withdrawn. A common access site is the iliac crest; however, the presence of stem cells within reamer-irrigator-aspirate provides an alternative methodology for marrow extraction.[20] In the most simple approach centrifugation produces a buffy coat layer containing the heterogeneous mononuclear cell fraction that can be used directly or purified further. Since MSCs comprise 0.001 to 0.01% of the total MNC population[13,14] (variations may be dependent on aspiration strategy[21]), and MSCs are plastic adherent, MNCs can be simply plated on to tissue culture plastic to enrich for MSCs. The use of flow cytometry, magnetic activated cell sorting (MACS), and other selection strategies may be advantageous for enrichment based on cell surface marker expression or adhesion characteristics of MSCs.[22,23] The exact location from which the stem cells are extracted has remained somewhat elusive, which may be due to difficulties concerning their analysis in vivo. Nonetheless, there is a growing body of literature that suggests MSCs reside in a vascular niche.[24]

9.2.2 Delivery Strategies

A significant advantage to the use of BM-MNCs or bone marrow aspirates containing BM-MNCs is that little manipulation is required. They can be used in an autologous approach applied on the same day of surgery. The combination of minimally manipulated BM-MNCs with FDA-approved materials significantly expedites clinical translation. For example, improvements in bone regeneration and mechanical strength have been observed when BM-MNCs were combined with PLLA scaffolds for the treatment of a cranial defect.[25] Another delivery strategy is to deliver via the circulation, taking advantage of the inherent homing ability of stem cells.[26] Regardless of the mode of delivery, the effect of injury and the health of the patient should be considered when utilizing BM-MNCs and other stem/progenitor cells in an autologous approach. Collectively, despite the heterogeneity and low stem cell content within BM-MNCs, they represent a relatively straightforward and noninvasive approach to improving bone regeneration.

From a purely scientific standpoint the combination of BM-MNCs with scaffolds is relatively infrequent for bone tissue engineering. Scientists quite often opt for utilizing MSCs; for the sake of experimental practicality MSCs are usually culture-expanded (Table 9.1). As opposed to the heterogeneous population of MNCs, MSCs are unique in that since they have a low level of major histocompatibility complex (MHC) class I antigens, lack of MHC-II expression affords them the ability to bypass immune rejection and thus be used in an allogeneic fashion.[27] This feature provides significant

TABLE 9.1

Summary of Published Experiments Used to Test the Ability of Bone Marrow–Derived Mesenchymal Stem Cells (BM-MSCs) to Heal Bony Defects

Cell Type	Defect	Delivery	Outcome	Reference
MNC	8 mm rat calvaria	MNCs in fibrin glue in coralline HA or PLLA disks	MNCs delivered within fibrin glue on PLLA ↑ bone. MNCs on Coral HA n.s. formulation	25
MSC + HSC	Mouse ectopic	CaP cylinders	Synergistic actions of MSCs and HSCs may be beneficial	46
MSC	10 mm radial defect	24h culture (non-osteogenic media) in HAp cylinders	No improvement	30
MSCs	4 mm mouse calvaria	Systemic delivery/ collagen matrix	Homing to site of injury	28
MSCs	2x2 mm mouse mandible	Systemic delivery/ collagen matrix	Homing to site of injury	28
MSCs	4 mm mouse calvaria	PEG-RGD	Improvement	49
MSCs	8 mm rat femoral defect	MSCs loaded in HAp/TCP cylinders	Complete healing of the defect	50
MSCs	3 cm sheep tibia defect	MSCs loaded in mineralized collagen	MSCs from bone marrow healed better than MSCs from adipose tissue	51

flexibility when considering their combination with biomaterials suitable for bone regeneration. Although MSCs are typically procured following culture expansion, this period may be exploited if preconditioning strategies are employed. Li et al. demonstrated improved survivability of BMDSCs exposed to hypoxia, a finding correlated with an improved Bcl-2/Bax ratio and decreased caspase-3 activation.[28] There are a number of clinical studies supporting their safety. Possibly one of the most dramatic demonstrations of the immunomodulatory capacity of MSCs and of their safety is their application for the treatment of inflammatory diseases,[29] of which graft versus host disease has been the most well studied. It seems an important consideration when delivering MSCs is the conditions in which they are maintained prior to their delivery. One of the conditions that influence their potential for bone regeneration could be whether or not they are treated with osteogenic induction media prior to their application. Several studies have demonstrated significant improvements in bone regeneration when MSCs were induced prior to implantation. Conversely, the same improvements were not observed when non-induced MSCs were used to treat rat femur and rabbit radius defects.[30,31] However, with the rapidly advancing field of tissue engineering will likely come the development of scaffolds capable of circumventing this limitation. In addition to the delivery of MSCs within the site of injury, the ability of MSCs to home to areas in need of repair has been exploited.[28] A limitation thus far has been the entrapment of MSCs in filter organs.[32] However, this can be at least partially avoided when other injection routes are used.

9.2.3 Mechanism of Action

The differentiation of stem cells into a committed, differentiated cell within a given tissue was previously thought to be the primary function of stem cells. This was intuitive given the potential for stem cells to take on the characteristics of a differentiated cell when induced toward a specific lineage in vitro. For example, MSCs derived from the bone marrow could be induced toward adipogenic, chondrogenic, and osteogenic lineages when exposed to appropriate induction media.[9,33,34] In vivo, the labelling of BM-MSCs demonstrated the incorporation of exogenously delivered cells into mature osteocytes.[35] The osteogenic capacity of stem cells can further be augmented when they are genetically manipulated and/or encouraged to progress down the osteogenic lineage when exposed to osteogenic factors.[36] A large number of studies have demonstrated significant improvements in bone regeneration when MSCs were cultured in osteogenic induction media prior to their delivery as discussed above. Presumably this "primes" MSCs toward a more osteogenic phenotype prior to their application. Conversely, the delivery of MSCs in the absence of induction media has been demonstrated to have little or no effect when expanded in standard expansion media. There is an abundance of literature supporting the ability of stem cells to directly contribute to osteogenesis through their differentiation; however, the capabilities of MSCs have expanded to include their effects on the microenvironment, which may indirectly contribute to improved bone regeneration and hence osteogenesis. When considering the use of BM-MSCs for osteogenesis it is important to take into account their decline in osteogenic capacity with age.[13]

More recently it has become accepted that stem cells are more than simply building blocks, but that they also play the role of orchestrating regeneration through the modulation of the microenvironment. Perhaps one of the most convincing pieces of evidence that MSCs secrete factors that improve healing are the experiments where stem cell conditioned media were effective.[37] It is not surprising that one of the targets of the paracrine factors secreted by MSCs may be the vasculature, given its importance in bone repair. For example, bone healing after injury is mediated by a steady blood supply of nutrients and growth factors from the vasculature. When tissue engineered scaffolds do not develop adequate vascularization, the nutrient supply is limited and cell death can easily occur.[38] Moreover, lack of vascularization also means that the arrival of hormones and growth factors by cells and removal of toxic byproducts is inhibited.[39] Conversely, creating a more suitable environment for bone regeneration through enhanced angiogenesis encourages bone growth. The effect of BMSCs on angiogenesis for bone healing has been supported by a number of in vitro and in vivo experiments. The mechanism whereby MSCs improve angiogenesis may not occur directly through differentiation, but may be due to the effects of MSCs on the microenvironment. MSCs secrete a number of critical growth factors for favorable regeneration, including VEGF, a growth factor widely accepted to play a role in angiogenesis.[40–42] In this regard, the use of purified MSCs may be better than BM-MNCs, since MSCs produced a greater angiogenic response when used in a model of hindlimb ischemia.[43] Similarly, when considering the role of MSCs on the microenvironment, their immunomodulatory capacity should not be overlooked. MSCs possess the ability to modulate the immune system, for example, through their effects on dendritic and T cells, thereby inducing a local immunosuppressive environment.[44,45] Given that the inflammatory response is such an integral part of the bone healing cascade, it is intuitive that stem cell therapies may exert their effects through it.

Determining the mechanism(s) through which the heterogeneous populations of BM-MNCs exert their effects is not straightforward. The beneficial effects of delivering more than one cell type isolated from the bone marrow may have its advantages. The co-transplantation of HSCs and MSCs results in greater vascularization and bone formation in vivo than achieved with MSCs alone.[46] In addition, the presence of endothelial progenitor cells within bone marrow and their therapeutic value is worth mentioning.[15,47,48] Collectively, the presence of multiple stem cell types, and the positive effects realized when even unpurified isolates of bone marrow are used, suggest that bone marrow is a rich source of stem cells that extends beyond that of MSCs alone.

9.3 Adipose Tissue

One of the most exciting advances concerning the use of stem cells for tissue engineering and regenerative medicine is the effective isolation of stem cells from adipose tissue.[7] Analogous to the MSC comprising a small component of the overall BM-MNC population from bone marrow aspirate, there are MSCs that can be derived from adipose tissue as they comprise a small percentage of cells within the stromal vascular fraction (SVF) (Figure 9.1). Also, like bone marrow, the cell derived from adipose tissue most commonly utilized therapeutically is the adipose-derived mesenchymal stem cell (ASC). In fact, the explosion of research directed toward ASC research likely benefited from the years of work directed to better understanding bone marrow–derived mesenchymal stem cells. Although relatively minor differences exist, there are a number of factors in common between BM-MSCs and ASCs.[52] Stem cells derived from adipose tissue have several characteristics in common with BMSCs, including their potential to differentiate into a number of cell types within the mesenchymal lineage and the commonality of several cell surface markers, in addition to the use of a number of different names.[12,53]

9.3.1 Isolation and Delivery

A particularly unique advantage of adipose tissue is their ease of isolation and the number of MSCs that can be obtained. For example, it has been estimated that ~18% of nucleated cells are typically derived from the bone marrow, versus ~24% of cells from adipose tissue.[54] A likely explanation for this abundance is the high vascularity of adipose tissue, and the vascular residence of MSCs.[24]

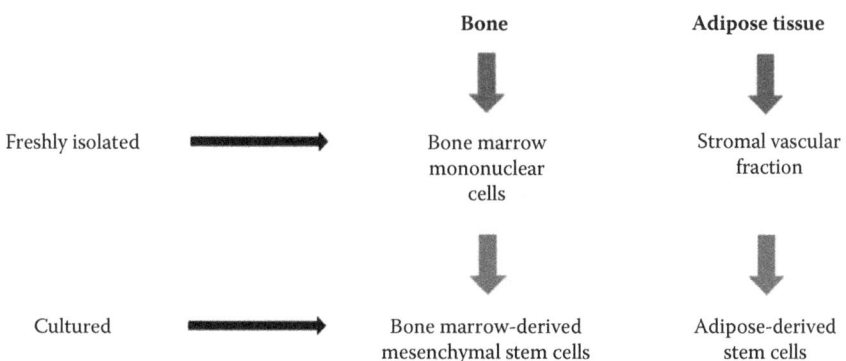

FIGURE 9.1
Schematic comparing the similarities found between bone marrow–derived mesenchymal stem cells (BM-MSCs) and adipose tissue–derived stem cells (ASCs). Bone marrow is harvested from bone, from which BM-MSCs are harvested; similarly adipose tissue is harvested during liposuction to yield ASCs.

ASCs can be isolated during a simple liposuction aspiration; therefore, morbidity associated with their extraction is minimal. Adipose tissue is digested, typically with collagenase, and subjected to centrifugation to separate the stromal vascular fraction from adipocytes. At this point, similar to BM-MNCs, the stromal vascular fraction represents a heterogeneous mixture of cells, which contains a variety of cells with hematopoietic markers, preadipocytes, fibroblasts, and erythrocytes, to name a few.[55,56] The clinical use of devices capable of isolating the SVF in the operating room is occurring in Asia and Europe, but is not currently approved in the United States. ASCs have been used clinically to augment an autologous bone graft to repair a critically sized defect in a pediatric patient.[57] Analogous to the purification of MSCs from the BM-MNC population, the goal is to isolate ASCs from the SVF and plate them on tissue culture plastic; the percentage of MSCs increases accordingly over time in vitro.[55] Given the many practical and logistical advantages, investigations into the use of ASCs for bone injuries and potential for a useful alternative to BMSCs was a logical next step (Table 9.2). ASCs have been combined with

TABLE 9.2

Summary of Published Experiments Used to Test the Ability of Adipose Tissue–Derived Stem Cells (ASCs) to Heal Bony Defects

Cell Type	Defect	Delivery	Outcome	Reference
ASCs	4 mm mouse calvaria	PEG-RGD	Improvement	49
ASCs	0.5 mm mouse femur	Passage 2-3 systemic delivery	Improved healing	46
ASCs	4 mm mouse calvaria	24h culture (non-osteogenic media) on apatite-coated PLGA	Improved healing	58
ASCs	Bilateral 9 mm diameter cylinder in dog mandible	48h incubation in Collatamp—3 wks between harvest and surgery	No differences seen between cell free and ASC-seeded Collatamp	68
ASCs	8 mm rat calvaria	Osteogenic-induced ASCs in demineralized bone matrix	Osteogenic regeneration enhanced in osteoinducted ASCs	69
ASCs	3.4 × 3.7 cm human mandible defect	Passages 3-4 in β-TCP granules and BMP-2	Promising therapy that circumvents need for ectopic bone formation	70
ASCs	10 × 10 mm rabbit craniotomy	Passage 4 in demineralized bone matrix	ASCs and DBM have positive bone regeneration effect, but not significantly better than DBM alone	71

a number of scaffolds in animal models of bone regeneration. Interestingly, human ASCs seeded on PLGA scaffolds improved the healing of mouse calvarial defects, even in the absence of pre-differentiation.[58] Currently, whether they are as effective as BMSCs is equivocal. A direct comparison of porcine,[59] sheep,[51] and rat[60] BMSCs and ASCs have demonstrated an increased,[51,59] and equivalent[60] osteogenic capacity. A direct comparison of BMSCs and ASCs also showed an improved survival of BMSCs during calvarial bone healing in mice.[49] As with BMSCs, ASCs have been delivered systemically and safely in humans[61,62] and their ability to home around bone defects has been demonstrated to be an effective strategy to augment bone healing.[63]

9.3.2 Mechanism of Action

ASCs have been shown to improve bone growth in vivo, and as discussed above, their osteogenic differentiation may contribute to this. A number of studies in other animal models have demonstrated the ability of ASCs to encourage angiogenesis,[64] a concept applicable for bone regeneration that can be augmented with the use of VEGF overexpression.[65] Like with BM-MSCs, their immunomodulatory capacity has been documented, and in some cases is superior,[66,67] which seems logical and may also exert an effect through this mechanism.

Given their logistical and practical advantages with regards to their procurement, ASCs are indeed a stem cell with great promise for clinical improvements. However, similar to that of BMSCs, it is plausible to conjecture that a number of other stem cells will be isolated from adipose tissue in the future. If the vasculature is indeed the primary source of mesenchymal stem cells, it is likely that other cells of the vasculature may provide a fruitful avenue for research in the future.

9.4 Other Cell Types

There is an abundance of literature utilizing stem cells derived from bone marrow or adipose tissue, particularly, mesenchymal stem cells derived from these tissues. As stated above, MSCs have been isolated from virtually every organ.[1] The features of MSCs, including differentiation capacity, immunomodulatory capacity, and secretory profile, are relatively consistent whether they are taken from bone marrow or adipose tissue. The use of skeletal muscle as a source of cells for bone regeneration is not as common. However, when taking into consideration the proximity of skeletal muscle to bone and the importance of skeletal muscle in fracture healing of composite injuries, the concept becomes more intuitive. For example, fracture healing is significantly impaired in composite injuries where there is a concomitant loss of skeletal muscle, which suggests that skeletal muscle may contain cells beneficial to fracture healing. Also, the finding that cells of MyoD-lineage (indicating a myogenic origin) contribute to fracture healing, especially in the absence of an intact periosteum, supports this contention.[72] The hypothesis that cells derived from skeletal muscle have osteogenic potential is supported by the frequent use of a skeletal muscle–derived cell line (C2C12) for osteogenic differentiation.[73–75] Collectively, this suggests that skeletal muscle may represent a source of cells beneficial for the improvement of bone repair.

9.4.1 Isolation and Delivery

Similar to adipose tissue, skeletal muscle represents an abundant source of tissue from which stem cells can be extracted. The digestion of muscle biopsies with collagenase liberates a heterogeneous mixture of cells. An alternative means to obtain skeletal muscle is from the use of discarded tissue.[76] The type of stem cell isolated from skeletal muscle is dependent on the selection strategy. The most thoroughly studied stem cell from skeletal muscle is the satellite cell, which can be obtained in high purity through the elimination of fibroblasts using a pre-plate method. Despite their reported osteogenic potential, the use of the satellite cell for bone regeneration has received little attention. Conversely, other purified fractions from skeletal muscle exist, in particular MDSCs, which are selected based on their late adherence to plastic using the pre-plate method. Their origin in vivo, similar to that of the MSC, may be vascular. Their human counterpart, which can be isolated using flow cytometry, are referred to as myogenic endothelial cells (MECs),[77] and demonstrate significant osteogenic potential.[78] Both MDSCs and MECs have been combined with scaffolds resulting in improved regeneration in vivo (Table 9.3).

TABLE 9.3

Summary of Published Experiments Used to Test the Ability of Muscle-Derived Stem Cells (MDSCs) and Endothelial Progenitor Cells to Heal Bony Defects and/or Regenerate Bone

Cell Type	Defect	Delivery	Outcome	Reference
MDSCs	5 mm mouse calvaria	BMP-4 transduced in thrombin etc.	Improvement	81
MDSCs	6 mm mouse calvaria	VEGF and/or BMP-4 transduced seeded on Gelfoam	Improved healing	80
MDSCs	Subcutaneous implant	Freshly isolated cells and osteogenic factor mixed in chitosan	MDSCs demonstrated potential to create bone in vivo	83
MDSCs	5 mm mouse calvaria	Freshly isolated BMP-4 transduced cells in Gelfoam, bovine collagen gel, and fibrin sealant	MDSCs in Gelfoam regenerated much more bone	84

(Continued)

TABLE 9.3 (*Continued*)

Summary of Published Experiments Used to Test the Ability of Muscle-Derived Stem Cells (MDSCs) and Endothelial Progenitor Cells to Heal Bony Defects and/or Regenerate Bone

Cell Type	Defect	Delivery	Outcome	Reference
MDSCs	5 mm mouse calvaria	Human MDSCs in fibrin sealant	MDSCs are as good as BM-MSCs when BMP is genetically added	85
MDSCs	5 mm mouse calvaria	Mouse MDSCs transduced in BMP-4 and seeded in collagen sponge	MDSCs include stem cells and can be used in gene therapy to deliver BMP-2	86
EPCs	5 mm rat femur	Cultured 7-10 days on Gelfoam	Improved healing	48
EPCs	5 mm rat femur	Cultured 7-10 days on Gelfoam	Improved healing	15
EPCs	Rigid dome model above rat calvaria	β-TCP granules coated with fibronectin	The addition of cells showed a significant increase in bone formation	87
EPCs	5 mm rat femur	EPCs and BM-MSCs in β-TCP scaffold	EPCs promote directly and indirectly early vascularization of MSC-stimulated bone formation	88

9.4.2 Mechanisms of Action

The osteogenic potential of MDSCs has been demonstrated and they provide a straightforward mechanism of action.[79] The genetic manipulation of MDSCs with VEGF and BMP-4 produces greater bone regeneration than without.[80] MDSCs have the potential to successfully form ectopic bone and improve cranial defect healing in vivo,[81] a scenario that is enhanced in the presence of the sustained release of BMP-2.[82]

9.5 Summary

There are many factors to consider when choosing the most appropriate source for healing bone, not the least of which is your intended application. For example, clinicians may have fewer options for patient care when considering cell-based applications (e.g., bone marrow) than basic scientists exploring the limits of various cell types from less obvious tissues (e.g., skeletal muscle). Another important consideration when comparing cells derived from various sources and the experimental results are the conditions in which they are applied (scaffold type, number, culture status). Regardless of the experimental or clinical applications, it is exciting to consider that regardless of whether MSCs are derived from bone marrow or adipose tissue, their ability to heal bone defects has been established, and the number of delivery strategies available is similar.

References

1. da Silva Meirelles, L., P.C. Chagastelles, and N.B. Nardi, Mesenchymal stem cells reside in virtually all post-natal organs and tissues. *J Cell Sci*, 2006. 119 (Pt 11): 2204–13.
2. Friedenstein, A.J., S. Piatetzky, II, and K.V. Petrakova, Osteogenesis in transplants of bone marrow cells. *J Embryol Exp Morphol*, 1966. 16(3): 381–90.
3. Friedenstein, A.J., R.K. Chailakhyan, N.V. Latsinik, et al., Stromal cells responsible for transferring the microenvironment of the hemopoietic tissues. Cloning in vitro and retransplantation in vivo. *Transplantation*, 1974. 17(4): 331–40.
4. Friedenstein, A.J., K.V. Petrakova, A.I. Kurolesova, et al., Heterotopic of bone marrow. Analysis of precursor cells for osteogenic and hematopoietic tissues. *Transplantation*, 1968. 6(2): 230–47.
5. Sacchetti, B., A. Funari, S. Michienzi, et al., Self-renewing osteoprogenitors in bone marrow sinusoids can organize a hematopoietic microenvironment. *Cell*, 2007. 131(2): 324–36.
6. Majumdar, M.K., M.A. Thiede, J.D. Mosca, et al., Phenotypic and functional comparison of cultures of marrow-derived mesenchymal stem cells (MSCs) and stromal cells. *J Cell Physiol*, 1998. 176(1): 57–66.
7. Zuk, P.A., M. Zhu, H. Mizuno, et al., Multilineage cells from human adipose tissue: Implications for cell-based therapies. *Tissue Eng*, 2001. 7(2): 211–28.
8. Koc, O.N. and H.M. Lazarus, Mesenchymal stem cells: Heading into the clinic. *Bone Marrow Transplant*, 2001. 27(3): 235–9.
9. Pittenger, M.F., A.M. Mackay, S.C. Beck, et al., Multilineage potential of adult human mesenchymal stem cells. *Science*, 1999. 284(5411): 143–7.
10. Caplan, A.I., Mesenchymal stem cells. *J Orthop Res*, 1991. 9(5): 641–50.
11. Friedenstein, A.J., R.K. Chailakhyan, and U.V. Gerasimov, Bone marrow osteogenic stem cells: In vitro cultivation and transplantation in diffusion chambers. *Cell Tissue Kinet*, 1987. 20(3): 263–72.
12. Dominici, M., K. Le Blanc, I. Mueller, et al., Minimal criteria for defining multipotent mesenchymal stromal cells. The International Society for Cellular Therapy position statement. *Cytotherapy*, 2006. 8(4): 315–7.
13. Stolzing, A., E. Jones, D. McGonagle, et al., Age-related changes in human bone marrow-derived mesenchymal stem cells: Consequences for cell therapies. *Mech Ageing Dev*, 2008. 129(3): 163–73.
14. Martins, A.A., A. Paiva, J.M. Morgado, et al., Quantification and immunophenotypic characterization of bone marrow and umbilical cord blood mesenchymal stem cells by multicolor flow cytometry. *Transplant Proc*, 2009. 41(3): 943–6.
15. Li, R., K. Atesok, A. Nauth, et al., Endothelial progenitor cells for fracture healing: A microcomputed tomography and biomechanical analysis. *J Orthop Trauma*, 2011. 25(8): 467–71.

16. Roncalli, J., F. Mouquet, C. Piot, et al., Intracoronary autologous mononucleated bone marrow cell infusion for acute myocardial infarction: Results of the randomized multicenter BONAMI trial. *Eur Heart J*, 2011. 32(14): 1748–57.

17. van Ramshorst, J., J.J. Bax, S.L. Beeres, et al., Intramyocardial bone marrow cell injection for chronic myocardial ischemia: A randomized controlled trial. *Jama*, 2009. 301(19): 1997–2004.

18. Rosenzweig, A., Cardiac cell therapy—Mixed results from mixed cells. *N Engl J Med*, 2006. 355(12): 1274–7.

19. Umemura, T., K. Nishioka, A. Igarashi, et al., Autologous bone marrow mononuclear cell implantation induces angiogenesis and bone regeneration in a patient with compartment syndrome. *Circ J*, 2006. 70(10): 1362–4.

20. Porter, R.M., F. Liu, C. Pilapil, et al., Osteogenic potential of reamer irrigator aspirator (RIA) aspirate collected from patients undergoing hip arthroplasty. *J Orthop Res*, 2009. 27(1): 42–9.

21. Muschler, G.F., C. Boehm, and K. Easley, Aspiration to obtain osteoblast progenitor cells from human bone marrow: The influence of aspiration volume. *J Bone Joint Surg Am*, 1997. 79(11): 1699–709.

22. Jamous, M., A. Al-Zoubi, M.N. Khabaz, et al., Purification of mouse bone marrow-derived stem cells promotes ex vivo neuronal differentiation. *Cell Transplant*, 2010. 19(2): 193–202.

23. Ramakrishnan, A., B. Torok-Storb, and M.M. Pillai, Primary marrow-derived stromal cells: isolation and manipulation. *Methods Mol Biol*, 2013. 1035: 75–101.

24. Crisan, M., S. Yap, L. Casteilla, et al., A perivascular origin for mesenchymal stem cells in multiple human organs. *Cell Stem Cell*, 2008. 3(3): 301–13.

25. Kretlow, J.D., P.P. Spicer, J.A. Jansen, et al., Uncultured marrow mononuclear cells delivered within fibrin glue hydrogels to porous scaffolds enhance bone regeneration within critical-sized rat cranial defects. *Tissue Eng Part A*, 2010. 16(12): 3555–68.

26. van der Bogt, K.E., A.A. Hellingman, M.A. Lijkwan, et al., Molecular imaging of bone marrow mononuclear cell survival and homing in murine peripheral artery disease. *JACC Cardiovasc Imaging*, 2012. 5(1): 46–55.

27. Ryan, J.M., F.P. Barry, J.M. Murphy, et al., Mesenchymal stem cells avoid allogeneic rejection. *J Inflamm (Lond)*, 2005. 2: 8.

28. Li, S., Q. Tu, J. Zhang, et al., Systemically transplanted bone marrow stromal cells contributing to bone tissue regeneration. *J Cell Physiol*, 2008. 215(1): 204–9.

29. Newman, R.E., D. Yoo, M.A. LeRoux, et al., Treatment of inflammatory diseases with mesenchymal stem cells. *Inflamm Allergy Drug Targets*, 2009. 8(2): 110–23.

30. Rai, B., J.L. Lin, Z.X. Lim, et al., Differences between in vitro viability and differentiation and in vivo bone-forming efficacy of human mesenchymal stem cells cultured on PCL-TCP scaffolds. *Biomaterials*, 2010. 31(31): 7960–70.

31. Rathbone, C.R., T. Guda, B.M. Singleton, et al., Effect of cell-seeded hydroxyapatite scaffolds on rabbit radius bone regeneration. *J Biomed Mater Res A*, 2013. 102(5): 1458–66.

32. Gao, J., J.E. Dennis, R.F. Muzic, et al., The dynamic in vivo distribution of bone marrow-derived mesenchymal stem cells after infusion. *Cells Tissues Organs*, 2001. 169(1): 12–20.

33. Jiang, Y., B.N. Jahagirdar, R.L. Reinhardt, et al., Pluripotency of mesenchymal stem cells derived from adult marrow. *Nature*, 2002. 418(6893): 41–9.

34. Villa-Diaz, L.G., S.E. Brown, Y. Liu, et al., Derivation of mesenchymal stem cells from human induced pluripotent stem cells cultured on synthetic substrates. *Stem Cells*, 2012. 30(6): 1174–81.
35. Park, B.W., E.J. Kang, J.H. Byun, et al., In vitro and in vivo osteogenesis of human mesenchymal stem cells derived from skin, bone marrow and dental follicle tissues. *Differentiation*, 2012. 83(5): 249–59.
36. Carpenter, R.S., L.R. Goodrich, D.D. Frisbie, et al., Osteoblastic differentiation of human and equine adult bone marrow-derived mesenchymal stem cells when BMP-2 or BMP-7 homodimer genetic modification is compared to BMP-2/7 heterodimer genetic modification in the presence and absence of dexamethasone. *J Orthop Res*, 2010. 28(10): 1330–7.
37. Ando, Y., K. Matsubara, J. Ishikawa, et al., Stem cell-conditioned medium accelerates distraction osteogenesis through multiple regenerative mechanisms. *Bone*, 2014. 61: 82–90.
38. Brighton, C.T. and R.M. Hunt, Histochemical localization of calcium in the fracture callus with potassium pyroantimonate. Possible role of chondrocyte mitochondrial calcium in callus calcification. *J Bone Joint Surg Am*, 1986. 68(5): 703–15.
39. Grellier, M., L. Bordenave, and J. Amedee, Cell-to-cell communication between osteogenic and endothelial lineages: Implications for tissue engineering. *Trends Biotechnol*, 2009. 27(10): 562–71.
40. Ferrara, N., Role of vascular endothelial growth factor in regulation of physiological angiogenesis. *Am J Physiol Cell Physiol*, 2001. 280(6): C1358–66.
41. Hoeben, A., B. Landuyt, M.S. Highley, et al., Vascular endothelial growth factor and angiogenesis. *Pharmacol Rev*, 2004. 56(4): 549–80.
42. Byrne, A.M., D.J. Bouchier-Hayes, and J.H. Harmey, Angiogenic and cell survival functions of vascular endothelial growth factor (VEGF). *J Cell Mol Med*, 2005. 9(4): 777–94.
43. Iwase, T., N. Nagaya, T. Fujii, et al., Comparison of angiogenic potency between mesenchymal stem cells and mononuclear cells in a rat model of hindlimb ischemia. *Cardiovasc Res*, 2005. 66(3): 543–51.
44. Di Nicola, M., C. Carlo-Stella, M. Magni, et al., Human bone marrow stromal cells suppress T-lymphocyte proliferation induced by cellular or nonspecific mitogenic stimuli. *Blood*, 2002. 99(10): 3838–43.
45. Jiang, X.X., Y. Zhang, B. Liu, et al., Human mesenchymal stem cells inhibit differentiation and function of monocyte-derived dendritic cells. *Blood*, 2005. 105(10): 4120–6.
46. Moioli, E.K., P.A. Clark, M. Chen, et al., Synergistic actions of hematopoietic and mesenchymal stem/progenitor cells in vascularizing bioengineered tissues. *PLoS One*, 2008. 3(12): e3922.
47. Palladino, M., I. Gatto, V. Neri, et al., Combined therapy with sonic hedgehog gene transfer and bone marrow-derived endothelial progenitor cells enhances angiogenesis and myogenesis in the ischemic skeletal muscle. *J Vasc Res*, 2012. 49(5): 425–31.
48. Li, R., A. Nauth, C. Li, et al., Expression of VEGF gene isoforms in a rat segmental bone defect model treated with EPCs. *J Orthop Trauma*, 2012. 26(12): 689–92.
49. Degano, I.R., M. Vilalta, J.R. Bago, et al., Bioluminescence imaging of calvarial bone repair using bone marrow and adipose tissue-derived mesenchymal stem cells. *Biomaterials*, 2008. 29(4): 427–37.

50. Kadiyala, S., N. Jaiswal, and S.P. Bruder, Culture-expanded, bone marrow-derived mesenchymal stem cells can regenerate a critical-sized segmental bone defect. *Tissue Engineering*, 1997. 3(2): 173–185.

51. Niemeyer, P., K. Fechner, S. Milz, et al., Comparison of mesenchymal stem cells from bone marrow and adipose tissue for bone regeneration in a critical size defect of the sheep tibia and the influence of platelet-rich plasma. *Biomaterials*, 2010. 31(13): 3572–9.

52. Strioga, M., S. Viswanathan, A. Darinskas, et al., Same or not the same? Comparison of adipose tissue-derived versus bone marrow-derived mesenchymal stem and stromal cells. *Stem Cells Dev*, 2012. 21(14): 2724–52.

53. Bourin, P., B.A. Bunnell, L. Casteilla, et al., Stromal cells from the adipose tissue-derived stromal vascular fraction and culture expanded adipose tissue-derived stromal/stem cells: A joint statement of the International Federation for Adipose Therapeutics and Science (IFATS) and the International Society for Cellular Therapy (ISCT). *Cytotherapy*, 2013. 15(6): 641–8.

54. Vishnubalaji, R., M. Al-Nbaheen, B. Kadalmani, et al., Comparative investigation of the differentiation capability of bone-marrow- and adipose-derived mesenchymal stem cells by qualitative and quantitative analysis. Cell Tissue Res, 2012. 347(2): 419–27.

55. McIntosh, K., S. Zvonic, S. Garrett, et al., The immunogenicity of human adipose-derived cells: Temporal changes in vitro. *Stem Cells*, 2006. 24(5): 1246–53.

56. Mitchell, J.B., K. McIntosh, S. Zvonic, et al., Immunophenotype of human adipose-derived cells: Temporal changes in stromal-associated and stem cell-associated markers. *Stem Cells*, 2006. 24(2): 376–85.

57. Lendeckel, S., A. Jodicke, P. Christophis, et al., Autologous stem cells (adipose) and fibrin glue used to treat widespread traumatic calvarial defects: case report. *J Craniomaxillofac Surg*, 2004. 32(6): 370–3.

58. Levi, B., A.W. James, E.R. Nelson, et al., Human adipose derived stromal cells heal critical size mouse calvarial defects. *PLoS One*, 2010. 5(6): e11177.

59. Monaco, E., M. Bionaz, S. Rodriguez-Zas, et al., Transcriptomics comparison between porcine adipose and bone marrow mesenchymal stem cells during in vitro osteogenic and adipogenic differentiation. *PLoS One*, 2012. 7(3): e32481.

60. Peng, L., Z. Jia, X. Yin, et al., Comparative analysis of mesenchymal stem cells from bone marrow, cartilage, and adipose tissue. *Stem Cells Dev*, 2008. 17(4): 761–73.

61. Ra, J.C., I.S. Shin, S.H. Kim, et al., Safety of intravenous infusion of human adipose tissue-derived mesenchymal stem cells in animals and humans. *Stem Cells Dev*, 2011. 20(8): 1297–308.

62. Fang, B., Y. Song, L. Liao, et al., Favorable response to human adipose tissue-derived mesenchymal stem cells in steroid-refractory acute graft-versus-host disease. *Transplant Proc*, 2007. 39(10): 3358–62.

63. Lee, S.W., P. Padmanabhan, P. Ray, et al., Stem cell-mediated accelerated bone healing observed with in vivo molecular and small animal imaging technologies in a model of skeletal injury. *J Orthop Res*, 2009. 27(3): 295–302.

64. Planat-Benard, V., J.S. Silvestre, B. Cousin, et al., Plasticity of human adipose lineage cells toward endothelial cells: Physiological and therapeutic perspectives. *Circulation*, 2004. 109(5): 656–63.

65. Jabbarzadeh, E., T. Starnes, Y.M. Khan, et al., Induction of angiogenesis in tissue-engineered scaffolds designed for bone repair: A combined gene therapy-cell transplantation approach. *Proc Natl Acad Sci U S A*, 2008. 105(32): 11099–104.

66. Ivanova-Todorova, E., I. Bochev, M. Mourdjeva, et al., Adipose tissue-derived mesenchymal stem cells are more potent suppressors of dendritic cells differentiation compared to bone marrow-derived mesenchymal stem cells. *Immunol Lett*, 2009. 126(1–2): 37–42.

67. Bochev, I., G. Elmadjian, D. Kyurkchiev, et al., Mesenchymal stem cells from human bone marrow or adipose tissue differently modulate mitogen-stimulated B-cell immunoglobulin production in vitro. *Cell Biol Int*, 2008. 32(4): 384–93.

68. Haghighat, A., A. Akhavan, B. Hashemi-Beni, et al., Adipose derived stem cells for treatment of mandibular bone defects: An autologous study in dogs. *Dent Res J (Isfahan)*, 2011. 8(Suppl 1): S51–7.

69. Kim, H.P., Y.H. Ji, S.C. Rhee, et al., Enhancement of bone regeneration using osteogenic-induced adipose-derived stem cells combined with demineralized bone matrix in a rat critically-sized calvarial defect model. *Curr Stem Cell Res Ther*, 2012. 7(3): 165–72.

70. Sándor, G.K., V.J. Tuovinen, J. Wolff, et al., Adipose stem cell tissue-engineered construct used to treat large anterior mandibular defect: A case report and review of the clinical application of good manufacturing practice-level adipose stem cells for bone regeneration. *J Oral Maxillofac Surg*, 2013. 71(5): 938–50.

71. Han, D.S., H.K. Chang, J.H. Park, et al., Consideration of bone regeneration effect of stem cells: Comparison between adipose-derived stem cells and demineralized bone matrix. *J Craniofac Surg*, 2014. 25(1): 189–95.

72. Liu, R., O. Birke, A. Morse, et al., Myogenic progenitors contribute to open but not closed fracture repair. *BMC Musculoskelet Disord*, 2011. 12: 288.

73. Yu, S., Q. Geng, F. Sun, et al., Osteogenic differentiation of C2C12 myogenic progenitor cells requires the Fos-related antigen Fra-1—A novel target of Runx2. *Biochem Biophys Res Commun*, 2013. 430(1): 173–8.

74. Shi, K., J. Lu, Y. Zhao, et al., MicroRNA-214 suppresses osteogenic differentiation of C2C12 myoblast cells by targeting Osterix. *Bone*, 2013. 55(2): 487–94.

75. Khayat, G.R., D.H. Rosenzweig, Z. Khavandgar, J. Li, et al., Low-frequency mechanical stimulation modulates osteogenic differentiation of C2C12 Cells. *ISRN Stem Cells*, 2013. 2013(2013): 9.

76. Nesti, L.J., W.M. Jackson, R.M. Shanti, et al., Differentiation potential of multipotent progenitor cells derived from war-traumatized muscle tissue. *J Bone Joint Surg Am*, 2008. 90(11): 2390–8.

77. Zheng, B., B. Cao, M. Crisan, et al., Prospective identification of myogenic endothelial cells in human skeletal muscle. *Nat Biotechnol*, 2007. 25(9): 1025–34.

78. Zheng, B., G. Li, W.C. Chen, et al., Human myogenic endothelial cells exhibit chondrogenic and osteogenic potentials at the clonal level. *J Orthop Res*, 2013. 31(7): 1089–95.

79. Payne, K.A., L.B. Meszaros, J.A. Phillippi, et al., Effect of phosphatidyl inositol 3-kinase, extracellular signal-regulated kinases 1/2, and p38 mitogen-activated protein kinase inhibition on osteogenic differentiation of muscle-derived stem cells. *Tissue Eng Part A*, 2010. 16(12): 3647–55.

80. Peng, H., V. Wright, A. Usas, et al., Synergistic enhancement of bone formation and healing by stem cell-expressed VEGF and bone morphogenetic protein-4. *J Clin Invest*, 2002. 110(6): 751–9.

81. Meszaros, L.B., A. Usas, G.M. Cooper, et al., Effect of host sex and sex hormones on muscle-derived stem cell-mediated bone formation and defect healing. *Tissue Eng Part A*, 2012. 18(17–18): 1751–9.

82. Li, H., N.R. Johnson, A. Usas, et al., Sustained release of bone morphogenetic protein 2 via coacervate improves the osteogenic potential of muscle-derived stem cells. *Stem Cells Transl Med*, 2013. 2(9): 667–77.

83. Kim, K.S., J.H. Lee, H.H. Ahn, et al., The osteogenic differentiation of rat muscle-derived stem cells in vivo within in situ-forming chitosan scaffolds. *Biomaterials*, 2008. 29(33): 4420–8.

84. Usas, A., A.M. Ho, G.M. Cooper, et al., Bone regeneration mediated by BMP4-expressing muscle-derived stem cells is affected by delivery system. *Tissue Eng Part A*, 2009. 15(2): 285–93.

85. Gao, X., A. Usas, Y. Tang, et al., A comparison of bone regeneration with human mesenchymal stem cells and muscle-derived stem cells and the critical role of BMP. *Biomaterials*, 2014. 35(25): 6859–70.

86. Lee, J.Y., D. Musgrave, D. Pelinkovic, et al., Effect of bone morphogenetic protein-2-expressing muscle-derived cells on healing of critical-sized bone defects in mice. *J Bone Joint Surg Am*, 2001. 83-a(7): 1032–9.

87. Zigdon-Giladi, H., T. Bick, D. Lewinson, et al., Mesenchymal stem cells and endothelial progenitor cells stimulate bone regeneration and mineral density. *J Periodontol*, 2014. 85(7): 984–90.

88. Seebach, C., D. Henrich, K. Wilhelm, et al., Endothelial progenitor cells improve directly and indirectly early vascularization of mesenchymal stem cell-driven bone regeneration in a critical bone defect in rats. *Cell Transplant*, 2012. 21(8): 1667–77.

Part IV

Clinical Considerations

10

Bone Graft and Bone Graft Alternatives in Spine Surgery: From Bench to Bedside

Joshua A. Parry and Michael J. Yaszemski

CONTENTS

10.1 Spine Fusion

Spine fusions are responsible for a majority of the bone grafting procedures performed in the United States.[1] In 2008, there were an estimated 400,000 spine fusions, representing a 2.4 fold increase over the previous decade.[2] For these reasons, the field of spine surgery is heavily vested in bone graft and bone graft alternatives.

Fusion of the spine can restores stability, reduce pain, and increase function for a number of common pathologies, including curve deformities, tumors, infections, traumatic injuries, and age-related degenerative changes like degenerative disc disease.[3–5] The success of spinal surgery, whether dealing with a large multi-segment defects or single-level fusions, depends heavily on successful union of bony elements. Implanted instrumentation, such as metal rods, screws, plates, and cages, can provide stability and load-bearing temporarily, but will ultimately fail over time if the spine does not fuse.[6] Failure to fuse can result in a fibrous union, referred to as a pseudoarthrosis, which can be unstable, painful, and disabling, requiring additional surgeries with increasing morbidity.[6–8]

Three major types of spine fusions exist—anterior, posterior, or a combined anterior and posterior fusion (circumferential fusion) (Figure 10.1).[9] The type of fusion performed varies considerably depending on the indication, pathology, and other situation specific factors. Fusion of the anterior spine, or vertebral bodies, benefits from a rich blood supply, wide-surface area, and compressive loading.[10] The posterior spine, consisting of the lamina, pedicles, spinous processes, transverse processes, and facet joints, has more difficulty fusing secondary to decreased vascularity, less surface area, and tensile loading.

For anterior spine fusions the intervertebral disc is removed and replaced with a structural bone graft or artificial fusion cage made of metal or plastic, which is then filled with cancellous bone graft, in a process referred to as interbody fusion.[11] This can be done from an anterior, posterior, transforaminal,

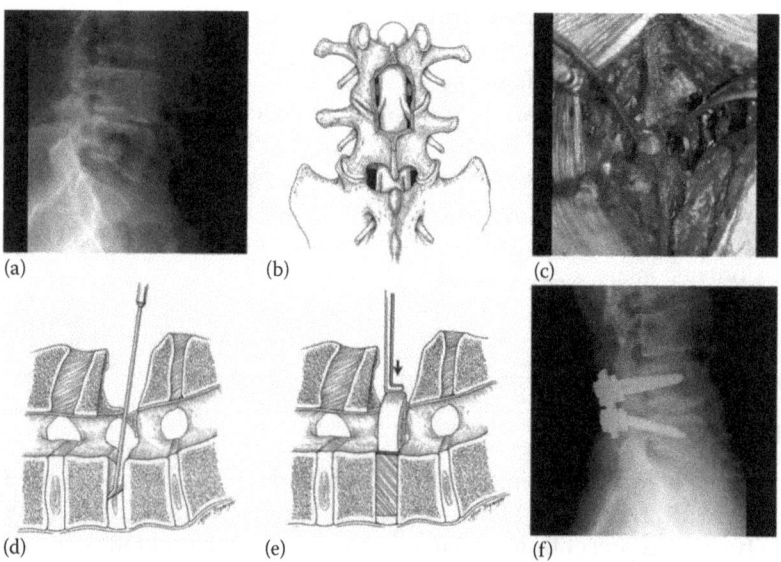

(a)   (b)   (c)

(d)   (e)   (f)

FIGURE 10.1

Posterior lumbar interbody fusion (PLIF). (a) Preoperative lateral radiograph of the lumbar spine demonstrating severe degenerative disk disease at L4-5 and significant loss of intervertebral disk height in a 56-year-old woman. (b) Posterior element resection during the exposure phase of PLIF. (c) Intraoperative photograph of the same patient as in panel (a) demonstrating wide resection. Medial retraction of the nerve roots allows visualization and resection of the L4-5 disk. (d) Disk resection can be done with a combination of curets, rongeurs, and shavers. (e) After preparing the end plates, the bone graft is inserted. (f) Postoperative radiograph of the same patient as in panel (a) demonstrating disk space reconstruction and neuroforaminal distraction. (Panels (b), (d), and (e) adapted with permission from Simmons J: Posterior lumbar interbody fusion, in Frymoyer JW [ed]: *The Adult Spine: Principles and Practice.* Philadelphia, PA: Lippincott Williams & Wilkins, 1991, pp 1961–1977.)

or transpsoas approach. For larger defects structural bone graft can be used as strut grafting or a longer fusion cage can be implanted.[9,10]

Posterior spine fusions can involve the lamina, facet joints, and the spinous and transverse processes. The area of bone to be fused must be decorticated to expose the stem cell-rich porous matrix and vascular supply below. Bone graft is directly applied to the decorticated area.[10]

Stability is necessary for successful fusion. To obtain a rigid construct the spine segments undergoing fusion are commonly fixed with instrumentation, like plates, rods, and screws, to provide stability to the construct until successful fusion, occurring on average of 6 to 12 months later.[10,12–14] However, fusion rates vary widely depending on surgical approach, location, instrumentation, graft source, and method of evaluation with rates ranging from 40 to 98%.[6,15,16]

The goal of the following chapter is to review the bone graft and bone graft alternatives currently available for spine fusion, including those technologies currently being investigated for future use.

10.2 Autograft

Bone autograft, or bone harvested and implanted into the same individual, is the gold standard adjunct for promoting spine fusion.[17] Bone graft can consist of cortical bone, cancellous bone, or a combination of the two. Cortical bone is the dense peripheral layer of bone that endows the skeleton with mechanical strength.[9,17] Cancellous bone is the highly porous, mechanically weak, inner layer of bone, rich in cells. Cortical bone acts as a structural graft, providing immediate stability; it takes years to slowly incorporate with host bone. Cancellous bone is a non-structural graft that acts as a porous scaffold, able to rapidly incorporate with host bone. Corticocancellous grafts consist of both bone types, available as a tri-cortical graft, a horseshoe shaped ring of cortical bone, or as cylindrical grafts.[9,10]

Iliac crest bone graft (ICBG) is an easily accessible source of cancellous or corticocancellous bone, and the single most common source of autograft in spine surgery, excluding the small amount of local bone graft taken from surgery site.[6] In a retrospective study of 5000 posterolateral lumbar fusions with ICBG, Dimar et al.[16] found a fusion rate of 87%, a rate supported by the literature.[15,18] ICBG is not without significant downsides, including donor site morbidities like chronic pain, wound complications, numbness, and limited function.[3,19–21] In the same study by Dimar et al.[16] 60% of patients still suffered from graft site pain two years postoperatively.

The Dimar et al.[16] retrospective study highlighted another major weakness of ICBG: its limited supply. On average they harvested only 36 cm^3 from each patient. For large defects or spine fusions a greater amount of bone graft is usually needed. Despite the issues with ICBG it is still heavily utilized. Recent studies have reevaluated the donor site morbidity associated with its harvest and found that the incidence of chronic pain is less than once thought, with rates as low as 14%.[17,22,23] However, donor site morbidities continue to be an issue leading spine surgeons to search elsewhere for equally efficacious sources of bone graft.

Local bone graft is the most obvious source of autograft; taken from the operative site at the time of surgery, it avoids further donor site complications. Like ICBG, its quantity is limited, especially in cases of infection and tumors.[24-26]

With advances in microsurgery techniques, vascularized bone grafts, including fibular and rib-strut grafts, are viable options for instances where non-vascularized autograft results in poor fusion rates, like multi-segment spinal reconstructions in areas of soft-tissue compromise.[27-29] Vascularized autografts are limited by the same factors as ICBG including limited availability, donor site morbidity, and increased operative times.

The ability of autograft to promote spine fusion stems from three properties—osteoinduction, osteogenesis, and osteoconduction.[17,30,31] Osteoinductive materials contain molecules or growth factors that recruit stem cells, promoting osteoblastic differentiation, and thus bone formation. Osteogenic materials contain osteoprogenitor cells that participate directly in new bone formation. Osteoconductive materials act as a scaffold for the ingrowth of new bone.[17,30,31] Due to the limitations of autograft, extensive research has been performed to develop an autograft alternative with similar osteogenic, osteoinductive, and osteoconductive capabilities.[17,31]

Bone graft alternatives are used in three major roles—as bone graft substitutes, extenders, or enhancers.[32] Bone graft substitutes completely replace bone graft, enhancers are added to a normal volume of bone graft to increase the fusion rate, and expanders are added to a smaller-than-usual volume of bone graft to increase the amount available.

Currently available bone graft alternatives used in spine surgery include osteoconductive allografts and ceramics, osteoinductive agents like bone morphogenetic protein (BMP) and demineralized bone matrix (DBM), and osteogenic bone marrow derivatives. To date none of these alternatives have been proven to be superior to autograft (Table 10.1).[30,32-34]

Future directions in bone graft alternatives include osteogenic techniques like the implantation of mesenchymal stem cells (MSCs) or gene therapy, both of which have had success in small animal spine fusion models, but their use in humans has not yet been investigated.[31,35]

Despite extensive research and development of bone graft alternatives, autograft remains the gold standard adjunct in spine fusions. The ideal graft would be cost-effective, readily available, and low risk, with the same osteoinductive, osteogenic, and osteoconductive properties of autograft. The formula for this ideal alternative in spinal fusion may ultimately be a combination of current technologies or future technologies not yet explored.

TABLE 10.1

Advantages/Disadvantages of Bone Graft and Bone Graft Alternatives

	Advantages	Disadvantages
Graft		
Iliac crest	Gold standard	Donor morbidity
Local autograft	Osteoinductive	Limited quantity
	Osteoconductive	
	Osteogenic	
Allograft		
Fresh-frozen	Large availability, low cost, growth factors	Disease transmission
Freeze-dried	Large availability, low cost	No growth factors
DBM	Large availability, low cost	Few growth factors
Ceramics	Structurally sound, no immunogenicity	Requires osteoinductive cells
β-TCP	Porosity; mineral structure like bone	Structurally weak
CHA	Structurally sound	Slow resorption
Silicate-substituted Calcium phosphate	Structurally sound	Cost
Calcium sulfate	Resorbable; biocompatible	Wound drainage
rhBMP-2/7	Growth factors	Cost
AGF	Growth factors	Cost; efficacy?
BMA	Live cells, growth factors, low cost	Osteoinductive only
Vitoss	Structurally sound, osteoinductive w/BMA	Cost; bovine antigenicity?
Healos	Structurally sound, osteoinductive w/BMA	Cost; bovine antigenicity?

10.3 Osteoconductive Materials

10.3.1 Allograft

Bone allograft refers to processed cadaveric bone that is used in a different individual. It is commonly used to facilitate spine fusion both as a graft extender, where it is mixed with autograft to increase the total amount of graft material available, or as a graft substitute.[17] Advantages of allograft include its unlimited availability and avoidance of donor site morbidity.[9,17,31]

Disadvantages of allograft are that processing removes the osteoinductive and osteogenic properties inherent to fresh autograft, making it primarily an osteoconductive scaffold in the clinical setting.[17] Processing is done by freezing or freeze-drying. Both techniques remove the donor's cells and thus any osteogenic capability.[36] Fresh-frozen grafts have the advantage of preserving osteoinductive molecules but also retain immunogenicity and the ability to transmit infectious disease like HIV and hepatitis. The risk of transmittable diseases is exceedingly rare with modern screening and testing, with nine documented cases of HIV ever being reported, all of which were implanted before modern HIV testing was available.[37] In contrast, freeze-drying (lyophilization) has a lower risk immunogenicity and infection, but also results in the removal of any osteoinductive properties.[36,38] For this reason fresh-frozen allografts result in higher fusion rates than freeze-dried allografts.[39,40]

Like autograft, the efficacy of allograft as a bone graft substitute or extender in spine fusion varies depending on the type of allograft, surgical procedure, age of patient, and location. For instance, posterior lumbar spine fusions using cancellous allograft have generally been shown to have inferior fusion rates compared to autograft.[17,31,40–43] An et al.[39] performed a prospective study on 20 patients undergoing posterolateral lumbar fusions, directly comparing cancellous autograft on one side of the spine to either cancellous fresh-frozen allograft, freeze-dried allograft, or a mixture of autograft and allograft on the opposite side. The autograft side reached solid fusion in 80% of cases, compared to 50% with the mixed autograft/allograft, and there were no solid fusions with allograft alone. This is in contrast to Bendo et al.,[44] who found that fresh-frozen femoral head structural allografts resulted in successful fusion in 95% of lumbar interbody fusions. Allograft has also been shown to have comparable fusion rates to autograft when used for cervical interbody fusions and posterior fusions in adolescent scoliosis.[45–47]

When used in the right setting, allograft, either as a bone graft extender or substitute, has comparable efficacy as autograft in spine fusions while avoiding the downsides of donor site morbidity and limited availability. Allograft is limited by the risk of transmittable diseases, slower incorporation times, immune-mediated resorption, and limited efficacy in certain situations.[36,38,48]

10.3.2 Ceramics (Synthetic Bone Graft)

Calcium sulfate, beta-tricalcium phosphate (β-TCP), and hydroxyapatite (HA) are commercially available calcium-based synthetics commonly used as bone graft extenders or substitutes. Ceramics are suitable osteoconductive scaffolds because they can be manufactured to have similar pore sizes, porosity, and compressive modulus as bone.[17,49]

Ceramics have the advantage of being absorbed over time, eventually being replaced by bone. β-TCP is resorbed over a period of months, while HA can take years.[49] A combination of β-TCP and HA is most commonly used in the clinical setting.[49,50] Calcium sulfate is resorbed in a matter of weeks.[49] This rate of degradation has been associated with inflammatory reactions that lead to wound problems, limiting its use in spine fusions.

Advantages of ceramic synthetic bone grafts include their biocompatibility, unlimited availability, and non-immunogenicity.[49] However, ceramics are brittle, requiring protection from load-bearing with instrumentation until fusion is complete.[50]

Like allograft, ceramics are purely osteoconductive, lacking osteogenic and osteoinductive properties. When ceramics are combined with local autograft or bone marrow aspirate fusion rates approach that of ICBG, while avoiding donor site complications.[32] In a prospective randomized study assessing single-level instrumented posterolateral lumbar fusions with either β-TCP and local bone graft or ICBG alone, fusion was observed in all cases.[51] The only difference in clinical outcomes consisted of donor site pain in the ICBG group. Epstein et al.[52] retrospectively reviewed 79 single-level instrumented lumbar fusions with β-TCP and local autograft and found a 94% fusion rate at six months. In another prospective study 28 patients undergoing posterior spinal fusions for adolescent idiopathic scoliosis were randomized to receive autograft mixed with allograft or autograft mixed with β -TCP.[53] No pseudoarthrosis was noted in either group. There were no significant differences in the density of the bone comprising the fusion mass between the two groups.

Synthetic bone grafts play a similar role as allograft in spine fusions, acting as an osteoconductive scaffold that can be combined with osteoinductive and osteogenic substrates to achieve similar fusion rates without the risk of infectious disease transmission, immune-mediated resorption, or delayed incorporation. However, few randomized prospective comparisons exist; whether the increased costs of synthetic bone graft outweigh its advantages over allograft remains unknown.[32]

10.3.3 Interbody Fusion Cages

Interbody cages were developed to prevent the collapse, subsidence, and expulsion of bone graft that is often seen with intervertebral spine fusions.[9,54] These three-dimensional cages, originally made of stainless steel, are placed in between two vertebral bodies to facilitate their fusion, while also maintaining the space's height and participating in load-bearing. Cages currently available for use consist of titanium, trabecular metal, carbon fiber, or polyetheretherketone (PEEK) (Figure 10.2). They can be filled with bone graft and bone graft substitute, as well as osteoinductive factors to increase the rate of fusion.[6,54]

The stiffness of metallic interbody cages are greater than vertebral bone, which result in stress-shielding at the fusion site that can interfere with bone formation.[55,56] Stainless steel and titanium have an elastic modulus of 200 GPa and 110 GPa respectively, greatly exceeding that of cortical bone, 2.4 GPa; this mismatch has prompted the development of cages with lower elastic moduli.[55]

Trabecular metal (TM) is a highly porous tantalum metal that is biocompatible, osteoconductive, and shares an elastic modulus similar to trabecular, or cancellous, bone.[57] Despite these theoretical advantages its use in interbody fusion has had mixed outcomes.[58–60] Kasliwal et al.[58] performed a prospective, randomized, multicenter study with 39 patients comparing anterior cervical decompression and fusion (ACDF) with either a TM cage filled with autograft,

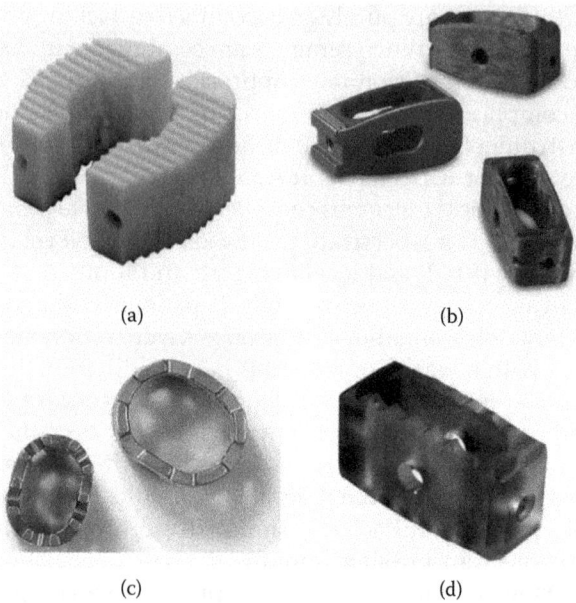

(a)   (b)

(c)   (d)

FIGURE 10.2
Interbody devices specifically designed for posterior lumbar interbody fusion. All are capable of accepting threaded instrumentation (note the hole in each implant), which allows precise seating. (a) Commercially manufactured allograft. (b) Carbon cages. (c) Titanium cages. (d) Bioabsorbable interbody spacer. (Reproduced with permission from Medtronic Sofamor Danek USA, Inc., Minneapolis, MN.)

a solid TM block, or a tricortical ICBG control. The study was stopped due to poor fusion rates in the two TM groups. The fusion rate at two years was 44% in the TM groups versus 100% in the autograft group. The inferior fusion rate of TM cages in ACDF may be improved with the added stability of anterior plate fixation. A prospective randomized study of 50 patients undergoing ACDF with allograft or porous tantalum with additional anterior plate and screw fixation found no difference in radiographic union, 86% versus 90% respectively, or clinical outcomes between the two groups.[60]

Radiopaque metal cages made from titanium or TM make the assessment of bony union difficult on both radiographs and computed tomography (CT). Radiolucent cages made of polymers like polyetheretherketone (PEEK) and carbon fiber make it much easier to monitor the progress of fusions; they also have an elastic modulus similar to bone, potentially reducing stress-shielding and increasing fusion rates.[54]

Several studies have reported success with carbon-fiber cages. In one prospective study, 40 patients undergoing ACDF were randomized to either carbonfiber cages filled with autograft or anterior plating with allograft.[61] The fusion rate was 100% in both groups at two years with no significant differences in complications or clinical outcomes. These results are supported by another randomized study of 42 cervical interbody fusions with either tricortical autograft or a carbon fiber cage.[62] The authors concluded that although fusion rates were similar, the carbon fiber cages were more expensive and associated with higher rates of pain. Few randomized comparative studies documenting the effectiveness of carbon-fiber cages currently exist.

Polyaryletherekeketone (PEEK) is a radiolucent non-resorbable polymer used in spine surgery for multiple different applications including interbody cages and spinal rods.[9,63] Its elastic modulus is 8.3 GPa, much closer to the 2.4 GPa of vertebral bone.[55,64] The use of PEEK has resulted in successful fusions in several studies and is commonly used in clinical practice. Cho et al.[65] performed a randomized control study of multilevel anterior cervical fusions in a 130 patients and found that PEEK cages had higher fusion rates (100% versus 87%) and fewer complications than tricortical ICBG. In a follow-up study, the same author compared PEEK cages filled with a biphasic calcium phosphate ceramic or ICBG, and found 100% fusion rate in both groups.[66]

Despite the advantages of radiolucent PEEK and carbon fiber over titanium and TM interbody cages, a recent systematic review of the literature failed to demonstrate any significant differences in the clinical or radiographic outcomes between the different cages and bone graft, with similar rates of fusion, subsidence, and migration in all groups.[54]

To improve the bioactivity and cell attachment of PEEK, which is biologically inert, surface coatings and composite mixtures have been investigated, including HA, titanium, gold, and carbon.[64,67–69] Difficulties exist with both approaches. Surface coatings become unstable over time. Composite mixtures increase the elastic modulus, making PEEK prone to fracture. Due to these issues, modified PEEK materials have not yet been applied in clinical applications.[64]

Bioabsorbable polymer interbody cages, like the non-absorbable polymer PEEK, are radiolucent and have a low elastic modulus.[70,71] The gradual resorption of polymer cages would theoretically result in a larger area for potential bone formation and decrease stress-shielding and migration over time. Instead, the reduced strength inherent to bioabsorable cages leads to high incidences of subsidence and fracture.[70] The breakdown of the polymer was also associated with aseptic inflammatory reactions, which is well documented with degradable polymers in other orthopedic applications.[71–73]

Jiya et al.[74] compared bioabsorbable poly-L-lactide-co-D,L-lactide (PLDLLA) to PEEK cages for posterior lumbar fusion in 26 patients. At two years the clinical parameters were significantly increased in all patients in the PEEK group while there were no significant improvements in the PLDLLA group. The fusion rate was 92% in the PEEK group compared to 50% in the PLDLLA group. The PLDLLA cages were associated with a higher rate of subsidence and osteolysis. The inferiority of PLDLLA cages seen in this study, including their association with complications like osteolysis and mechanical failure, has been well established.[71,75] Their use is not recommended.

Interbody cages are available in a wide variety of materials. Depending on the surgical indications, approach, type of material, and use of bone graft or bone graft substitute, these cages have clinical results and fusion rates similar to bone graft. Carbon fiber and PEEK cages have a theoretical advantage over traditional metal cages because they eliminate imaging artifacts and decrease stress shielding. These advantages have not yet been shown to result in superior clinical results. Bioabsorbable polymer cages are associated with a high rate of fracture, subsidence, and osteolysis; their use is currently not advised.

10.4 Osteoinductive Agents: Bone Morphogenetic Proteins

Bone morphogenetic proteins (BMP) are non-collagenous glycoproteins with osteoinductive abilities.[76] Osteoinductive agents are able to induce the differentiation of pluripotent mesenchymal cells into chondroblasts and osteoblasts—cells that participate in bone formation.[17] This protein was originally discovered in 1965 after the observation that demineralized bone matrix implanted into the muscle of rabbits resulted in ectopic bone formation.[76] There are a total of 20 BMPs that have been described. BMP-2 and BMP-7, also referred to as osteogenic protein-1 (OP-1), have the greatest osteoinductive effect of all the BMPs.[76] Subsequently, recombinant-human BMP-2 (rhBMP-2) and rhBMP-7 (rhOP-1) have been approved for use in spine fusions in the United States. Specifically, rhBMP-2 is approved for anterior interbody lumbar fusion in combination with threaded titanium cage, while rhBMP-7 has a humanitarian exemption for use in posterolateral lumbar fusions in refractory nonunions or in settings of multiple comorbidities where autograft is unavailable or unlikely to work.[9,17,76,77]

One of the early prospective clinical trials studying rhBMP-2 for use in anterior lumbar fusions compared 136 fusions with titanium cages filled with ICBG to 143 titanium cages filled with collagen sponges soaked in rhBMP-2. The fusion rates at two years were similar between groups, 89% with ICBG and 95% with rhBMP-2, with no significant difference in clinical outcomes.[78] Subsequent trials have failed to demonstrate a clear benefit of rhBMP-2 over bone graft.[77,79,80] In one prospective trial of 51 anterior lumbar fusions PEEK interbody cages were divided into two compartments: one compartment contained ICBG and the other contained a rhBMP-2 collagen matrix.[79] They found significantly higher fusion rates on the side with ICBG (89%) versus the side with rhBMP-2 (71%). These results are consistent with a systematic review of 13 randomized control trials and 31 cohort studies by Fu et al.,[33] who compared rhBMP-2 to ICBG for spine fusions. They found no difference in fusions, clinical outcome measures, or complication rates. They did find that rhBMP-2 was associated with an increased risk of retrograde ejaculation, urogenital complications, wound complications, dysphagia, and cancer.

In 2002, when rhBMP-2 was approved for clinical use, it was used in 0.7% of all spine fusions; this rate increased quickly to 25% in 2006.[81] Its off-label use increased as well, with estimates of up to 85% of its total use.[76] As the use of rhBMP-2 became more widespread, especially its off-label use, complications became more apparent, ranging from 20% to 70%.[77] Reported complications ranged from uncontrolled bone formation, osteoclast resorption, local reactions, nerve reactions, and carcinogenicity. In 2006, the Federal Drug Administration (FDA) released a warning that use of rhBMP-2 in the anterior cervical spine could result in life-threatening swelling and severe dysphagia.[33,77] In a systematic review of early industry-sponsored study data, Caragee et al.[77] concluded that true risk of complications from rhBMP-2 was 10 to 50 times that originally reported.

The monetary cost of rhBMP-2 was investigated by Dagostino et al.[82] through a large population study. They examined thoracolumbar and lumbar fusions performed between 2002, when rh-BMP-2 first came on the market, to 2008, when it was used in over 25% of spine fusions. No net change in autograft use was seen during this time. They found that rhBMP-2 significantly increased hospital charges by more than $13,000, resulting in over $900 million hospital charges in that time period.

In 2004, rh-BMP-7 (rhOP-1) was approved by the FDA for humanitarian exemption, which limited its use to fewer than 4000 people per year; as a result its use has been studied to a lesser extent than rhBMP-2.[83–85] A small study of 18 patients undergoing posterolateral lumbar fusion with either rhOP-1 putty or ICBG found no significant differences in radiographic fusion, clinical measures, or complications between the two treatments.[84] In 2009 the FDA voted against the approval of rhOP-1 due to concerns of complications seen with rhBMP-2 and its lack of clinical benefit over bone graft.[86] Its use remains limited under a humanitarian exemption.

BMPs are osteoinductive glycoproteins whose ability to stimulate bone formation is well documented. Early industry-sponsored studies supported the use of rhBMP-2 as a low-risk potent bone graft alternative in spine fusion. Mounting evidence has failed to show a clear benefit of rhBMP-2 over bone graft; its use is also associated with concerning adverse side effects and substantial costs.

10.5 Demineralized Bone Matrix

Demineralized bone matrix (DBM) consists of decalcified cadaveric bone that retains non-collagenous proteins, collagen, and osteoinductive like BMPs.[30] Many formulations exist for use in spine fusions, including gels, sheets, and puttys. DBM is used as a bone graft enhancer or expander. The concentrations of osteoinductive growth factors found in different DBM products are limited and range widely, depending upon the individual donors and particular product.[87] Concentrations of BMP-2 and BMP-7 in DBM range from 20 to 200 ng/g, a million times less than doses of rhBMP-2 used for lumbar fusions.[49]

In a randomized control trial of 28 patients undergoing single-level instrumented posterior lumbar fusion with either DBM and local bone graft (LBG) or ICBG alone, no significant difference in fusion rate or clinical outcomes was demonstrated at two years. The fusion rate was 86% in the DBM and LBG group compared to 92% in the ICBG group.[88]

Cammisa et al.[89] performed another randomized prospective study with 120 patients receiving instrumented posterolateral lumbar fusions with DBM and ICBG in a 2:1 ratio on one side of the spine versus ICBG alone on the other side. Both sides had the same volume of graft material placed. At two years the fusion rates were 52% on the DBM:ICBG side and 54% on the side with only ICBG. They concluded that DBM can be used successfully as a bone graft extender. No adverse events were associated with the use DBM.

Only four randomized control trials currently exist comparing DBM and ICBG. In a systematic review of DBM's use as a bone graft extender or enhancer, fusion rates were determined to be similar to bone graft alone.[90] No evidence exists for the use of DBM alone as a stand-alone bone graft substitute.

10.6 Autologous Platelet Concentrate

Platelets contain osteoinductive growth factors such as platelet-derived growth factor (PDGF), tumor growth factor-beta (TGF-B), and vascular endothelial growth factor (VEGF), factors known for their role in stimulating fracture healing.[91] Autologous platelet concentrate (APC), also commonly known as platelet-rich plasma (PRP), is used in a wide range of orthopedic applications for its theoretical ability to stimulate healing.[92] APC is obtained from a preoperative blood draw before the surgery; this has the disadvantage of increased time and medical costs, but has the benefit of providing a source of non-immunogenic osteoinductive growth factors. The blood undergoes centrifugation to obtain concentrated level of platelets two to five times that of whole blood.[93] APC is usually applied via thrombin gel or in combination with bone graft or bone graft substitute.

Autologous growth factor concentrate (AGF) (Interpore Cross, Irvine, CA) is the proprietary name of a method that uses ultrafiltration to reach a super-concentrated level of platelets, eight to ten times that of whole blood.[94]

The evidence for APC in spine surgery is controversial. It use has been associated with both increased and decreased fusion rates.[7,94,95] Jenis et al.[94] performed a prospective study comparing lumbar interbody fusions of 57 levels using either AGF and allograft versus ICBG alone. At two years the fusion rate was 89% in the AGF group and 85% in the autograft group. They found no significant differences in fusion rates or measured clinical outcomes between the two groups. In contrast, a retrospective study of 76 patients receiving instrumented posterolateral lumbar fusions with both ICBG and AGF versus ICBG alone found that at two years the AGF group had a nonunion rate of 25%, an increase from 17% in the control group.[96] The authors concluded that AGF added expense while not affecting fusion rates, recommending against its use. Acebal-Cortina et al.[95] performed a prospective study on 117 patients who received posterolateral lumbar fusions with a combination of β-TCP/HA, AGF, and local bone graft versus the same combination without AGF. Pseudoarthrosis developed in 25% of patients in the AGF group versus 7.5% in the control group, which was determined to be significantly different. Nine patients in the AGF group required reoperation versus two patients in the control group.

One reason attributed to the failure of AGF and other APCs in clinical studies is the potential instability of its delivery.[96] AGF is most commonly delivered in a fibrin clot that is subject to rapid degradation, which may lead to a sudden release of all the growth factors. Other issues include variability in growth factor concentrations from donor to donor, variability in platelet concentration techniques, and the presence of factors in AGF that may actually inhibit bone formation.[94]

10.7 Osteogenic Agents: Mesenchymal Stem Cells

Pluripotent mesenchymal stem cells have the ability to differentiate into osteoprogenitor (OPs) cells, ultimately becoming osteoblasts and directly participating in bone formation.[97] Bone marrow is the largest and most accessible source of OPs in the body. Spine surgeons commonly use bone marrow aspirate (BMA) as a way to deliver osteogenic cells and osteoinductive factors to fusion sites.[98,99] The addition of bone marrow aspirate to osteoconductive grafts like allograft and ceramics has been shown to result in similar fusion rates as ICBG.[100–102] Bone marrow can be extracted from the iliac crest or locally at the operative site; its aspiration has a lower risk of pain and adverse events compared to ICBG harvesting.[98,103]

In a study of 30 patients receiving instrumented posterolateral lumbar fusions with BMA and HA/B-TCP porous scaffolds on one side of the spine and ICBG alone on the other side, all levels fused successfully except for one on the autograft side, showing that BMA could enhance the fusion rates of purely osteoconductive scaffolds.[100]

Taghavi et al.[104] retrospectively reviewed 62 patients (125 levels) after posterolateral lumbar fusions with either a rhBMP-2 collagen matrix, BMA with allograft, or ICBG. They found that all three groups achieved 100% union for single-level fusions. However, when they compared multilevel fusions, BMA with allograft resulted in an inferior fusion rate of 63% compared to 100% in the BMP-2 and ICBG group.

The efficacy of BMA as a bone graft enhancer is still being investigated. In a systematic review of BMA's use in spine fusions there was insufficient evidence to make any conclusion about the efficacy of BMA.[105]

BMA's ability to promote spine fusion may be limited by the amount of OPs and osteoinductive agents present in the bone marrow, which has been shown to vary significantly from person to person.[99] OPs make up a very small proportion of cells found in BMA, anywhere from 0.001 to 0.01%; therefore, increasing the concentration of OPs delivered to the fusion site may increase its efficacy.

Bone marrow aspirate concentrate (BMAC) is one method used to increase the number of OPs delivered to the fusion site. Perioperative centrifugation can increase the number of OPs by three to four times.[97,106] The success of BMAC to promote fusion has been linked directly to the concentration of cells. Hernigue et al.[107] injected BMAC into tibial nonunions and found that the only nonunions that persisted were injected with BMAC with concentrations of OPs less than 1500 cells/cm^3. In a prospective randomized study of BMAC's use in spine fusions, 25 patients underwent posterolateral lumbar fusions with BMAC combined with allograft on one side and ICBG alone on the other side.[106] The measured concentration of OPs in the BMAC used was three to four times that of BMA. They demonstrated a positive trend between the number of OPs and radiographic fusion, but this did not reach significance. No difference in fusion rates was seen between the two sides.

Ex vivo culture expansion of MSCs is one technique described to increase the number of OPs. The injection of MSCs after undergoing expanded ex-vivo culture was shown to result in fusion rates superior to autograft in a lumbar fusion sheep model.[108] However, ex vivo expansion of human MSCs faces difficult hurdles before it can be used in clinical applications, including high costs, culture times, sterility management, and regulatory issues. No human studies have been attempted at this time.

The ability of BMA to enhance fusion rates is thought to be tied to its concentration of OPs. There is clinical evidence to support its use as a bone graft enhancer in spine fusions, however the evidence is currently insufficient. Early studies evaluating BMAC in spine fusions are promising and may offer superior results secondary to the increased concentration of osteogenic cells. Investigations into the delivery of high concentrations of OPs via ex vivo expanded MSCs have demonstrated potential in animal models, but this has not yet been applied clinically.

10.8 Gene Therapy

Gene therapy describes a process where a gene encoding a certain protein is inserted into the DNA sequence of a target cell via a vector, giving that cell the ability to produce the protein.[109] Vectors can be derived from viruses or non-viral sources, like liposomes and plasmids. This process was first successful in 1990 when a girl, suffering from a rare immunodeficiency disorder, had her white blood cells transfected with a gene encoding the enzyme she lacked, temporarily restoring her immunity.[110]

In the context of spine fusion, gene therapy may provide a stable and lasting source of osteoinductive factors by implanting cells with genes encoding bone-promoting proteins like BMP-2.[111] By delivering stable concentrations of osteoinductive molecules at the area of interest over a longer period of time, gene therapy could offer increased efficacy compared to the local delivery of short-lived factors currently utilized today.

Small animal studies have demonstrated the potential of this gene therapy technology. In a rat spine fusion model, bone marrow cells transfected with a viral vector encoding BMP-2 resulted in superior fusion rates compared to bone marrow cells alone.[112] In another rat model adipose derived stem cells (ASCs) transfected with a rhBMP-6-encoding plasmid were injected into spinal defects, resulting in twice the bone formation of a fibrin-glue control.[113]

Gene therapy has theoretical potential in spine surgery for the delivery of osteoinductive agents to stimulate bone formation, but at this time no human studies have been attempted. The clinical use of gene therapy faces considerable obstacles; its issues include short-lived effects, host-immune responses, and unpredictable vectors that can be toxic, infective, and even mutagenic if inserted into the wrong sequence of DNA.[109]

10.9 Conclusion

Currently there is not an ideal substitute for autograft, the gold standard adjunct in spine fusion procedures. A diverse group of bone graft alternatives exist, but none have been able to reproduce the osteogenic, osteoinductive, and osteoconductive capabilities of autograft. Composite grafts, combining osteoconductive bone graft substitutes with osteoinductive and osteogenic agents, show promise in many clinical studies. Current bone graft alternatives avoid the donor site morbidity and limited availability of autograft but are limited by efficacy, cost, and safety issues. Future research may ultimately identify a combination of current technologies or future technologies that result in excellent fusion rates and clinical outcomes.

References

1. Boden SD. Overview of the biology of lumbar spine fusion and principles for selecting a bone graft substitute. *Spine (Phila PA 1976)*. 2002;27(16 Suppl 1):S26–31.
2. Rajaee SS, Bae HW, Kanim LEA, Delamarter RB. Spinal fusion in the United States: Analysis of trends from 1998 to 2008. *Spine (Phila PA 1976)*. 2012;37(1):67–76.

3. Cheng LM, Wang JJ, Zeng ZL, et al. Pedicle screw fixation for traumatic fractures of the thoracic and lumbar spine. *Cochrane Database Syst Rev.* 2013;31(5):6–9.

4. Franzin FJ, Gotfryd AO, Neto NJC, et al. Radiographic and functional evaluation of the iliac bone graft in the treatment of adolescent idiopathic scoliosis. *J Pediatr Orthop B.* 2014;23(4):307–311.

5. Jacobs W, Willems PC, Kruyt M, et al. Systematic review of anterior interbody fusion techniques for single- and double-level cervical degenerative disc disease. *Spine (Phila PA 1976).* 2011;36(14):E950–960.

6. Raizman NM, O'Brien JR, Poehling-Monaghan KL, Yu WD. Pseudarthrosis of the spine. *Journal of the American Academy of Orthopaedic Surgeons.* August 1, 2009 2009;17(8):494–503.

7. Carreon L, Glassman SD, Campbell MJ. Treatment of anterior cervical pseudoarthrosis: Posterior fusion versus anterior revision. *Spine J.* 2006;6(2):154–156.

8. Martin BI, Mirza SK, Comstock BA, Gray DT, Kreuter W, Deyo RA. Reoperation rates following lumbar spine surgery and the influence of spinal fusion procedures. *Spine (Phila PA 1976).* 2007;32(3):382–387.

9. Lebow R, Tom Yao, Charles B. Stevenson, Joseph S. Cheng. Bone graft options, bone graft substitutes, and bone harvest techniques. In: Winn HR, ed. *Youmans Neurological Surgery, Sixth Edition.* Philadelphia, PA: Elsevier; 2011; pp. 2992–2998.

10. Devlin V. *Spine Secrets Plus.* St. Louis, MO: Elsevier/Mosby; 2012.

11. Enker P, Steffee AD. Interbody fusion and instrumentation. *Clin Orthop Relat Res.* 1994(300):90–101.

12. Kornblum MB, Fischgrund JS, Herkowitz HN, Abraham DA, Berkower DL, Ditkoff JS. Degenerative lumbar spondylolisthesis with spinal stenosis: A prospective long-term study comparing fusion and pseudarthrosis. *Spine (Phila PA 1976).* 2004;29(7):726–733; discussion 733–724.

13. Fraser JF, Härtl R. Anterior approaches to fusion of the cervical spine: A meta-analysis of fusion rates. *J Neurosurg Spine.* 2007;6(4):298–303.

14. Fischgrund JS, Mackay M, Herkowitz HN, Brower R, Montgomery DM, Kurz LT. 1997 Volvo Award winner in clinical studies. Degenerative lumbar spondylolisthesis with spinal stenosis: A prospective, randomized study comparing decompressive laminectomy and arthrodesis with and without spinal instrumentation. *Spine (Phila PA 1976).* 1997;22(24):2807–2812.

15. Bono CM, Lee CK. Critical analysis of trends in fusion for degenerative disc disease over the past 20 years: Influence of technique on fusion rate and clinical outcome. *Spine (Phila PA 1976).* 2004;29(4):455–463; discussion Z455.

16. Dimar JR, Glassman SD, Burkus JK, Pryor PW, Hardacker JW, Carreon LY. Two-year fusion and clinical outcomes in 224 patients treated with a single-level instrumented posterolateral fusion with iliac crest bone graft. *Spine J.* 2009;9(11):880–885.

17. Grabowski G, Cornett CA. Bone graft and bone graft substitutes in spine surgery: Current concepts and controversies. *J Am Acad Orthop Surg.* 2013;21(1):51–60.

18. Suratwala SJ, Pinto MR, Gilbert TJ, Winter RB, Wroblewski JM. Functional and radiological outcomes of 360 degrees fusion of three or more motion levels in the lumbar spine for degenerative disc disease. *Spine (Phila PA 1976).* 2009;34(10):E351–358.

19. Kim DH, Rhim R, Li L, et al. Prospective study of iliac crest bone graft harvest site pain and morbidity. *Spine J.* 2009;9(11):886–892.

20. Sasso RC, LeHuec JC, Shaffrey C, Group SIR. Iliac crest bone graft donor site pain after anterior lumbar interbody fusion: A prospective patient satisfaction outcome assessment. *J Spinal Disord Tech.* 2005;18 Suppl:S77–81.
21. Schwartz CE, Martha JF, Kowalski P, et al. Prospective evaluation of chronic pain associated with posterior autologous iliac crest bone graft harvest and its effect on postoperative outcome. *Health Qual Life Outcomes.* 2009;7:49.
22. Delawi D, Dhert WJA, Castelein RM, Verbout AJ, Oner FC. The incidence of donor site pain after bone graft harvesting from the posterior iliac crest may be overestimated: A study on spine fracture patients. *Spine (Phila PA 1976).* 2007;32(17):1865–1868.
23. Howard JM, Glassman SD, Carreon LY. Posterior iliac crest pain after posterolateral fusion with or without iliac crest graft harvest. *Spine J.* 2011;11(6):534–537.
24. Ohtori S, Suzuki M, Koshi T, et al. Single-level instrumented posterolateral fusion of the lumbar spine with a local bone graft versus an iliac crest bone graft: A prospective, randomized study with a 2-year follow-up. *Eur Spine J.* 2011;20(4):635–639.
25. Sengupta DK, Truumees E, Patel CK, et al. Outcome of local bone versus autogenous iliac crest bone graft in the instrumented posterolateral fusion of the lumbar spine. *Spine (Phila PA 1976).* 2006;31(9):985–991.
26. Witoon N, Tangviriyapaiboon T. Clinical and radiological outcomes of segmental spinal fusion in transforaminal lumbar interbody fusion with spinous process tricortical autograft. *Asian Spine J.* 2014;8(2):170–176.
27. Ackerman DB, Rose PS, Moran SL, Dekutoski MB, Bishop AT, Shin AY. The results of vascularized-free fibular grafts in complex spinal reconstruction. *J Spinal Disord Tech.* 2011;24(3):170–176.
28. Shin AY, Dekutoski MB. The role of vascularized bone grafts in spine surgery. *Orthop Clin North Am.* 2007;38(1):61–72, vi.
29. Wilden JA, Moran SL, Dekutoski MB, Bishop AT, Shin AY. Results of vascularized rib grafts in complex spinal reconstruction. *J Bone Joint Surg Am.* 2006;88(4):832–839.
30. Aghdasi B, Montgomery SR, Daubs MD, Wang JC. A review of demineralized bone matrices for spinal fusion: The evidence for efficacy. *Surgeon.* 2013;11(1):39–48.
31. Wang S, Yaszemski MJ, Knight AM, Gruetzmacher JA, Windebank AJ, Lu L. Photo-crosslinked poly(epsilon-caprolactone fumarate) networks for guided peripheral nerve regeneration: Material properties and preliminary biological evaluations. *Acta Biomater.* 2009;5(5):1531–1542.
32. Alsaleh KAM, Tougas CA, Roffey DM, Wai EK. Osteoconductive bone graft extenders in posterolateral thoracolumbar spinal fusion: A systematic review. *Spine (Phila PA 1976).* 2012;37(16):E993–1000.
33. Fu R, Selph S, McDonagh M, et al. Effectiveness and harms of recombinant human bone morphogenetic protein-2 in spine fusion: A systematic review and meta-analysis. *Ann Intern Med.* 2013;158(12):890–902.
34. Simmonds MC, Brown JVE, Heirs MK, et al. Safety and effectiveness of recombinant human bone morphogenetic protein-2 for spinal fusion: A meta-analysis of individual-participant data. *Ann Intern Med.* 2013;158(12):877–889.
35. Werner BC, Li X, Shen FH. Stem cells in preclinical spine studies. *Spine J.* 2014;14(3):542–551.

36. Mroz TE, Joyce MJ, Lieberman IH, Steinmetz MP, Benzel EC, Wang JC. The use of allograft bone in spine surgery: Is it safe? *Spine J.* 2009;9(4):303–308.
37. Hinsenkamp M, Muylle L, Eastlund T, Fehily D, Noël L, Strong DM. Adverse reactions and events related to musculoskeletal allografts: Reviewed by the World Health Organisation Project NOTIFY. *Int Orthop.* 2012;36(3):633–641.
38. Ehrler DM, Vaccaro AR. The use of allograft bone in lumbar spine surgery. *Clin Orthop Relat Res.* 2000(371):38–45.
39. An HS, Lynch K, Toth J. Prospective comparison of autograft vs. allograft for adult posterolateral lumbar spine fusion: Differences among freeze-dried, frozen, and mixed grafts. *J Spinal Disord.* 1995;8(2):131–135.
40. Buttermann GR, Glazer PA, Bradford DS. The use of bone allografts in the spine. *Clin Orthop Relat Res.* 1996(324):75–85.
41. Jorgenson SS, Lowe TG, France J, Sabin J. A prospective analysis of autograft versus allograft in posterolateral lumbar fusion in the same patient. A minimum of 1-year follow-up in 144 patients. *Spine (Phila PA 1976).* 1994;19(18):2048–2053.
42. Miyazaki M, Tsumura H, Wang JC, Alanay A. An update on bone substitutes for spinal fusion. *Eur Spine J.* 2009;18(6):783–799.
43. Urrutia J, Molina M. Fresh-frozen femoral head allograft as lumbar interbody graft material allows high fusion rate without subsidence. *Orthop Traumatol Surg Res.* 2013;99(4):413–418.
44. Bendo JA, Spivak JM, Neuwirth MG, Chung P. Use of the anterior interbody fresh-frozen femoral head allograft in circumferential lumbar fusions. *J Spinal Disord.* 2000;13(2):144–149.
45. Lansford TJ, Burton DC, Asher MA, Lai S-M. Radiographic and patient-based outcome analysis of different bone-grafting techniques in the surgical treatment of idiopathic scoliosis with a minimum 4-year follow-up: Allograft versus autograft/allograft combination. *Spine J.* 2013;13(5):523–529.
46. Miller LE, Block JE. Safety and effectiveness of bone allografts in anterior cervical discectomy and fusion surgery. *Spine (Phila PA 1976).* 2011;36(24):2045–2050.
47. Samartzis D, Shen FH, Matthews DK, Yoon ST, Goldberg EJ, An HS. Comparison of allograft to autograft in multilevel anterior cervical discectomy and fusion with rigid plate fixation. *Spine J.* 2003;3(6):451–459.
48. Epstein NE. Iliac crest autograft versus alternative constructs for anterior cervical spine surgery: Pros, cons, and costs. *Surg Neurol Int.* 2012;3(Suppl 3):S143–156.
49. Rihn JA, Kirkpatrick K, Albert TJ. Graft options in posterolateral and posterior interbody lumbar fusion. *Spine (Phila PA 1976).* 2010;35(17):1629–1639.
50. Park JJ, Hershman SH, Kim YH. Updates in the use of bone grafts in the lumbar spine. *Bull Hosp Jt Dis (2013).* 2013;71(1):39–48.
51. Dai L-Y, Jiang L-S. Single-level instrumented posterolateral fusion of lumbar spine with beta-tricalcium phosphate versus autograft: A prospective, randomized study with 3-year follow-up. *Spine (Phila PA 1976).* 2008;33(12):1299–1304.
52. Epstein NE. Beta tricalcium phosphate: Observation of use in 100 posterolateral lumbar instrumented fusions. *Spine J.* 2009;9(8):630–638.
53. Muschik M, Ludwig R, Halbhübner S, Bursche K, Stoll T. Beta-tricalcium phosphate as a bone substitute for dorsal spinal fusion in adolescent idiopathic scoliosis: Preliminary results of a prospective clinical study. *Eur Spine J.* 2001;10 Suppl 2:S178–184.
54. Kersten RFMR, van Gaalen SM, de Gast A, Oner FC. Polyetheretherketone (PEEK) cages in cervical applications: A systematic review. *Spine J.* 2013;1;15(6):1446–1460.

55. Smit TH, Müller R, van Dijk M, Wuisman PIJM. Changes in bone architecture during spinal fusion: three years follow-up and the role of cage stiffness. *Spine (Phila PA 1976)*. 2003;28(16):1802–1808; discussion 1809.
56. van Dijk M, Smit TH, Sugihara S, Burger EH, Wuisman PI. The effect of cage stiffness on the rate of lumbar interbody fusion: An in vivo model using poly (l-lactic acid) and titanium cages. *Spine (Phila PA 1976)*. 2002;27(7):682–688.
57. Levine BR, Sporer S, Poggie RA, Della Valle CJ, Jacobs JJ. Experimental and clinical performance of porous tantalum in orthopedic surgery. *Biomaterials*. 2006;27(27):4671–4681.
58. Kasliwal MK, Baskin DS, Traynelis VC. Failure of porous tantalum cervical interbody fusion devices: Two-year results from a prospective, randomized, multicenter clinical study. *J Spinal Disord Tech*. 2013;26(5):239–245.
59. Löfgren H, Engquist M, Hoffmann P, Sigstedt B, Vavruch L. Clinical and radiological evaluation of Trabecular Metal and the Smith-Robinson technique in anterior cervical fusion for degenerative disease: A prospective, randomized, controlled study with 2-year follow-up. *Eur Spine J*. 2010;19(3):464–473.
60. Schoettle T, Standard S, Lanford G, Abram S, Robertson D, Robie BH. Successful use of a modern porous tantalum (Trabecular Metal) device for cervical interbody fusion: Results from a prospective, randomized multi-center clinical study: Poster #11. *Spine Journal Meeting Abstracts*. 2005(7):178–179.
61. Ryu SI, Mitchell M, Kim DH. A prospective randomized study comparing a cervical carbon fiber cage to the Smith-Robinson technique with allograft and plating: Up to 24 months follow-up. *Eur Spine J*. 2006;15(2):157–164.
62. Siddiqui AA, Jackowski A. Cage versus tricortical graft for cervical interbody fusion. A prospective randomised study. *J Bone Joint Surg Br*. 2003;85(7):1019–1025.
63. Kurtz SM, Devine JN. PEEK biomaterials in trauma, orthopedic, and spinal implants. *Biomaterials*. 2007;28(32):4845–4869.
64. Ma R, Tang T. Current strategies to improve the bioactivity of PEEK. *Int J Mol Sci*. 2014;15(4):5426–5445.
65. Cho D-Y, Lee W-Y, Sheu P-C. Treatment of multilevel cervical fusion with cages. *Surg Neurol*. 2004;62(5):378–385, discussion 385–376.
66. Cho D-Y, Lee W-Y, Sheu P-C, Chen C-C. Cage containing a biphasic calcium phosphate ceramic (Triosite) for the treatment of cervical spondylosis. *Surg Neurol*. 2005;63(6):497–503; discussion 503–494.
67. Briem D, Strametz S, Schröder K, et al. Response of primary fibroblasts and osteoblasts to plasma treated polyetheretherketone (PEEK) surfaces. *J Mater Sci Mater Med*. 2005;16(7):671–677.
68. Barkarmo S, Wennerberg A, Hoffman M, et al. Nano-hydroxyapatite-coated PEEK implants: A pilot study in rabbit bone. *J Biomed Mater Res A*. 2013;101(2):465–471.
69. Yao C, Storey D, Webster TJ. Nanostructured metal coatings on polymers increase osteoblast attachment. *Int J Nanomedicine*. 2007;2(3):487–492.
70. Madigan L, Vaccaro AR, Lim MR, Lee JY. Bioabsorbable interbody spacers. *J Am Acad Orthop Surg*. 2007;15(5):274–280.
71. Smith AJ, Arginteanu M, Moore F, Steinberger A, Camins M. Increased incidence of cage migration and nonunion in instrumented transforaminal lumbar interbody fusion with bioabsorbable cages. *J Neurosurg Spine*. 2010;13(3):388–393.

72. Böstman OM. Intense granulomatous inflammatory lesions associated with absorbable internal fixation devices made of polyglycolide in ankle fractures. *Clin Orthop Relat Res.* 1992(278):193–199.

73. Apostolopoulos A, Nikolopoulos D, Polyzois I, Liarokapis S, Rossas C, Michos I. Pretibial cyst formation after anterior cruciate ligament reconstruction with poly-L acid screw fixation: A case report presentation and review of the literature. *J Surg Orthop Adv.* 2012;21(3):151–156.

74. Jiya TU, Smit T, van Royen BJ, Mullender M. Posterior lumbar interbody fusion using non-resorbable poly-ether-ether-ketone versus resorbable poly-L-lactide-co-D,L-lactide fusion devices. Clinical outcome at a minimum of 2-year follow-up. *Eur Spine J.* 2011;20(4):618–622.

75. Frost A, Bagouri E, Brown M, Jasani V. Osteolysis following resorbable poly-L-lactide-co-D, L-lactide PLIF cage use: A review of cases. *Eur Spine J.* 2012;21(3):449–454.

76. Even J, Eskander M, Kang J. Bone morphogenetic protein in spine surgery: Current and future uses. *J Am Acad Orthop Surg.* 2012;20(9):547–552.

77. Carragee EJ, Hurwitz EL, Weiner BK. A critical review of recombinant human bone morphogenetic protein-2 trials in spinal surgery: Emerging safety concerns and lessons learned. *Spine J.* 2011;11(6):471–491.

78. Burkus JK, Gornet MF, Dickman CA, Zdeblick TA. Anterior lumbar interbody fusion using rhBMP-2 with tapered interbody cages. *J Spinal Disord Tech.* 2002;15(5):337–349.

79. Flouzat-Lachaniette C-H, Ghazanfari A, Bouthors C, Poignard A, Hernigou P, Allain J. Bone union rate with recombinant human bone morphogenic protein-2 versus autologous iliac bone in PEEK cages for anterior lumbar interbody fusion. *Int Orthop.* 2014;38(9):2001–2007.

80. Haid RW, Branch CL, Alexander JT, Burkus JK. Posterior lumbar interbody fusion using recombinant human bone morphogenetic protein type 2 with cylindrical interbody cages. *Spine J.* 2004;4(5):527–538; discussion 538–529.

81. Cahill KS, Chi JH, Day A, Claus EB. Prevalence, complications, and hospital charges associated with use of bone-morphogenetic proteins in spinal fusion procedures. *JAMA.* 2009;302(1):58–66.

82. Dagostino PR, Whitmore RG, Smith GA, Maltenfort MG, Ratliff JK. Impact of bone morphogenetic proteins on frequency of revision surgery, use of autograft bone, and total hospital charges in surgery for lumbar degenerative disease: Review of the Nationwide Inpatient Sample from 2002 to 2008. *Spine J.* 2014;14(1):20–30.

83. Delawi D, Dhert WJA, Rillardon L, et al. A prospective, randomized, controlled, multicenter study of osteogenic protein-1 in instrumented posterolateral fusions: Report on safety and feasibility. *Spine (Phila PA 1976).* 2010;35(12):1185–1191.

84. Vaccaro AR, Whang PG, Patel T, et al. The safety and efficacy of OP-1 (rhBMP-7) as a replacement for iliac crest autograft for posterolateral lumbar arthrodesis: minimum 4-year follow-up of a pilot study. *Spine J.* 2008;8(3):457–465.

85. Stryker.com. OP-1/BMP-7 - OP-1 Implant for Fracture. 2016; Retrieved October 15, 2016, from http://www.stryker.com/cn/products/Orthobiologicals /Osteoinductive/OP-1/OP-1Implant/020210.

86. Healio.com. FDA advisory committee votes 6-1 against approval of OP-1 Putty | Orthopedics. 2013; http://www.healio.com/orthopedics/business-of-orthopedics /news/online/%7Bca821eb5-b3db-490b-922d-08432ca1bc21%7D/fda-advisory -committee-votes-6-1-against-approval-of-op-1-putty. Accessed May 7, 2014.

87. Bae H, Zhao L, Zhu D, Kanim LE, Wang JC, Delamarter RB. Variability across ten production lots of a single demineralized bone matrix product. *J Bone Joint Surg Am*. 2010;92(2):427–435.

88. Kang J, An H, Hilibrand A, Yoon ST, Kavanagh E, Boden S. Grafton and local bone have comparable outcomes to iliac crest bone in instrumented single-level lumbar fusions. *Spine (Phila PA 1976)*. 2012;37(12):1083–1091.

89. Cammisa FP, Lowery G, Garfin SR, et al. Two-year fusion rate equivalency between Grafton DBM gel and autograft in posterolateral spine fusion: A prospective controlled trial employing a side-by-side comparison in the same patient. *Spine (Phila PA 1976)*. 2004;29(6):660–666.

90. Tilkeridis K, Touzopoulos P, Ververidis A, Christodoulou S, Kazakos K, Drosos GI. Use of demineralized bone matrix in spinal fusion. *World J Orthop*. 2014;5(1):30–37.

91. Kaplan KL, Broekman MJ, Chernoff A, Lesznik GR, Drillings M. Platelet alpha-granule proteins: Studies on release and subcellular localization. *Blood*. 1979;53(4):604–618.

92. Hsu WK, Mishra A, Rodeo SR, et al. Platelet-rich plasma in orthopaedic applications: Evidence-based recommendations for treatment. *J Am Acad Orthop Surg*. 2013;21(12):739–748.

93. Castillo TN, Pouliot MA, Kim HJ, Dragoo JL. Comparison of growth factor and platelet concentration from commercial platelet-rich plasma separation systems. *Am J Sports Med*. 2011;39(2):266–271.

94. Jenis LG, Banco RJ, Kwon B. A prospective study of autologous growth factors (AGF) in lumbar interbody fusion. *Spine J*. 2006;6(1):14–20.

95. Acebal-Cortina G, Suárez-Suárez MA, García-Menéndez C, Moro-Barrero L, Iglesias-Colao R, Torres-Pérez A. Evaluation of autologous platelet concentrate for intertransverse lumbar fusion. *Eur Spine J*. 2011;20 Suppl 3:361–366.

96. Carreon LY, Glassman SD, Anekstein Y, Puno RM. Platelet gel (AGF) fails to increase fusion rates in instrumented posterolateral fusions. *Spine (Phila PA 1976)*. 2005;30(9):E243–246; discussion E247.

97. Gan Y, Dai K, Zhang P, Tang T, Zhu Z, Lu J. The clinical use of enriched bone marrow stem cells combined with porous beta-tricalcium phosphate in posterior spinal fusion. *Biomaterials*. 2008;29(29):3973–3982.

98. McLain RF, Fleming JE, Boehm CA, Muschler GF. Aspiration of osteoprogenitor cells for augmenting spinal fusion: Comparison of progenitor cell concentrations from the vertebral body and iliac crest. *J Bone Joint Surg Am*. 2005;87(12):2655–2661.

99. Muschler GF, Boehm C, Easley K. Aspiration to obtain osteoblast progenitor cells from human bone marrow: The influence of aspiration volume. *J Bone Joint Surg Am*. 1997;79(11):1699–1709.

100. Bansal S, Chauhan V, Sharma S, Maheshwari R, Juyal A, Raghuvanshi S. Evaluation of hydroxyapatite and beta-tricalcium phosphate mixed with bone marrow aspirate as a bone graft substitute for posterolateral spinal fusion. *Indian J Orthop*. 2009;43(3):234–239.

101. Kitchel SH. A preliminary comparative study of radiographic results using mineralized collagen and bone marrow aspirate versus autologous bone in the same patients undergoing posterior lumbar interbody fusion with instrumented posterolateral lumbar fusion. *Spine J*. 2006;6(4):405–411; discussion 411–402.

102. Moro-Barrero L, Acebal-Cortina G, Suárez-Suárez M, Pérez-Redondo J, Murcia-Mazón A, López-Muñiz A. Radiographic analysis of fusion mass using fresh autologous bone marrow with ceramic composites as an alternative to autologous bone graft. *J Spinal Disord Tech.* 2007;20(6):409–415.

103. Hyer CF, Berlet GC, Bussewitz BW, Hankins T, Ziegler HL, Philbin TM. Quantitative assessment of the yield of osteoblastic connective tissue progenitors in bone marrow aspirate from the iliac crest, tibia, and calcaneus. *J Bone Joint Surg Am.* 2013;95(14):1312–1316.

104. Taghavi CE, Lee K-B, Keorochana G, Tzeng S-T, Yoo JH, Wang JC. Bone morphogenetic protein-2 and bone marrow aspirate with allograft as alternatives to autograft in instrumented revision posterolateral lumbar spinal fusion: A minimum two-year follow-up study. *Spine (Phila PA 1976).* 2010;35(11):1144–1150.

105. Khashan M, Inoue S, Berven SH. Cell based therapies as compared to autologous bone grafts for spinal arthrodesis. *Spine (Phila PA 1976).* 2013;38(21):1885–1891.

106. Johnson RG. Bone marrow concentrate with allograft equivalent to autograft in lumbar fusions. *Spine (Phila PA 1976).* 2014;39(9):695–700.

107. Hernigou P, Mathieu G, Poignard A, Manicom O, Beaujean F, Rouard H. Percutaneous autologous bone-marrow grafting for nonunions. Surgical technique. *J Bone Joint Surg Am.* 2006;88 Suppl 1 Pt 2:322–327.

108. Gupta MC, Theerajunyaporn T, Maitra S, et al. Efficacy of mesenchymal stem cell enriched grafts in an ovine posterolateral lumbar spine model. *Spine.* 2007;32(7):720–726.

109. Misra S. Human gene therapy: A brief overview of the genetic revolution. *J Assoc Physicians India.* 2013;61(2):127–133.

110. Blaese RM. Development of gene therapy for immunodeficiency: Adenosine deaminase deficiency. *Pediatr Res.* 1993;33(1 Suppl):S49–53; discussion S53–45.

111. Barba M, Cicione C, Bernardini C, et al. Spinal fusion in the next generation: Gene and cell therapy approaches. *ScientificWorldJournal.* 2014;2014:406159.

112. Miyazaki M, Sugiyama O, Tow B, et al. The effects of lentiviral gene therapy with bone morphogenetic protein-2-producing bone marrow cells on spinal fusion in rats. *J Spinal Disord Tech.* 2008;21(5):372–379.

113. Sheyn D, Kallai I, Tawackoli W, et al. Gene-modified adult stem cells regenerate vertebral bone defect in a rat model. *Mol Pharm.* 2011;8(5):1592–1601.

11

Bone Grafts for Craniofacial Applications

Sergio A. Montelongo, Teja Guda, and Joo Ong

CONTENTS

11.1 Introduction

The skull is the most distinct and complex array of bones in the craniofacial region. Divided into the cranial bones and the facial bones, the bones of the skull come with different shapes and functions and thus are expected to exhibit different mechanical properties. Studies done to test these mechanical properties are usually limited to cadaveric samples and are subjected to individual variations. Additionally, when analyzing the mechanical data for bones, it is also important to note that the mechanical properties in bone vary greatly at the hierarchical level and are very much dependent on whether the testing is performed at the macroscale, microscale, or nanoscale level.[1] As such, there is then not one value that will simplify the mechanical properties of bone, but rather, ranges of values that describe the mechanical response of bone under different testing circumstances.

The cranial bones are made up of the frontal bone, parietal bone, temporal bone, occipital bone, sphenoid bone, and ethmoid bone.[2] These bones are subject to mechanical loads resulting from orofacial functions. The cranial bones are diploic, that is, two cortical plates sandwiching a thin layer of trabecular bone. Differences in bone density, elastic modulus, and cortical thickness have been observed between and within bones, and these values are generally highest at the occipital bone and intermediate at parietal and frontal bones.[3] Studies correlating mechanical properties and loading rate have shown that cranial bones are heavily influenced by their loading rates. It was also reported that testing speed, strain rate, cranial sampling position, and intercranial variation have significant effects on some mechanical parameters. Motherway et al. reported the modulus to be 7.56 GPa, 10.77 GPa, and 15.54 GPa for slow loading rate, intermediate loading rate, and fast loading rate, respectively; and the frontal bone to be less porous, have a higher bone volume, and be able to absorb higher energy before failure when compared to the parietal bone.[4]

Unlike the frontal bone, parietal bone, temporal bone, occipital bone, sphenoid bone, and ethmoid bone, the mandible bone and zygomatic bone are collectively classified as facial bones. Studies have shown that different regions in the mandible exhibit different mechanical properties, with the anterior of the mandibular bone exhibiting significantly higher density, elastic modulus, and ultimate compressive strength when compared to the middle and distal regions of the mandibular bone.[5] A mean elastic modulus of 96 MPa was reported when pooling together all regions of the mandible, including the outer cortical bone, whereas a mean elastic modulus of 56 MPa was observed after removing the cortical bone.[6] In the same study, the elastic modulus of 431 MPa observed for the trabecular bone on the mandibular condyle was in the range of bones such as the femur and tibia. With other studies reporting a mandibular bone density of 0.35 g/cm^3, these mechanical values are important when considering placing implants in edentulous patients.[7]

In comparison to the parietal and frontal bones, zygomatic bones are reported to have lower thickness (2.2 mm), density (1.6 g/cm^3), and modulus (10.8 GPa). The zygoma has a relatively dense core of trabecular bone and is suggested to play a more significant structural role than the proportionately lesser amounts of trabecular bone in most other craniofacial bones.[3]

It is important to note that the mechanical characteristics of the different craniofacial bones are involved with various functions, including the protection of the brain, mastication, breathing, hearing, and speech, and thus play an important role in a person's quality of life due to the major role of facial esthetics in social acceptance8 and in a person's self-esteem.[9,10] As a result, any congenital malformations or traumatic injuries such as trauma and cancer can be devastating to many patients. Repair of these malformations or injuries in the craniofacial skeletons can be challenging and successful treatment is dependent on different factors including the size of the defect, the quality of bone tissue surrounding the defect, and the choice of reconstructive method.[11] In many instances, bone grafting procedures are necessary to stimulate bone-healing and to fill large bone defects. Since there are many available graft options, ranging from autogenous grafts to synthetic grafts, this chapter will summarize the main types of bone grafting that have been used to repair bone defects in the craniofacial region.

11.2 Clinical Need

Craniomaxillofacial (CMF) injuries can be a threat to a person's quality of life since these injuries can interfere with the person's vital functions. The incidents causing these injuries range from traffic accidents, assaults and sports, to battlefield injuries.[12] According to a study most craniofacial fractures occur in the mandible (~50% of craniomaxillofacial fractures), followed by the zygomatic bone (~20% of CMF fractures), and maxillary bone (~13% of CMF fractures).[13]

Armed conflict CMF injuries have historically represented 16% to 21% of injuries to U.S. armed forces, with fractures adding up to 24% of all CMF injuries.[14,15] However, with the percentage of CMF injuries increasing to 29% during the more recent conflicts of Operation Iraqi Freedom (OIF) and Operation Enduring Freedom (OEF), the rate of craniofacial fractures also increased to 27%.[16] The greatest contributor to these CMF injuries was the use of explosive devices, which in turn can potentially leave open fractures and wounds exposed to contaminating factors.[17]

For civilians as well as armed forces, the orbit is particularly susceptible to fractures, due both to its position and its thin bones.[18] Typically observed during physical assault and traffic accidents, blunt periorbital trauma, particularly of the zygomatico-orbital complex, can compromise the orbital floor structure, thereby resulting in fractures.[19,20] Defined as a blow-out fracture of the orbit, fractures involving the orbital wall and/or floor orbital have a wide range of severity and extension that may result in functional and aesthetic issues such as residual dystopia, diplopia (double vision), enophthalmos (posterior displacement of the eyeball), and reduced vision.

11.3 Autogenous Bone Graft Sources

Depending on the presence of an anastomosis or an alternate blood supply to the donor site, vascularized bone grafts are highlly successful, with some studies reporting success rates of greater than 90%.[21,22] It has also been reported that the vasculature is independent of the recipient site.[23] In addition to the successful reconstruction of the bone, some investigators have also observed improvements of the vascularization at the recipient site, improving the likelihood of success for successive non-vascularized grafts in areas with close proximity to the recipient site as well as for soft tissue reconstruction.[24,25] It has also been suggested that vascularized bone grafts generally have slower resorption and therefore are used for primary bone reconstruction as opposed to using non-vascularized grafts.[26] However, vascularized grafts are more delicate to work with and require special equipment and special techniques, and they take a longer time to harvest. In addition, the amount of vascularized grafts harvested is generally smaller in comparison to the harvesting of non-vascularized grafts, with patients requiring longer recovery time in the hospital, thereby significantly increasing the patient's financial burden.[21,27] Among the bone sources used to harvest vascularized grafts are the scapula, vascularized iliac crest,[28] vascularized rib,[24] vascularized radius, vascularized fibula,[22] and vascularized skull.[29,30] The following subsections discuss some of the bone sources that are generally used to harvest grafts for craniofacial bone reconstructions.

11.3.1 Iliac Crest

The iliac crest is one of the most common donor sites for bone grafts since large segments of the cortical or cancellous bone can quickly be obtained.[31] A full-thickness iliac crest graft can closely resemble the thickness and height of a mandibular bone. It has been reported that iliac crest grafts showed reasonable long-term survival, with an approximate 70% success rate in filling mandibular defects up to 6 cm in size and a declining success with defects exceeding 6 cm in size.[21,27] These grafts can be obtained from both the posterior and anterior iliac crest, although grafts obtained from the posterior iliac crest have been reported to exhibit higher morbidity (25%) at the donor site when compared to grafts obtained from the anterior iliac crest (18%).[32,33] In comparison to the success rate in mandibular defects, iliac crest grafts also have comparable success rate when used for reconstructing alveolar clefts.[34]

11.3.2 Calvarial Graft

Another source of autografts for maxillofacial reconstructions is the calvarium. Harvested for numerous craniofacial reconstructions, including nasal reconstruction,[35] maxillary ridge, sinus reconstruction,[36] maxillofacial reconstruction,[37] and skull defect reconstruction,[38] the calvarium is made up of two parallel cortical bone layers, separated by a thin cancellous bone layer. Curling off bones from the outer cortical bone plate with a sharp osteotome, the calvarial grafts can be harvested using the following techniques:

- Harvesting the partial thickness outer cortex, which can be used to sufficiently fill defects in children between the ages of 4 and 8 years.[39]

- Harvesting the full thickness outer cortex grafts, which are used mostly in adults whereby the full thickness of the outer layer is obtained.

- Harvesting the full thickness bicocortical grafts in instances where a large quantity of bone is needed and splitting the two cortices of the harvested grafts provides twice the graft surfaces for filling large defects.

The thickest and safest area on the calvarium that can be harvested for grafting is the parietal bone.[40,41] With an area of approximately 8 cm × 10 cm, this donor site is popular due to its mechanical properties and slow resorption rate.[41,42] Although calvarial grafts are highly biocompatible and are readily available as a graft source for different reconstructions and/or augmentations, lacerating the superior sagittal sinus or exposing the dura can be catastrophic during graft harvesting.[43] It is therefore important that anatomical structures such as emissary veins, the superior sagittal sinus, muscle attachment sites, dura exposure, and dura tears not be compromised during harvesting grafts from the calvarium.[41]

11.3.3 Chin and Retromolar Grafts

Bone areas of the chin and behind the third molar are also sources for bone grafts. By shaving the chin bone intraorally, the mandibular symphysis provides up to 3 cm² of cortical and corticoncellous bone.[31] Advantages of using grafts from the chin bone include ease of access, short healing periods, and minimal morbidity at the donor site.[44,45] However, the quantity of bone is not large and grafts from this donor site are limited to filling small defects as well as for the reconstruction of the alveolar process in children with cleft palate.[46] With grafts obtained from the bone area behind the third molar, also known as the retromolar region, the donor site has been reported to exhibit minimal morbidity by evaluating the superficial sensory function of the inferior alveolar and lingual nerves.[47] These grafts can be obtained from both the maxilla and mandible and are used for single tooth reconstruction, in conjunction with either ridge augmentation or crestal sinus floor elevation. In comparison to the grafts obtained from the chin bone, the amount of grafts available from the retromolar region is significantly smaller, approximately in the range of 0.75 cm² to 0.85 cm².[48] However, if the patient's third molar needs to be extracted, the possibility of grafting the retromolar region should be considered.[23]

11.3.4 Rib Graft

Grafts harvested from ribs 5 through 7 have also been used for mandibular segment reconstruction as well as treating children with cleft palate and defects in the ascending mandibular ramus and condylar region.[49] A relatively easy procedure with low morbidity, the costochondral graft harvested can be used as full thickness or split thickness.[50] Long-term studies with 15 years follow-up have reported no morbidity, with greater than 90% of patients that underwent nasal reconstruction using grafts harvested from the ribs indicating satisfaction and 86% reporting increased quality of life.[51,52] However, other studies have also reported complications from the use of rib grafts from the ribs, including chest wall pain, pleural injury,[53] and facial asymmetry due to graft overgrowth.[54–56] As a result of these complications as well as the availability of new graft sources for harvesting more and higher quality bone grafts, the use of grafts from the ribs has become less popular than 20 years ago.[31]

11.3.5 Mandibular Tori

For onlay bone graft augmentation as well as maxillary ridge augmentation, the bilateral mandibular tori have been used as a source of bone grafts.[57,58] While harvesting grafts from the mandibular tori has been successful with little donor site morbidity,[59] the tori are not an anatomical feature that is present in all humans. Present in less than a third of its population in the United States, such anatomical features are predominant in native inhabitants of the far north, that is, in Greenland and Alaska.[60]

11.3.6 Regional Pedicled Bone Grafts

Other popular sources of grafts are the pedicles. These grafts are osteomuscular flaps (with or without attached skin) in which the grafted bone is vascularized by means of the muscle.[61] Yielding mixed results, the source of pedicled grafts used for craniofacial reconstructions defects are pedicled rib, pedicled temporal bone, pedicled clavicle, and pedicled scapula.[27,62,63] The pedicled rib uses the pectoralis major, the latissimus dorsi, or the serratus anterior flaps as vascular sources.[31,62] All of those flaps permit the pedicled rib graft to reach only the bottom third of the face, thus making it suitable only for mandibular defects. However, as discussed earlier, the rib graft presents complications inherent to the costochondral graft, including exhibiting a high necrosis rate of the flaps[63] and the possibility of damage to the brachial plexus due to the position of the shoulder to access the latissimus dorsi muscle.[64] Similar to the pedicled ribs, the pedicled clavicle involves a flap of the sternocleidomastoid muscle and clavicular periosteum and/or bone segments from the clavicle.[65,66] Although the use of this flap permits a one-stage reconstruction of oropharyngeal defects, concerns with the use of this flap include its proximity to lymph nodes and thus the ability of cancer to metastasize to the sternocleidomastoid muscle.[67] Lastly, the temporalis flap has been used for paralyzed facial muscles and mid-facial full-thickness defect reconstructions or it can be paired with a partial or full thickness of temporal bone[68,69] as onlay graft for facial augmentation as well as for reconstructing craniofacial defects such as maxillary, orbital rim, palatal, orbital floor, and ascending mandibular ramus defects.[70,71] However, in addition to the complications associated with calvarial grafts, there are concerns with donor site morbidity as well as limitations in the patient opening his or her mouth when using grafts from the pedicled temporal bone.[23,31]

11.4 Alloplastic Bone Grafts

Demineralized bone matrix (DBM) is an alloplastic material that has been extensively used for craniofacial reconstruction.[72–75] In comparison to dry human cortical bone, which contains approximately 25% calcium by weight, the American Association of Tissue Banks defines demineralized bone as having no more than 8% residual calcium by weight.[76] Although there are different commercially available preparations of DBM[77] with different calcium content, most of them are devoid of calcium.[78] By extracting the mineral phase with 0.5 N to 0.6 N hydrochloric acid, this demineralization step acts as a viral inactivator, which decreases the risk of disease transfer.[79]

In addition to exhibiting both osteoconductive and osteoinductive properties,[80] the DBM also exhibits favorable mechanical properties, thus making it useful for reconstructing large cranial defects following cranioplasties.[81] Depending on the manufacturer, the bone growth potential of DMB is different for different commercially available products.[82] In addition, osteoinductivity of DMB is also highly dependent on the donor age group, with the highest osteoinductive potential displayed by female and male donors between 31 to 40 and 41 to 50 years of age, respectively.[80] However, extensive processing has been reported to deactivate the osteoinductive factors necessary for successful grafting as well as alter the mechanical properties and strength during preservation.[83] As a result, slower incorporation rates, together with slower and poorer vascularization and remodeling, were observed when DBM was used as a bone augmenting material, thereby resulting in a 25% failure rate and 30%–60% complication rate.[84] To accelerate the graft incorporation rates, investigators have coupled the use of growth factors such as bone morphogenetic proteins-2 to the DBM.[85,86]

11.5 Synthetic Bone Substitutes

In instances where large critical-sized bone injuries or malformation involves the pediatric population between the ages of 2 and 10 years old,[87] alloplastic reconstruction of large skull defects is least suited, with the greatest morbidity from autogenous bone graft sites[88] and the highest scarcity or inadequate availability of donor bone in this population.[89] In addition, the conventional surgical option of split calvarial grafts often explored in the adult population is not possible with the pediatric population because of the underdeveloped diploic space in children.[90] With allogenic bone grafts as a poorer substitute for autografts due to their risk of disease transmission, slower and poorer vascularization and remodeling, and higher failure and complication rates, there is an increasing clinical need for synthetic grafting materials, as the bone grafting procedures performed in the United States increased from 500,000 procedures in 2001[91] to 1.4 million procedures in 2007.[92]

From the field of tissue engineering, a vast number of synthetic bone grafts have emerged with the idea that these synthetic grafts will help to regenerate bone, thereby alleviating the conundrum of finding enough donor bone for grafting large defects. Among the many classes of synthetic biomaterials, families of calcium phosphate and calcium sulfate ceramics have been extensively studied for craniofacial reconstruction. Calcium phosphate cements, such as hydroxyapatite and tricalcium phosphate cements, have been used successfully to repair cerebral spinal fluid leaks,[93] obliterate the frontal sinus,[94] and augment and contour defects in the craniofacial skeleton in children and adults.[95] On the other hand, calcium sulfate hemihydrate, commonly known as plaster of paris, has been combined with porous hydroxyapatite granules to repair cranial defects.[96,97] Other craniofacial reconstruction procedures have included the use of composite materials in which degradable poly(DL-lactic-co-glycolic) acid or porous tri-calcium phosphate served as delivery vehicles for bone-inductive growth factors.[98] As in the DBM, growth factors are investigated with synthetic bone grafts to elicit favorable cellular responses, and these growth factors include the different bone morphogenetic proteins, transforming growth factor, vascular endothelial growth factor, and platelet-derived growth factor.[99,100]

11.6 Conclusions

As discussed in this chapter, there are different types of grafts that are used to either reconstruct, repair, or augment the craniofacial bones. While autogenous grafts offer the best path to ensure biocompatibility, there are issues with harvesting adequate amounts of bone, especially for large defects, as well as donor site morbidity issues and other complications. Additionally, rafts from popular donor sites like long bones are quickly resorbed in the craniofacial skeleton due to marked differences in their composition,[101] thus limiting the donor sites to craniofacial bones and the iliac crest. As an alternative to autogenous grafts, alloplastic and synthetic grafts are also available, but the current generation of these grafts is mostly used for filling small defects. There are also problems with the use of allogenic bone grafts, including risks in disease transmission, slower and poorer vascularization and remodeling, and higher failure and complication rates. Problems with the current synthetic grafts include their heavy dependence on biologic growth factors to elicit favorable outcomes. However, with the growing field of tissue engineering and the advent of favorable tissue-engineered solutions that are being commercialized, in the future dependence on autogenous and allogenic grafts for craniofacial bone reconstructions should be reduced.

References

1. Rho, J.-Y., L. Kuhn-Spearing, and P. Zioupos, Mechanical properties and the hierarchical structure of bone. *Medical Engineering & Physics*, 1998. 20(2): 92–102.
2. Sicher, H. and E.L. DuBrul, Temporomandibular articulation. *Oral Anatomy*. 5th edition. St. Louis, MO: CV Mosby, 1970.
3. Peterson, J. and P.C. Dechow, Material properties of the human cranial vault and zygoma. *The Anatomical Record Part A: Discoveries in Molecular, Cellular, and Evolutionary Biology*, 2003. 274(1): 785–797.
4. Motherway, J.A., P. Verschueren, G. Van der Perre, et al., The mechanical properties of cranial bone: The effect of loading rate and cranial sampling position. *Journal of Biomechanics*, 2009. 42(13): 2129–2135.
5. Misch, C.E., Z. Qu, and M.W. Bidez, Mechanical properties of trabecular bone in the human mandible: Implications for dental implant treatment planning and surgical placement. *Journal of Oral and Maxillofacial Surgery*, 1999. 57(6): 700–706.
6. Giesen, E.B.W., M. Ding, M. Dalstra, et al., Mechanical properties of cancellous bone in the human mandibular condyle are anisotropic. *Journal of Biomechanics*, 2001. 34(6): 799–803.
7. Van Oosterwyck, H., J. Duyck, J. Vander Sloten, et al., The influence of bone mechanical properties and implant fixation upon bone loading around oral implants. *Clinical Oral Implants Research*, 1998. 9(6): 407–418.
8. Adams, G.R., The effects of physical attractiveness on the socialization process. *Psychological Aspects of Facial Form. Craniofacial Growth Series Monograph*, 1981(11): 25–47.
9. Pertschuk, M.J. and L.A. Whitaker, Psychosocial adjustment and craniofacial malformations in childhood. *Plastic and Reconstructive Surgery*, 1985. 75(2): 177–182.
10. Levine, E., L. Degutis, T. Pruzinsky, et al., Quality of life and facial trauma: Psychological and body image effects. *Annals of Plastic Surgery*, 2005. 54(5): 502–510.
11. Tevlin, R., A. McArdle, D. Atashroo, et al., Biomaterials for craniofacial bone engineering. *Journal of Dental Research*, 2014. 93(12): 1187–1195.
12. Hussain, K., D.B. Wijetunge, S. Grubnic, et al., A comprehensive analysis of craniofacial trauma. *J Trauma*, 1994. 36(1): 34–47.
13. Ashfaq, A., W. Ahmed, S.G.A. Bukhari, et al., The maxillofacial trauma management trends at Armed Forces Institute of Dentistry, Rawalpindi. *Pakistan Oral & Dental Journal*, 2012. 32(2): 191–195.

14. Reister, F.A., *Battle Casualties and Medical Statistics: US Army Experience in the Korean War*. 1973. Washington, DC: Surgeon General, Dept. of the Army.
15. Beebe, G. and M. DeBakey, Location of hits and wounds. *Battle Casualties*, 1952. 314: 165–205.
16. Owens, B.D., et al., Combat wounds in operation Iraqi Freedom and operation Enduring Freedom. *Journal of Trauma and Acute Care Surgery*, 2008. 64(2): 295–299.
17. Lew, T.A., J.A. Walker, J.C. Wenke, et al., Characterization of craniomaxillofacial battle injuries sustained by United States service members in the current conflicts of Iraq and Afghanistan. *J Oral Maxillofac Surg*, 2010. 68(1): 3–7.
18. Gosau, M., M. Schöneich, F.G. Draenert, et al., Retrospective analysis of orbital floor fractures—Complications, outcome, and review of literature. *Clinical Oral Investigations*, 2011. 15(3): 305–313.
19. Hunsaker, D., Surgical correction of enophthalmos and diplopia. *Archives of Otolaryngology–Head & Neck Surgery*, 1989. 115(1): 13.
20. Nguyen, P. and P. Sullivan, Advances in the management of orbital fractures. *Clinics in Plastic Surgery*, 1992. 19(1): 87–98.
21. Pogrel, M., S. Podlesh, J.P. Anthony, et al., A comparison of vascularized and nonvascularized bone grafts for reconstruction of mandibular continuity defects. *Journal of Oral and Maxillofacial Surgery*, 1997. 55(11): 1200–1206.
22. Taylor, G.I., The current status of free vascularized bone grafts. *Clin Plast Surg*, 1983. 10(1): 185–209.
23. Ehrenfeld, M. and C. Hagenmaier (eds.), Autogenous bone grafts in maxillofacial reconstruction, in *Craniomaxillofacial Reconstructive and Corrective Bone Surgery*. 2002, New York, NY: Springer. pp. 295–309.
24. Serafin, D., R. Riefkohl, I. Thomas, et al., Vascularized rib-periosteal and osteocutaneous reconstruction of the maxilla and mandible: An assessment. *Plastic and Reconstructive Surgery*, 1980. 66(5): 718–727.
25. Hurwitz, D.J., Long-term results of vascularized cranial bone grafts. *Journal of Craniofacial Surgery*, 1994. 5(4): 237–241.
26. Bite, U., I.T. Jackson, H.W. Wahner, et al., Vascularized skull bone grafts in craniofacial surgery. *Annals of Plastic Surgery*, 1987. 19(1): 3–15.
27. Foster, R.D., J.P. Anthony, A. Sharma, et al., Vascularized bone flaps versus nonvascularized bone grafts for mandibular reconstruction: An outcome analysis of primary bony union and endosseous implant success. *Head & Neck*, 1999. 21(1): 66–71.
28. Modabber, A., M. Gerressen, M.B. Stiller, et al., Computer-assisted mandibular reconstruction with vascularized iliac crest bone graft. *Aesthetic Plastic Surgery*, 2012. 36(3): 653–659.
29. Jackson, I.T., G. Helden, and R. Marx, Skull bone grafts in maxillofacial and craniofacial surgery. *Journal of Oral and Maxillofacial Surgery*, 1986. 44(12): 949–955.
30. Jackson, I.T., M. Adham, U. Bite, et al., Update on cranial bone grafts in craniofacial surgery. *Annals of Plastic Surgery*, 1987. 18(1): 37–40.
31. Elsalanty, M.E. and D.G. Genecov, Bone grafts in craniofacial surgery. *Craniomaxillofacial Trauma & Reconstruction*, 2009. 2(3): 125.
32. Ahlmann, E., M. Patzakis, N. Roidis, et al., Comparison of anterior and posterior iliac crest bone grafts in terms of harvest-site morbidity and functional outcomes. *J Bone Joint Surg Am*, 2002. 84-A(5): 716–720.
33. Thorwarth, M., S. Srour, E. Felszeghy, et al., Stability of autogenous bone grafts after sinus lift procedures: A comparative study between anterior and posterior

aspects of the iliac crest and an intraoral donor site. *Oral Surgery, Oral Medicine, Oral Pathology, Oral Radiology, and Endodontology*, 2005. 100(3): 278–284.

34. Sindet-Pedersen, S. and H. Enemark, Mandibular bone grafts for reconstruction of alveolar clefts. *Journal of Oral and Maxillofacial Surgery*, 1988. 46(7): 533–537.

35. Romo, T., 3rd and R.D. Jablonski, Nasal reconstruction using split calvarial grafts. *Otolaryngology–Head & Neck Surgery*, 1992. 107(5): 622–630.

36. Bastos, A.S., R. Spin-Neto, N. Conte-Neto, et al., Calvarial autogenous bone graft for maxillary ridge and sinus reconstruction for rehabilitation with dental implants. *Journal of Oral Implantology*, 2014. 40(4): 469–478.

37. Hunter, D., S. Baker, and S.M. Sobol, Split calvarial grafts in maxillofacial reconstruction. *Otolaryngology–Head and Neck Surgery*, 1990. 102(4): 345–350.

38. Agrawal, A. and L.N. Garg, Split calvarial bone graft for the reconstruction of skull defects. *J Surg Tech Case Rep*, 2011. 3(1): 13–16.

39. Frodel, J.L., Calvarial bone graft harvest in children. *Otolaryngology–Head and Neck Surgery*, 1999. 121(1): 78–81.

40. Sahoo, N.K. and M. Rangan, Role of split calvarial graft in reconstruction of craniofacial defects. *J Craniofac Surg*, 2012. 23(4): e326–31.

41. Frodel, J.L., Jr., L.J. Marentette, V.C. Quatela, et al., Calvarial bone graft harvest. Techniques, considerations, and morbidity. *Archives of Otolaryngology–Head & Neck Surgery*, 1993. 119(1): 17–23.

42. Bauer, T.W. and G.F. Muschler, Bone graft materials. An overview of the basic science. *Clin Orthop Relat Res*, 2000(371): 10–27.

43. Cannella, D.M. and L.N. Hopkins, Superior sagittal sinus laceration complicating an autogenous calvarial bone graft harvest: Report of a case. *J Oral Maxillofac Surg*, 1990. 48(7): 741–743.

44. Joshi, A., An investigation of post-operative morbidity following chin graft surgery. *Br Dent J*, 2004. 196(4): 215–218.

45. Weibull, L., G. Widmark, C.-J. Ivanoff, et al., Morbidity after chin bone harvesting—A retrospective long-term follow-up study. *Clinical Implant Dentistry and Related Research*, 2009. 11(2): 149–157.

46. Borstlap, W.A., K.L. Heidbuchel, H.P.M. Freihofer, et al., Early secondary bone grafting of alveolar cleft defects: A comparison between chin and rib grafts. *Journal of Cranio-Maxillofacial Surgery*, 1990. 18(5): 201–205.

47. Nkenke, E., M. Radespiel-Troger, J. Wiltfang, et al., Morbidity of harvesting of retromolar bone grafts: A prospective study. *Clin Oral Implants Res*, 2002. 13(5): 514–521.

48. Cremonini, C.C., M. Dumas, C. Pannuti, et al., Assessment of the availability of bone volume for grafting in the donor retromolar region using computed tomography: A pilot study. *International Journal of Oral & Maxillofacial Implants*, 2010. 25(2): 374–378.

49. Perrott, D.H., H. Umeda, and L.B. Kaban, Costochondral graft construction/reconstruction of the ramus/condyle unit: Long-term follow-up. *International Journal of Oral and Maxillofacial Surgery*, 1994. 23(6): 321–328.

50. Johnson, P.E. and I. Raftopoulos, In situ splitting of a rib graft for reconstruction of the orbital floor. *Plastic and Reconstructive Surgery*, 1999. 103(6): 1709–1711.

51. Gurley, J.M., T. Pilgram, C.A. Perlyn, et al., Long-term outcome of autogenous rib graft nasal reconstruction. *Plastic and Reconstructive Surgery*, 2001. 108(7): p. 1895–1905; discussion 1906–1907.

52. Paul D. Sawin, Vincent C. Traynelis, and Arnold H. Menezes, A comparative analysis of fusion rates and donor-site morbidity for autogeneic rib and iliac

crest bone grafts in posterior cervical fusions. *Journal of Neurosurgery*, 1998. 88(2): 255–265.

53. Figueroa, A.A., B.J. Gans, and S. Pruzansky, Long-term follow-up of a mandibular costochondral graft. *Oral Surgery, Oral Medicine, Oral Pathology, Oral Radiology, and Endodontology*, 1984. 58(3): 257–268.

54. Guyuron, B. and C.I. Lasa Jr, Unpredictable growth pattern of costochondral graft. *Plastic and Reconstructive Surgery*, 1992. 90(5): 880–886.

55. Peltomäki, T. and K. Isotupa, The costochondral graft: A solution or a source of facial asymmetry in growing children. A case report. *Proceedings of the Finnish Dental Society. Suomen Hammaslaakariseuran Toimituksia*, 1990. 87(1): 167–176.

56. Ko, E.W.-C., C.-S. Huang, and Y.-R. Chen, Temporomandibular joint reconstruction in children using costochondral grafts. *Journal of Oral and Maxillofacial Surgery*, 1999. 57(7): 789–798.

57. Ganz, S.D., Mandibular tori as a source for onlay bone graft augmentation: A surgical procedure. *Pract Periodontics Aesthet Dent*, 1997. 9: 973–982.

58. Barker, D., A. Walls, and J. Meechan, Case report: Ridge augmentation using mandibular tori. *British Dental Journal*, 2001. 190(9): 474–476.

59. Proussaefs, P., Clincal and histologic evaluation of the use of mandibular tori as donor site for mandibular block autografts: Report of three cases. *International Journal of Periodontics and Restorative Dentistry*, 2006. 26(1): 43.

60. Sonnier, K.E., G.M. Horning, and M.E. Cohen, Palatal tubercles, palatal tori, and mandibular tori: Prevalence and anatomical features in a U.S. population. *Journal of Periodontology*, 1999. 70(3): 329–336.

61. Lam, K., W. Wei, and K. Siu, The pectoralis major costomyocutaneous flap for mandibular reconstruction. *Plastic and Reconstructive Surgery*, 1984. 73(6): 904–910.

62. Cuono, C.B. and S. Ariyan, Immediate reconstruction of a composite mandibular defect with a regional osteomusculocutaneous flap. *Plastic and Reconstructive Surgery*, 1980. 65(4): 477–483.

63. Biller, H., Y. Krespi, W. Lawson, et al., A one-stage flap reconstruction following resection for stomal recurrence. *Otolaryngology–Head and Neck Surgery*, 1979. 88(4): 357–360.

64. Logan, A. and M. Black, Injury to the brachial plexus resulting from shoulder positioning during latissimus dorsi flap pedicle dissection. *British Journal of Plastic Surgery*, 1985. 38(3): 380–382.

65. Conley, J. and P.J. Gullane, The sternocleidomastoid muscle flap. *Head & Neck Surgery*, 1980. 2(4): 308–311.

66. Alagöz, M.S., A.Ç. Uysal, E. Tüccar, et al., How cranial could the sternocleidomastoid muscle be split? *Journal of Craniofacial Surgery*, 2005. 16(2): 201–204.

67. Ariyan, S. and C.B. Cuono, Myocutaneous flaps for head and neck reconstruction. *Head & Neck Surgery*, 1980. 2(4): 321–345.

68. Koranda, F.C., M.F. McMahon, and V.R. Jernstrom, The temporalis muscle flap for intraoral reconstruction. *Archives of Otolaryngology–Head & Neck Surgery*, 1987. 113(7): 740–743.

69. Antonyshyn, O., R. Colcleugh, L. Hurst, et al., The temporalis myo-osseous flap: An experimental study. *Plastic and Reconstructive Surgery*, 1986. 77(3): 406–413.

70. Cheney, M.L. and M. Urken, Regional flaps. In *Atlas of Regional and Free Flaps for Head and Neck Reconstruction*, Urken, M.L. et al. (eds.), 1995, Philadelphia, PA: Lippincott Williams & Wilkins, p. 65.

71. Renner, G., W.E. Davis, and J. Templer, Temporalis pericranial muscle flap for reconstruction of the lateral face and head. *The Laryngoscope*, 1984. 94(11): 1418–1422.
72. Salyer, K.E., E. Gendler, J.L. Menendez, et al., Demineralized perforated bone implants in craniofacial surgery. *Journal of Craniofacial Surgery*, 1992. 3(2): 55–62.
73. Chen, T.M. and H.J. Wang, Cranioplasty using allogeneic perforated demineralized bone matrix with autogenous bone paste. *Annals of Plastic Surgery*, 2002. 49(3): 272–279.
74. Chao, M.T., S. Jiang, D. Smith, et al., Demineralized bone matrix and resorbable mesh bilaminate cranioplasty: A novel method for reconstruction of large-scale defects in the pediatric calvaria. *Plastic and Reconstructive Surgery*, 2009. 123(3): 976–982.
75. Salyer, K.E., J. Bardach, C.A. Squier, et al., Cranioplasty in the growing canine skull using demineralized perforated bone. *Plastic and Reconstructive Surgery*, 1995. 96(4): 770–779.
76. Banks, A.A.o.T., J.E. Woll, and D.O. Kasprisin, *Standards for Tissue Banking.* McLean, VA: American Association of Tissue Banks, 2001.
77. Mah, J., J. Hung, J. Wang, et al., The efficacy of various alloplastic bone grafts on the healing of rat calvarial defects. *The European Journal of Orthodontics*, 2004. 26(5): 475–482.
78. Pietrzak, W., S. Miller, D. Kucharzyk, et al., Demineralized bone graft formulations: Design, development, and a novel example. *Proceedings of the Pittsburgh Bone Symposium*, Pittsburgh, PA, August, 2003: 19–23.
79. Eppley, B.L., W.S. Pietrzak, and M.W. Blanton, Allograft and alloplastic bone substitutes: A review of science and technology for the craniomaxillofacial surgeon. *Journal of Craniofacial Surgery*, 2005. 16(6): 981–989.
80. Zhang, M., R.M. Powers Jr, and L. Wolfinbarger Jr, Effect(s) of the demineralization process on the osteoinductivity of demineralized bone matrix. *Journal of Periodontology*, 1997. 68(11): 1085–1092.
81. Salyer, K.E., E. Gendler, and C.A. Squier, Long-term outcome of extensive skull reconstruction using demineralized perforated bone in Siamese twins joined at the skull vertex. *Plastic and Reconstructive Surgery*, 1997. 99(6): 1721–1726.
82. Acarturk, T.O. and J.O. Hollinger, Commercially available demineralized bone matrix compositions to regenerate calvarial critical-sized bone defects. *Plastic and Reconstructive Surgery*, 2006. 118(4): 862–873.
83. Voggenreiter, G., R. Ascherl, G. Blümel, et al., Effects of preservation and sterilization on cortical bone grafts. *Archives of Orthopaedic and Trauma Surgery*, 1994. 113(5): 294–296.
84. Zara, J.N., R.K. Siu, X. Zhang, et al., High doses of bone morphogenetic protein 2 induce structurally abnormal bone and inflammation in vivo. *Tissue Engineering Part A*, 2011. 17(9-10): 1389–1399.
85. Elsalanty, M.E., Y.-C. Por, D.G. Genecov, et al., Recombinant human BMP-2 enhances the effects of materials used for reconstruction of large cranial defects. *Journal of Oral and Maxillofacial Surgery*, 2008. 66(2): 277–285.
86. Cheng, H., W. Jiang, F.M. Phillips, et al., Osteogenic activity of the fourteen types of human bone morphogenetic proteins (BMPs). *J Bone Joint Surg Am*, 2003. 85(8): 1544–1552.
87. Cooper, G.M., M.P. Mooney, A.K. Gosain, et al., Testing the "critical-size" in calvarial bone defects: Revisiting the concept of a critical-sized defect (CSD). *Plastic and Reconstructive Surgery*, 2010. 125(6): 1685.

88. Langer, R. and J.P. Vacanti, Tissue Engineering. *Science*, 1993. 260(5110): 920–926.
89. Oppenheimer, A.J., J. Mesa, and S.R. Buchman, Current and emerging basic science concepts in bone biology: Implications in craniofacial surgery. *Journal of Craniofacial Surgery*, 2012. 23(1): 30–36.
90. DeCesare, G.E., F.W. Deleyiannis, and J.E. Losee. Reconstruction of osteomyelitis defects of the craniofacial skeleton. In *Seminars in Plastic Surgery*, Hollier, L.H., (ed), New York, NY: Thieme Medical Publishers, 2009.
91. Greenwald, A.S., S.D. Boden, V.M. Goldberg, et al., Bone-graft substitutes: Facts, fictions and applications, In *American Academy of Orthopaedic Surgeons*. San Fransisco, CA: AAOS, 2008, pp. 1–6.
92. Engelhardt, S.A., Bone graft materials in orthopaedics: 50+ companies vie for a piece of the $1.9BB pie, in U.S. *Orthopaedic Product News* 2008, May/June: 50–62.
93. Costantino, P.D., D.H. Hiltzik, C. Sen et al., Sphenoethmoid cerebrospinal fluid leak repair with hydroxyapatite cement. *Archives of Otolaryngology–Head & Neck Surgery*, 2001. 127(5): 588.
94. Petruzzelli, G.J. and J.A. Stankiewicz, Frontal sinus obliteration with hydroxyapatite cement. *The Laryngoscope*, 2002. 112(1): 32–36.
95. Baker, S.B., J. Weinzweig, R.E. Kirschner, et al., Applications of a new carbonated calcium phosphate bone cement: Early experience in pediatric and adult craniofacial reconstruction. *Plastic and Reconstructive Surgery*, 2002. 109(6): 1789–1796.
96. Costantino, P.D., D. Hiltzik, S. Govindaraj, et al., Bone healing and bone substitutes. *Facial Plastic Surgery: FPS*, 2002. 18(1): 13–26.
97. Pou, A.M., Update on new biomaterials and their use in reconstructive surgery. *Current Opinion in Otolaryngology & Head and Neck Surgery*, 2003. 11(4): 240–244.
98. Desilets, C.P., L.J. Marden, A.L. Patterson, et al., Development of synthetic bone-repair materials for craniofacial reconstruction. *Journal of Craniofacial Surgery*, 1990. 1(3): 150–157.
99. Vaccaro, A.R., The role of the osteoconductive scaffold in synthetic bone graft. *Orthopedics*, 2002. 25(5): S571–S578.
100. Reddi, A.H. and N.S. Cunningham, Initiation and promotion of bone differentiation by bone morphogenetic proteins. *Journal of Bone and Mineral Research*, 1993. 8(S2): S499–S502.
101. Van den Bos, T., D. Speijer, R. Bank, et al., Differences in matrix composition between calvaria and long bone in mice suggest differences in biomechanical properties and resorption: Special emphasis on collagen. *Bone*, 2008. 43(3): 459–468.

Part V

Translational Pathways for Bone Graft Development

12

Preclinical Models: A "Bedside-to-Bench" Directive

Larry D. Swain and David L. Carnes, Jr.

CONTENTS

12.1 Introduction

The objective of musculoskeletal tissue engineering is to facilitate and improve patient outcomes with concomitant reduction in morbidity, complication, and expense. Researchers can maximize preclinical animal-model predictive value by testing in multiple mammalian species, lowering the risk of new tissue engineering approaches. A strong understanding and knowledge of the intended clinical goal will inform preclinical design, scientifically rigorous methods, product parameters, and clarify regulatory-pathway strategies. AOVET, the veterinary specialty group of the AO Foundation, the AO Research Institute, and the European Academy for the Study of Scientific and Technological Advance, have sought to establish standards and guidelines on the use and design of musculoskeletal animal-research models (see Auer et al., 2007) with the overall goal of enhanced outcome performance. "It is better not to do the experiment than to do it using the wrong model" (Alini et al., 2008).

Our purpose then, in this chapter, is to discuss the current status of pre-clinical animal models with respect to musculoskeletal tissue-engineering research and means to enhance successful translation to clinical trial, approval, and adoption. Although we will, by way of example, review some technical advances and recently published adaptive applications of established and new animal models, our main interest is to suggest that expedited clinical translation can be achieved through judicious choice of model and analytic techniques. Central to our thesis is that in appropriately planned and executed studies:

- Clinical goals, based on relevance, prevalence and need, guide pre-clinical strategies.
- Study conditions mimic targeted clinical conditions.
- Assessment methods accurately measure defined outcome parameters.
- Materials and methods reflect clinical application requirements.

The above collectively depict a "modus operandi" of "bedside-to-bench" progressive decision making focused on achieving bone tissue-engineering translational research goals of differentiated clinical outcome. Ultimately, the long-term objective is enhanced public health policy (Jiang et al., 2013).

12.1.1 Opportunity and Need Do Not Predict Success

Numerous skeletal tissue-engineering efforts, employing widely variant strategies, are underway (Amini et al., 2012), driven primarily by clinical needs with respect to large segmental defects, non-healing craniofacial and appendicular defects, bone-soft tissue interfaces, and spine fusion. A National Institutes of Health sponsored workshop "Bone Tissue Engineering and Regeneration: From Discovery to the Clinic" assessed the state of the art and barriers to clinical translation (O'Keefe et al., 2011). Workshop participants succinctly delineated the enormous opportunity presented the tissue-engineering field as "approximately 15 million fractures annually ($45B); 1.6 million patients with trauma with hospital admission ($27B); 2 million osteoporotic fractures ($24B); 500,000 knee, 350,000 hip replacements, and 90,000 revision arthroplasty procedures ($30B); 300,000 spinal fusions, 20,000 revision spine fusions ($18B) ..." Of note, the number of bone-defect repairs is expected to double by 2020 (Baroli, 2009).

Nevertheless, skeletal tissue engineering has failed to significantly impact clinical practice, given the limited gains in health outcomes despite immense investment in basic and translational science (Kelley et al., 2012) and 12,000+ published papers (Hollister et al., 2011). Musculoskeletal reconstruction requires controlled delivery or placement of biomaterials, bioactive molecules, genes, or cells in temporally dynamic environments, but we do not really know how to best control these parameters. For instance, significant questions concerning rhBMP-2 outcomes are increasing (Cahill et al., 2009) and use of high dose BMP-2 induces multiple unintended side effects, including heterotopic bone formation (Wong et al., 2008) and central and peripheral nervous system side effects (Dmitriev et al., 2011). Dauntingly, a cascade of multiple molecular events support the wound-healing environment, with more than 6500 genes differentially regulated during healing progression (Rundle et al., 2006). The significant barriers to clinically translating single biologics suggest that for multi-biologic constructs even greater challenges will demand more clinically relevant and predictive preclinical models. Henderson et al. (2013), following a systematic review of preclinical research, conclude that the "vast majority of medical interventions introduced into clinical development prove unsafe or ineffective" and that variable preclinical research is a major contributor, as for example, acute-induction preclinical models often do not characterize or reflect chronic human disease progression and outcome.

12.1.2 Challenges to Industry and Academia

There are no set requirements for preclinical studies, and as such, each should be tailored to end-use therapy-specific factors. Using the intended clinical application to inform preclinical design and methods is fundamental to our premise, additionally shedding light on regulatory pathway strategies. Major animal model selection criteria include species, immunocompetence, disease status, and prototype mode-of-use considerations that inform clinical-trial design endpoints as well (Frey-Vasconcells et al., 2012). Model choice and design must closely represent critical features of the projected indication, recognizing that multiple animal models are likely required to satisfactorily address safety and efficacy considerations. A large-animal model may be more representative of the human condition, as for orthopedic indications, where large-animal joint anatomy and load-bearing function more closely simulate human equivalents.

Evans (2011a) posits "At what point is it best to stop tweaking and move forward to the next phase of development?" An enormous number of scaffolds, for example, are described in the literature and each can be endlessly modified (Woolfson et al., 2010). Is it best to select the most promising and advance to the next phase of development? Contrary to this perspective, however, academia evaluates faculty performance largely on publication rate, a deterrent to late-stage preclinical translation. Industry considers working with the

FDA one of the major obstacles hampering commercial product development and tailoring research to address market/commercialization requirements is a significant stumbling block in the academic environment. Nevertheless, a project formulated from the beginning with regulatory requirements in mind has a greater chance of clinical approval than attempted guideline placation post-development (Johnson et al., 2011).

The Tissue Engineering and Regenerative Medicine International Society–North America recently established an Industry Committee to study the issue of commercialization (Hellman et al., 2011). Industry challenges to translational success include regulatory approval, product development, physician acceptance, and payer reimbursement, all requiring products tailored to specific clinical indications and unmet needs. Ultimately, industry must assess risk/benefit ratios that consider large-animal preclinical studies, clinical trials, and manufacturing implementation requiring regulatory approval pathways years in duration and incurring onerous financial burden. Pursuing technologies where, at minimum, proof-of-concept has been established is, therefore, increasingly important. By way of example, scientists developing new osteoinductive stem cell therapies, biomaterials, or growth factor-laden constructs would be well served to demonstrate the inductive properties in models of ectopic bone formation (Scott et al., 2012). Likewise, testing in vivo biomaterial-inflammatory reactions (Markel et al., 2012) may also serve as a component of early-stage development strategy. In vivo data, in addition to basic characterization, elevates perceived value of a technology and substantially allays industry proof-of-concept expectations and risk/benefit considerations. There is definitive need for greater balance between basic science and translational research, as 90%–95% of resources are allocated toward basic research. Hollister et al. (2011) succinctly summarize this funding-distribution dilemma as "innovative discoveries are of limited value if they cannot be used in clinical applications, and it is clear that substantial innovation is needed to overcome the hurdles to clinical translation."

12.2 Translational Research

Translational research can be characterized as a temporal process moving from basic to clinical to post-clinical research with public health impact the ultimate objective (Trochim et al., 2011). Ideally, this flow of research is bidirectional, fluidly moving either direction between basic science and clinical implementation, each informing the other. Meslin et al. (2013) have described translating knowledge from biomedical science into clinical applications as crossing a valley of death, further inhibited by science policies as well. Stem cell science is a prime example of success impeded by recalcitrant policy challenges. Additionally, barriers exist between research and clinical medicine training programs, limiting student exposure to human pathophysiology instruction and mentors.

Members of the Evaluation Committee of the Association for Clinical Research Training (ACRT) concluded that translational research fosters multidirectional and multidisciplinary integration of research programs (McGartland Rubio et al., 2010). The Howard Hughes Medical Institute has since initiated the "Med into Grad" graduate-training program to address such concerns and recommendations (Smith et al., 2013). The Clinical and Translational Science Awards (CTSA) and the National Center for Advancing Translational Sciences of the National Institutes of Health support translational efforts in academia, reflecting cost-sensitive and risk-averse medical-device industry preference for licensing technologies contingent on strong basic research, preclinical data, IP protection, product design, and a cogent regulatory strategy (Kleinbeck et al., 2012). Without question, systematic review of pertinent animal experiments would provide, as it were, a synthesis of evidence to aid in model/protocol selection informing proposed preclinical and clinical studies, yet systematic reviews of animal experiments occur at a ten fold lower rate compared to equivalent meta-analysis of human studies (Sandercock et al., 2002).

Publishing only positive data (publication bias), and therefore underreporting adverse outcomes, negatively impacts effective preclinical and clinical decision making. In reviewing publications for this chapter, only one paper surfaced reporting neutral data (Penteado et al., 2011), where extracorporeal shockwave therapy applied at the tibial insertion of rabbit patellar ligaments did not change vascularization as is thought the case in clinical application. Interestingly, the authors question if they used the most suitable model. Open access publishing of neutral/negative preclinical research would improve animal model predictability (Barkhordarian et al., 2013) and efforts to analyze systematic reviews and meta-analyses of in vivo preclinical studies are underway (Briel et al., 2013). In sharp contrast, Greek et al. (2013) purport that animal models fail as a predictive modality for human response and that even systematic reviews and meta-analyses of animal-based research do not salvage validity. The relevance of animal models to clinical progression is being questioned (Knight, 2008) and increasing stringency standards for evidence-based reporting of animal-study outcomes represents perhaps the most viable path forward.

The PLOS Medicine Editors (2013) endorse the ARRIVE guidelines for reporting animal research. ARRIVE (Animals in Research: Reporting In Vivo Experiments) guidelines define the minimum information that animal-based research publications should include (see Kilkenny et al., 2013). PLOS Medicine, in fact, now requires the ARRIVE checklist with manuscript submissions and promotes systematic reviews of animal research to enhance clinical-trial design (Hooijmans et al., 2013). Increasing the rate of biomedical research relevant to clinical innovation is a greater than ever concern of researchers and policy-makers worldwide (Vignola-Gagné et al., 2013).

12.3 General Guidelines for In Vivo Animal Experiments

In silico modeling and simulation can reduce the number of animals needed in early stage and preclinical research, as well as facilitate data translation into human clinical trial design. Reducing preclinical studies using mammalian animal models with a combination of in vitro assays, computer simulations, and noninvasive/minimally invasive human studies is a goal of both scientists and of course, animal rights activists. Nevertheless, computer simulations of physiological and pathophysiological processes are only as good as the data used to create them and they are of necessity, themselves, based on in vivo animal studies. The most sophisticated and advanced in vitro biochemical and cellular assay systems cannot serve as a surrogate to the biological complexity inherent in mammalian species. Data gained in vitro for example, differ from that in vivo with reference to scaffold performance (Karageorgiou et al., 2005).

It is essential that translational animal studies are as predictive of human clinical performance as possible. Scientific discovery to clinical utility (preclinical translation) relies on comparative animal models of injury and disease, the choice of which is multifactorial, taking into consideration species, mode of induction, whether acute or chronic in nature and how closely the model simulates targeted clinical maladies. Moving successfully from animal model to human application is onerous at best. Preclinical models are inconsistently predictive first and foremost because we understand relatively little about normal and disease biology. Preclinical studies, from which extrapolated data serve as the basis for clinical trials, are largely conducted using highly inbred animals that fundamentally fail to mimic the genetic and physiologic diversity of the human condition. Patient response is significantly more complex than in preclinical cohorts, due to genetic heterogeneity and variability of injury and comorbidities. We are as a species anything but homogenous and it is legitimate, though at the risk of offending status dogma, to question if non-purebred animals maintained under more natural conditions might yield study results more reflective of human response to therapeutic intervention. As noted by Zerhouni (2005), "it has also become clear that available animal models of human disease are often inadequate." Our proclivity toward study-design/model bias may well contribute to often seen discrepancies between stellar preclinical data and lackluster clinical performance (Muschler et al., 2010).

Additional factors that should be considered with reference to using animals for studying human disease include at minimum, differences in species developmental ontogeny, anatomy, loading and size differences, and of course mechanical, biochemical, and surgical interventions employed to induce the disease/defect model. Many induced animal models demonstrate only acute degeneration, which may be very different from chronic degeneration in humans. Patient comorbidities, such as fracture severity, cardiovascular health, diabetes, and advanced age are confounding factors. Patient use of therapeutics may further modulate musculoskeletal repair. For example, animal studies show that nonsteroidal anti-inflammatory drugs (NSAIDs) inhibit/delay fracture healing (Cottrell et al., 2010).

Animal age is extraordinarily relevant in that studies carried out using young, developing animals manifest outcomes unambiguously different than in a skeletally mature individual and possibly even more so in an older individual with comorbidity-modulated healing (Manolagas et al., 2010; Boskey et al., 2010). It is generally accepted that juveniles heal more quickly and efficiently than aged, concomitant with age-related loss of multipotent stem cells and regenerative capacity (Hasty et al., 2003). Ligament cells from skeletally immature pigs and sheep demonstrate greater cellular proliferation and migration than cells from adolescents or adults, suggesting that skeletal maturity influences biologic repair capacity (Mastrangelo et al., 2010). Cellular and growth factor release from equine pure-platelet rich plasma is similarly affected by intrinsic factors such as gender and age (Giraldo et al., 2013). By way of illustration, Xue et al. (2013) utilized an ex vivo articular cartilage model to demonstrate differential acute-injury healing-related gene expression between neonatal and adult ovine articular cartilage in response to mechanical trauma. Overlooking age-influenced robust-healing responses in young animal cohorts not only compromises study assumptions and biases study outcomes, but significantly contributes to unrealistic clinical-performance expectations and resultant translational failure.

12.3.1 Questions Basic to Tissue Engineering

Tissue engineering has at this point scarcely impacted patient care (Rustad et al., 2010). This results partly from as yet unresolved post-implantation construct/scaffold vascularization requirements (Rouwkema et al., 2008; Esther et al., 2011). In addressing questions of mass transport limitations pertinent to tissue engineered constructs, it is necessary to evaluate defects in which diffusion distances are clinically relevant. Liu et al. (2012) used bone marrow as a blood supply, delayed heparin release as an anticoagulant, and negative pressure therapy to promote scaffold blood-perfusion and vascularization. Swain et al. (2013) utilized a standard model in a novel way, demonstrating that negative pressure applied over scaffold-laden rabbit cranial critical-sized defects produces significant increases in scaffold cell-population/integration and defect closure, supporting the concept that the in situ environment can be manipulated to promote healing, independent of exogenous cells or factors. Creating heterotopic bone around existent vessels positioned in custom-made scaffolds may be a viable technique in reconstructive procedures. For example, Cai et al. (2013) have established an animal model for the study of heterotopic bone formation around vessels in New Zealand White rabbits: rhBMP-2 in a fibrin matrix, with a guided tissue regeneration membrane formed into a tube around a vessel bundle, separating the matrix/rhBMP-2 from skeletal muscle. Innovative adaptive application of established animal models, as above, supports our central thesis that judicious choice/use of preclinical models may expedite translation by addressing recognized hurdles to successful clinical extrapolation.

12.3.2 Impaired or Compromised Healing

The preponderance of animal models used in tissue engineering efforts involves uncontaminated, surgically created wounds, not reflective of most clinical conditions; yet, skeletal healing associated with comorbidities (infection, diabetes, smoking, glucocorticoid therapy) is attendant to increased risk of delayed union or nonunion, osteolysis, fixation failure, and diminished bone properties. Unfortunately, animal models of impaired bone healing are uncommon. Muschler et al. (2010) have provided extensive discussion of attributes that enhance predictive value and more effectively serve as clinically challenging wound-healing models. The authors validate the case for "an urgent need for more rigorous and more biologically relevant preclinical models." Admittedly, these factors are more difficult to consistently reproduce, but multiple-concomitant adverse biological factors more closely approximate recalcitrant clinical expediencies, enhancing clinical relevance and translational success while decreasing unexpected response and outcome.

12.4 Adaptive Application of Established and New Animal Models

A combination of different animal models of increasing stringency may be more representative and predictive, reflecting careful consideration of study and clinically focused hypotheses, with the understanding that no individual in vivo musculoskeletal-defect model stands out as singularly optimal (Horner et al., 2010). By way of example, the following models (reflecting primarily impaired and compromised healing) illustrate aspects of our "informed by clinical goals" thesis.

12.4.1 Craniofacial Models

Traumatic wound sites often entail substantial delay prior to reconstructive intervention, such as following battlefield evacuation and prioritized life-threating stabilization efforts. These delays unavoidably exacerbate reconstructive efforts, partly as a result of scar-tissue formation but also because as the trauma-induced bony hematoma subsides, so do its resident stem-cell populations (Park et al., 2002). To assess the efficiency of specific treatments in a challenging delayed versus immediate reconstruction model, bony defects were evaluated by Hussein et al. (2013). Treatment application was delayed for 4 weeks (rhBMP2/ACS) in periosteum-stripped canine mandibular critical-size segmental defects, substantially compromising the healing response and permitting clinically relevant assessment of possible functional rehabilitation. Barboza et al. (2004) reported that rhBMP2/ACS was effective in reconstructing canine chronic alveolar defects when applied 8 weeks post–defect creation, but the defects were not segmental and periosteum was preserved. Kinsella et al. (2012) reported successful bone regeneration in scarred and infected rabbit calvarial defects in which rhBMP2/ACS application was delayed 6 weeks, though the presence of the dura must be considered as a potentially osteogenic source. These studies demonstrate the utility of modifying preclinical design to more realistically reflect clinical reality, giving consideration to the profound impact of delayed intervention on healing outcome as well as potential treatment options.

Osteonecrosis of the jaw is an uncommon but serious side effect of intravenously administered high-dose bisphosphonate therapy, a standard component of specific cancer treatments (Hoff et al., 2008). Although uncommon, it is a major concern because millions take bisphosphonates for other skeletally targeted diseases (Khosla et al., 2007). Allen et al. (2011) investigated how bisphosphonate treatment affects bone in a post-extraction model in skeletally mature female beagles treated with intravenous zoledronic acid, prior to dental extraction, at doses similar to cancer patient protocol. μCT and dynamic (calcein) histomorphometric assessment demonstrated that extraction socket bone formation was not affected by bisphosphonate but subsequent remodeling was significantly suppressed. Control animals presented with a remodeling rate of approximately 50% per year while bisphosphonate-treated animals had a rate of less than 1%. This compromised osseous-healing model clearly serves to illustrate potential translational failure. If this common patient physiological variance (bisphosphonate altered remodeling rate) is not accounted for in the preclinical study design for new bone-targeted therapies, then predicted-clinical outcome may be dramatically off-the-mark with respect to patients on anti-resorptive therapy.

12.4.2 Long-Bone Models

Numerous animal models have been developed to investigate the etiology of bony nonunions (Niikura et al., 2006; Kokubu et al., 2003; Kratzel et al., 2008); several offer added clinical perspective and/or preclinical design possibilities. Gokhale et al. (2010) have developed a novel model to assess the effectiveness of therapeutic intervention of radiation-induced delayed bone wound healing in C57BL/6NHsd female mice tibiae manifesting combined fracture/irradiation injury. Irradiated bone wounds showed delayed healing but treatment with test articles accelerated healing. Of clinical significance, however, orthotopic Lewis lung carcinoma tumors were not protected from irradiation-induced suppression by the experimental treatment.

In a rat gap-osteotomy model of impaired bone healing, Preininger et al. (2013) demonstrated that proangiogenic progenitor cells isolated from peripheral blood facilitate tissue regeneration, circumventing bone marrow procurement-associated morbidity. The model accounts for major risk factors for impaired bone-healing (Preininger et al., 2012). In female ex-breeder Sprague-Dawley rats (age 12 months; minimum 3 litters) a mid-femoral osteotomy, with external fixator, was used to assess CD34(+) or CD133(+) loaded artificial blood clots; experimental clots improved healing in the aged rat osteotomy model. These observations are of product development and clinical application consequence, in that a limit to mesenchymal stem cell therapeutic use is the morbidity associated with marrow aspiration.

Dimitriou et al. (2012) have summarized experimental and clinical evidence on barrier membrane restoration of difficult-to-heal maxillofacial and orthopedic bone defects. Interestingly, the size of human segmental defects able to be bridged using membranes is not known. The paucity of promising preliminary human studies, though, suggest long-term observations in large animal models are required. Yet of 27 published preclinical studies for reconstruction of long bone defects, 21 used small animal models. Of 23 studies reporting the use of membranes in maxillo-facial reconstruction, 15 used small animal models. These data are indicative of the all too common failure to select animal models most germane to intended clinical goals, product parameters, and regulatory-pathway strategies. Many do not provide data that easily extrapolates to human implementation.

In silico mathematical modeling may prove to be of great value in preclinical-model design and development to promote translational implementation. Geris et al. (2010) used an in vivo model mimicking clinical nonunion and a mathematical model to examine nonunion progression. In silico simulations of periosteal stripping and marrow-canal curettage predicted nonunion. The prediction was confirmed in the subsequent in vivo study, demonstrating the potential value of in silico modeling as an aid to the design of experimental research parameters and protocols, potentially increasing their translational and predictive value.

12.4.3 Musculoskeletal Infection

Most in vivo bone tissue engineering efforts employ sterile, surgically created defects, but one can question the degree to which this reflects the clinically relevant circumstance of contaminated or scarred wounds associated with traumatic injury and delayed reconstruction (Nair et al., 2011). Treatment of infected segmental bone defects endures as a clinical problem, especially as regards infection control, while at the same time facilitating bone/tissue regeneration. To address bone regeneration in the infected environment, animal models must allow for the study of bone regeneration/

repair in the presence of clinically significant infection. The most common preclinical segmental bone-defect model is the rat femur, usually stabilized with fixation devices which exacerbate management problems in infected bone (Costerton et al., 1999; Donlan et al., 2002; Patel et al., 2009; Stinner et al., 2010). Fixation systems (external, internal, or intramedullary) may reflect clinical practice, basically achieved using load-bearing human implants in large-animal defect models (Harvey et al., 2011). Alternatively, scaled fixation devices may enable small-animal model utilization (Matthys et al., 2009; Garcia et al., 2008) and therefore opportunity to address molecular and cellular responses (Auer et al., 2007) in well-characterized murine models.

Interestingly, BMP-2 application concurrent with *S. aureus* inoculation prevents establishment of entrenched infection in critical-size segmental defects in the rat femur model of chronic osteomyelitis (Brick et al., 2009). The avidity with which microorganisms colonize implants, resist antibiotic treatment, and persist in contiguous tissues post–implant removal make prevention of paramount importance. Ideally, one would opt for a prophylactic approach, but there is no consensus *a propos* antibiotic timing. In a rat segmental defect model inoculated with *S. aureus,* Brown et al. (2010) demonstrated the importance of post-inoculation debridement/antibiotic-delivery timing, showing that infection rates significantly increase when antibiotic treatment is delayed 2–6 hours post-inoculation. Antoci et al. (2007) have tested vancomycin-modified titanium alloy rods in a rodent model of osteomyelitis. μCT analysis demonstrated bone resorption around control titanium alloy rods in infected femora, but in femora with vancomycin-modified titanium alloy rods, bone resorption was negligible. The model design allows for development and in vivo testing of more sophisticated metal-antibiotic-implant constructs to prevent implant biofilm formation (Hickok et al., 2012).

Infection resulting from open fracture is a pervasive concern, especially when associated with vascular trauma, as breakdown of the soft-tissue envelope can lead to infection-exacerbated nonunion and possible amputation (Johnson et al., 2007; Neubauer et al., 2006). Standard animal models for studying external traumatic-wound infections (rabbit, canine, sheep, goat) vary significantly in methodology. A comprehensive review of traumatic tibial and femoral open-fracture infection models (Dai et al., 2011) indicates most models use young animals corresponding to humans not yet adult; however, older patients are more susceptible to infection and manifest compromised healing capacity. In many studies, a single gender is used, even though animal gender may additionally impact study outcome. It is of special note, then, that an open-fracture model should closely mimic clinical actuality, involving bone, periosteum, and associated soft and vascular tissues (Buxton et al., 2005; Lindsey et al., 2010) as well as microorganisms often associated with clinical fracture infections, *S. aureus, A. baumannii,* and *P. aeruginosa* (Mody et al., 2009).

In cases of devastating trauma, notwithstanding aggressive antibiotic prophylaxis and delayed hardware placement, infection occurs frequently

(Mody et al., 2009; Moriarty et al., 2010). Orthopedic implants colonized by bacteria develop biofilm-augmented implant-associated pathologies and clinically represent a "train wreck" progression of surgical complications (Del Pozo et al., 2009; Zimmerli et al., 2004). Fixation-device infection can be mitigated so long as biofilm formation is prevented. A new knee prosthesis model of experimental implant-associated osteomyelitis that mimics human temporal progression has been established (Søe et al., 2013). With the prosthesis in situ, an inoculum of *S. aureus* is injected into the medullary canals of rat femur and tibia; the model appears to be effective and reproducible. Niska et al. (2012) have successfully combined in vivo bioluminescent and fluorescent optical imaging with X-ray and µCT in a mouse orthopedic-implant infection model that allows monitoring clinically relevant disease progression. LysEGFP mice, with EGFP-fluorescent neutrophils, were inoculated with bioluminescent *S. aureus*, affording whole body dynamic and temporal in vivo monitoring (Badr et al., 2011). Significantly, only 16 animals were utilized, an extraordinary case in point of the animal reduction possible with advanced in vivo imaging (Pribaz et al., 2012). The Niska et al. (2012) study is an excellent example of applying cutting-edge technologies to enhance the value and utility of a standard model.

The increasing number of diabetic cases is concomitant with increasing numbers of amputations (Cowie et al., 2010). Percutaneous-osseointegrated prostheses show promising clinical performance, but maintaining a skin seal around the implant interface to prevent infection is problematic (Le et al., 2011). A translational load-bearing ovine model to assess postoperative outcome following percutaneous-integrated implant placement has shown utility, with symmetric gait and weight-bearing function (Shelton et al., 2011). This model serves as a good example of a clinical condition/need guiding the design of a preclinical model to address a specific medical problem.

Nishioka et al. (1998) observed metaplasia of pulp connective tissue to bone-like tissue after tooth replantation in conventional and germ-free rats. Experimentally induced severe trauma damaged neurovascular tissues at the apical portion of the teeth, apparently inducing bone marrow cells to migrate into the dental canal/pulp. The absence of infection appears prerequisite to subsequent bony-tissue formation in the root canal space. Variant histologic responses, including intracanal bone, are observed in immature canine teeth with apical periodontitis following the use of antibiotic paste to disinfect the dental canals, substantiating a cause/effect relationship between trauma and infection with respect to specific tissue responses (Wang et al., 2010). All of the above demonstrate the complex healing responses attributable to the extraordinarily intricate interactions between trauma and infection. It is important to recognize in our preclinical assessments that delayed and compromised healing are not the only parameters associated with infection; non-intuitive tissue-specific responses may be induced or proscribed as well.

Diabetes is a complicit metabolic disease risk factor that increases the propensity for prosthetic-associated bacterial infections and its clinical occurrence is increasing (Boulton et al., 2004). Multiple animal models have shown that diabetes affects fracture healing, negatively impacting bone mineral density and biomechanical integrity (Von Herrath et al., 2009). The diabetic BB Wistar rat model, mimicking human type-1 diabetes, has successfully been used as a fracture model to study the effects of, and treatment modalities on, diabetic bone-wound healing (Sood et al., 2013). Implant-related infection in diabetic NOD/ShiLtJ mice, compared with non-diabetic CD1 mice, has proven successful as a model of *S. aureus* orthopedic infection after femur intramedullary pin placement (Lovati et al., 2013). In contrast to controls and CD1 mice, all *S. aureus*-challenged diabetic mice displayed severe implant-associated osteomyelitis. Just as localized trauma increases infection risk and exacerbates implant-associated pathologies, so too do systemic diseases, confounding successful clinical translation of otherwise encouraging preclinical-demonstrated therapeutic interventions. Animal models that manifest systemic disease may provide stringency standards that better screen treatment modalities targeting patient populations with significant incidences of systemic/metabolic maladies.

12.4.4 Cartilage Repair and Osteoarthritis

Articular cartilage repair is the greatest unmet musculoskeletal need/opportunity, with osteoarthritis the most prominent and rapidly growing contributing factor, approaching 2 million U.S. hospital documented cases per year (Hootman et al., 2006). Remarkably, research with respect to the 10,000–40,000 nonunion/malunion cases per year significantly outpaces osteoarthritis research efforts, prompting Parenteau et al. (2012) to suggest that "while bone-related research is appropriately supported, it includes little focus on arthritis and cartilage regeneration research, indicating a possible disconnect between research focus and medical need." This is perhaps the prominent example of where clinical need is not reflected in preclinical focus and effort.

A summary of preclinical osteoarthritis (OA) research highlights discrepancies between animal model and human OA, suggesting "the gold standard animal model has yet to be found" (Longo et al., 2012). There is even disagreement as to whether OA etiology stems from cartilage or bone-initiated pathologies. Nevertheless, recent reviews emphasize the critical role of preclinical models in developing effective treatments for cartilage injury and degeneration (Chu et al., 2010; Gregory et al., 2012; van den Berg et al., 2009). Rodent and rabbit models are cost effective and useful for pilot and proof-of-concept studies. Transgenic and knockout mice facilitate mechanistic studies and athymic mice and rats allow evaluation of human cells and tissues Limiting their translational value, however, are size, cartilage thickness, and intrinsic healing capacity. Large animal models, such as canine, caprine, and porcine (mini-pig), permit study of partial and full thickness chondral and osteochondral repair, but joint size and cartilage thickness are still significantly less than in humans. Based on the average human cartilage lesion size requiring treatment, comparable defects can best be studied in equine models. Although larger animals more closely approximate human clinical parameters, they do so at great financial cost and ethical consideration, especially canine and equine models. In the end, scientific and clinical applicability goals determine the most appropriate animal model (Ahern et al., 2009; Clar et al., 2005; Hunziker, 2002).

ACL surgical destabilization is the most widely used OA-induction method, but manifests onset and disease severity greater than in humans suffering similar injury. Though the ovine stifle joint is a standard model to investigate repair of articular cartilage defects (Osterhoff et al., 2011), patellar luxation is a frequent complication associated with medial parapatellar arthrotomy. A sheep mini-arthrotomy model that provides good exposure of the distal femoral trochlea without risk of postoperative patellar luxation has been developed (Orth et al., 2013a), enhancing the translational value and utility of this model.

Pan et al. (2012) quantified the permeability of the osteochondral interface in the knee joint of adult mice, introducing an innovative modification of a well-established OA model. The data suggest cross-talk between subchondral bone and articular cartilage is elevated in OA, consistent with the view that OA is a whole-joint disease (Goldring et al., 2010; Lories et al., 2011) with increased subchondral-bone turnover (Kwan et al., 2010). Contrast-enhanced EPIC-μCT and fluorescence imaging, employed to characterize articular cartilage, subchondral bone, and vascularization to monitor OA temporal progression in mono-iodoacetate (MIA)-induced OA in rats, has been reported (Xie et al., 2012). Knees of male 8-week old Wistar rats injected with MIA display femoral cartilage characteristics significantly altered in OA-induced knees, coincident with trabecular and subchondral bone loss. These animal models and image-intensive techniques appear to facilitate comprehensive evaluation of induced-OA degeneration, consistent with our concept of enhancing the translational-research value of recognized animal models.

Spontaneous OA models, in contrast with the above-described induction models, manifest disease onset and pace of development more reflective of the human condition, where disease progression is extremely variable (Poole et al., 2010). Age-related degenerative joint diseases, osteoarthritis, and intervertebral disc degeneration (IDD) contribute disproportionately to joint-related disabilities (Aigner et al., 2004). Vo et al. (2013) have recently reviewed causative mechanisms of these diseases and, more specifically, animal models of accelerated aging potentially useful for identifying clinically translatable therapies. ERCC1-deficient mice spontaneously develop osteoporosis and IDD within 6 months, manifesting age-related loss of disc height and degenerative vertebral structural changes (Vo et al., 2010). ERCC1-deficient mice stand out as a physiological exemplary model of accelerated aging for orthopedic research involving OA, IDD, and osteoporosis, mirroring numerous clinical-progression milestones.

Orth et al. (2013b) suggest a possible benefit of bilateral study designs to decrease sample size requirements for certain articular cartilage studies. Standardized osteochondral defects were created in the trochlear groove of rabbits: unilateral defects in 12 animals (n = 12 defects), bilateral defects in 6 animals (n = 12 defects). The unilateral design increased the required number of animals to detect discrete differences. Irrespective of statistical controversies surrounding this assumption, there are metabolic considerations as well. Great caution is urged with respect to the use of bilateral study design, as elevated cross-talk between subchondral bone and articular cartilage has been shown in OA (Pan et al., 2012; above) and bone injuries are known to have systemic influence on skeletal remodeling. Funk et al. (2009) histomorphometrically measured systemic effects of distraction osteogenesis on remodeling of the axial skeleton of mature Yucatan minipigs. A short period of distraction affected remote-site mineral apposition rate, presumably due to locally released growth factor circulation (Bab et al., 1994, 1985; Simmons, 1985; Muller et al., 1991). Systemic stimulation of bone metabolism following trauma is of concern with respect to the use of contralateral side controls (Bab et al., 1985). Interestingly, even stretching of soft tissues (muscle, nerve, skin, blood vessels) may also induce systemic bone-metabolic effects (Muller et al., 1992). More recently, circulating osteogenic precursor cells and their possible roles in bone remodeling have been reviewed (Pignolo et al., 2011). Evidence for such cells employed a parabiosis model whereby two animals share a common circulatory system: a parabiont mouse pair, one constitutively overexpressing green fluorescence protein (GFP) and a wild-type (WT) syngenic partner (Kumagai et al., 2008). After fibular fracture in the WT, GFP-labeled cells localized to the fracture site. Systemic effects of skeletal injury are thus well established. A unilateral design is a more stringent and demanding assessment, reflecting our stance pertaining to preclinical-model choice and rigorous study design.

More than 17 million shoulder rotator-cuff tendon tear injuries are reported yearly in the United States (Yamaguchi et al., 2006). Several in vivo shoulder models have been used to study tendon healing, tendinopathy, and joint instability; however, intrinsic differences among species make translation to clinical application difficult. Despite marked differences between quadruped and biped forelimb anatomy, most experimental animals are weight-bearing quadrupeds. The rat is appropriate to study the pathogenesis of rotator cuff disease or healing mechanisms of biologic treatments at the tendon–bone interface, but mechanical repair strategies are better studied in large animal models utilizing standard-of-care techniques in demanding mechanical-load environments (Longo et al., 2011). Derwin et al. (2010) have summarized ideal preclinical shoulder-model attributes. A true rotator cuff, however, is found only in advanced primates, functionally associated with overhead activity and non-sagittal plane upper limb use (Sonnabend et al., 2009). The baboon appears to best address animal model requirements to study rotator cuff repair (Sonnabend et al., 2010). The use of biomaterial scaffolds to guide host-tissue regeneration may be advantageous. Dickerson et al. (2013) reports the ovine in vivo assessment of a scaffold that facilitates regeneration of a bone–soft-tissue (tendon) interface, utilizing an existing model to test a new therapy to meet a specific clinical need.

12.4.5 Spine

The posterolateral fusion healing environment has been examined in a number of models and differs substantially from that of other bony sites (Boden, 2002). Spinal fusion in mice has been restricted to percutaneous injection of growth factors and mesenchymal stem cells into overlying musculature, precluding vertebral surgical exposure (Hasharoni et al., 2005; Alden et al., 1999); however, knockout and transgenic mice increasingly facilitate genetic and mechanistic studies of bone repair (Schindeler et al., 2009) and progressive diseases such as idiopathic scoliosis (Gao et al., 2007). A new surgical approach in C57BL6 mice suitable for genetically modified models more closely approximates clinical practice, and maximizes reproducibility and extrapolation of data (Bobyn et al., 2013). Studies of osteopenia in scoliotic animals suggest a relationship between adolescent idiopathic scoliosis and osteopenia. Dede et al. (2011) investigated the development of scoliosis in an established bipedal osteopenic rat model, whereby Sprague-Dawley rats are rendered bipedal by surgical intervention (Machida et al., 1999). Study results suggest that osteopenia may in fact contribute to emergent adolescent idiopathic scoliosis, but expose that bipedality itself may cause scoliosis in this model. We highlight this model in a precautionary vein; an established model (bipedality) later shown to manifest an unintended consequence (scoliosis); model choice, study design, and outcome are inexorably linked.

Yang et al. (2012) report the effects of a biphasic synthetic bone graft material implanted in cavities drilled into adjacent vertebrae of skeletally mature sheep to evaluate clinically relevant osteogenesis and remodeling applicable to osteoporotic-related vertebroplasty and kyphoplasty procedures. As an alternative Klein et al. (2013) have utilized a proximal tibia/distal femur sheep model for screening biomaterials for trabecular bone augmentation. They consider it a safe model that could serve as a basis for testing bone inducing or enhancing materials for vertebroplasty. The model also proved adequate for the study of material leakage sequelae such as pulmonary embolism. The sheep long-bone model represents a simpler, easier-to-use model as a possible surrogate for an established spine model.

There is need for preclinical models that approximate human osteoporosis characteristics and associated risk factors (Reinwald et al., 2008). The most studied animal model of osteoporosis is the ovariectomized rat, with cancellous bone remodeling similar to humans, but unlike humans, rats have open epiphyses and no Haversian systems. Bone mineral density (BMD) values from different animal studies are difficult to compare because of differing methods and equipment (Egermann et al., 2005). Additionally, mechanical strength parameters from different models are usually reported without normalizing for cross-sectional shape, and skeletal loading patterns differ substantially compared to humans. Using an established rat model of osteoporosis, Hoff et al. (2010) demonstrated changes in bone mineral with high sensitivity and spatial differentiation to identify local changes in bone mass. Nevertheless, BMD may not correctly predict fracture risk. Volumetric and fractal microarchitecture parameters demonstrate stronger correlation with bone strength than do BMD values (Topolinski et al., 2012). Further complicating clinical evaluations are analytical technical problems with respect to bone samples from humans treated with anti-resorptive bisphosphonates (Recker et al., 2011). These agents substantially reduce remodeling, skewing calculations of in vivo fluorochrome-labeled bone-remodeling dynamics (van Gaalen et al., 2010); specimens frequently contain minimal or no label, creating problems in analyzing histomorphometric parameters. Researchers are urged to consider altered metabolic-remodeling parameter differences between bisphosphonate treated patients and non-treated preclinical animals if the intent is translation to clinical application.

Degenerative disc disease continues to present significant clinical complications (Masuda et al., 2010), at times unresponsive to conventional, conservative interventional therapies. Based on radiological and anatomic similarities between goat and human cervical spines, Qin et al. (2012) implanted artificial vertebra/intervertebral joints in goat cervical spines and evaluated clinical, radiological, and biomechanical parameters to provide preclinical data for treating degenerative disc disease, verifying the model as appropriate for artificial vertebral-joint studies and to serve as a translational model leading to clinical trial study design.

12.5 Cell-Based Tissue Engineering

Clinical solutions to nonunion and osteoporotic fractures remain less than optimal (Kim et al., 2006). Five percent of scaphoid and ten percent of all fractures are nonunion, high morbidity injuries (Munk et al., 2004; Garrison et al., 2007) and a near one-third failure rate is associated with segmental bone-defect surgical management (Sorger et al., 2011), highlighting the challenge of bone regeneration in difficult healing scenarios (Bleich et al., 2012).

12.5.1 Gene Therapy

Osteogenic gene therapy shows great potential to successfully treat clinically challenging appendicular and craniofacial segmental defects caused by trauma or resection. Lazard et al. (2011) have examined bone healing and remodeling subsequent to heterotopic ossification (HO)-induced repair using an adenovirus gene-therapy approach in an exceptionally challenging repair-environment model. A fibula-diaphysis segmental defect was created in adult homozygous Athymic RNU Nude rats. The rodent fibula model is unique in that its proximal and distal ends are fused to the tibia, creating a non-weight-bearing environment, circumventing the need for fixation; the fibular fracture does not heal, but rather undergoes extensive resorption yielding a predictable ~10 mm non-healing gap defect. Significantly, HO induced via adenovirus-transformed cells introduced into a sutured muscle pocket heals critical-size defects even in this resorption-prone environment.

Rapid, cost-effective regenerative strategies are of great interest as economic burdens impede translation of most cell-based therapies. In the first published comparison of a cell-based bone repair technology and autologous bone grafting in a segmental defect model, Betz et al. (2013) compared bone healing capacities of gene-activated muscle grafts with bone grafting in syngeneic Fischer 344 rats. Muscle tissue from the hind limbs was incubated with an adenoviral vector carrying cDNA encoding BMP-2. Femoral bone defects were treated with either BMP-2 activated muscle tissue or autologous bone grafts, with similar results in each group. Routine harvest of muscle tissue is associated with negligible donor site morbidity (Chen et al., 1999). BMP-2 gene-activated muscle tissue could be a source for the augmentation of bone defects as gene-enhanced bone repair methods can be performed during a single surgery. A significant advantage of using a murine model is the availability of transgenic and knockout mouse models that provide the opportunity to advance therapeutic intervention, but the mouse femur-fracture model is technically demanding. To address this, Pelled et al. (2010) established a femoral-fracture mouse model, using internal fixation that permits biomaterial placement.

To assess the potential of gene therapies to impact clinical practice, they must be evaluated in animal models that best simulate clinical conditions (Evans, 2011b), but no "best" model exists. Transgenic mutant-mouse studies too often use single age/gender protocols, which can lead to gene-dependent inaccurate inferences. Clinically directed extrapolation is precarious, as mice manifest significant differences in mechanical loading and remodeling parameters (Elefteriou et al., 2011); yet data obtained in genetically modified mice nonetheless shed light on numerous complex biological interactions. Eventually, though, for gene-therapy strategies to secure broad regulatory approval and move beyond the proof-of-concept phase, they will likely require testing in larger animal models (Ishihara et al., 2008) over extended time periods. As an indication of the difficulties faced by gene-therapy interventions aimed at difficult-to-heal clinical indications, only one gene therapy product has reached the market: Gendicine, in China, for head and neck cancer (Wilson, 2009).

12.5.2 Stem Cells

Difficult-to-heal musculoskeletal defects and diseases are likewise being targeted by stem-cell based experiments and therapies. Topical publications, however, underscore the paucity of clinical utilization, as well as hazards and concerns of mesenchymal stem cell (MSC) use, even though numerous research milestones demonstrate their regenerative capacity (Steinert et al., 2012; Khan et al., 2010; Noth et al., 2010; Kuhn et al., 2010). For example, bone marrow stromal cells (BMSCs) are known to facilitate repair of cartilage and tendon injuries (Shenaq et al., 2010).

Recent studies serve to demonstrate our thesis that multiple animal models are likely needed to advance clinically relevant translational opportunities. Rodents are the *de facto* animal model for stem-cell research (Ren et al., 2012), indicative of the still early-stage nature of the field. A rat rotator-cuff acute tendon-repair surgical model (Gulotta et al., 2009, 2010, 2011) has proven valuable in examining the ability of transfected MSC to enhance tendon-bone refixation and tendon healing. Nevertheless, experimental application of stem cells in tendon repair has shown inconsistent results, with injury-site ectopic bone formation a very real possible consequence (Harris et al., 2004). To demonstrate that BMSCs home to non-osseous sites of ectopic bone formation, Song et al. (2013) used a sex-mismatched canine allogeneic transplantation model to demonstrate BMSC homing to osteoinductive biomaterial-induced ectopic bone-formation sites. Following total body irradiation to achieve immunosuppression in the females, BMSCs of male dogs were injected into female marrow cavities. Y-chromosomes in samples harvested from female dogs showed that bone marrow–derived osteoprogenitors home to sites of induced ectopic ossification. This is an excellent example of model development that provides clinically relevant results.

In treating critical-sized defects, Amorosa et al. (2013) suggested that under physiologic conditions human mesenchymal stem cells (hMSCs) modulate biomechanical characteristics of scaffold materials. Using a rat femoral-defect model, graft sites were treated with autograft, allograft, scaffold, or scaffold with hMSC. hMSC-seeded scaffolds enhanced bone formation and mimicked naive bone mechanical characteristics. Radiographic assessment, however, did not reflect mechanical properties of the repair; though allograft sites had radiographically superior callus bridging, they did not match the biomechanically stiffer hMSC-scaffold treated defects, which appeared radiographically less robust. As a precautionary note, radiographic evaluation may not accurately depict experimental or clinical fracture-healing quality; multiple evaluative techniques should be considered.

Jurgens et al. (2013) evaluated in vivo the osteochondral regenerative capacity of scaffolds seeded with freshly isolated adipose-derived stromal vascular fraction cells or cultured adipose stem cells and compared the results to acellular controls in goat-knee osteochondral defects. Cell-treated constructs exhibited higher levels of regenerated cartilage and mature subchondral bone, demonstrating the feasibility of a one-step surgical procedure for osteochondral-defect regeneration. Freshly isolated adipose stromal cells are at least equal to cultured adipose stem cells in this procedure, with the potential to reduce morbidity and cost by avoiding a second surgical intervention and in vitro expansion, coincident with reduced risk of infection.

Stem cell application, though, carries the risk of unexpected outcome. Regenerated bone tissue from human mandibular graft sites treated with dental pulp mesenchymal stem cells was completely different from control-site alveolar bone three years post-grafting. Analysis revealed that regenerated bone was uniformly vascularized and compact, rather than cancellous, with higher matrix density (Giuliani et al., 2013), possibly enhancing functional performance. While MSC application successfully repaired bone, consideration must be given when grafting stem cells; their differentiation fate and behavior may be affected by their site-specific origin as well as local treatment-area signals. It is known that mesenchymal stem cell differentiation potential is tied to and guided by tissue of origin/recipient site parameters (Porada et al., 2010). FDA guidelines relevant to the design of preclinical studies to assess cell therapy strategies are available (Halme et al., 2006). From a clinical perspective, however, teratoma-forming properties of stem cells and induced pluripotent cells (iPS) continue to be a major concern (Fink, 2009; Gutierrez-Aranda et al., 2010).

Political and economic pressures to keep down the costs of healthcare are dramatically accelerating. Bedside use of minimally manipulated autologous cells incurs few regulatory barriers compared to approaches requiring two invasive procedures and in vitro expansion (Evans et al., 2007). The most efficient and cost-effective progression to clinical success/adoption may preclude in vitro bioreactor expansion (Alman et al., 2011), recognizing that the best bioreactor is the in vivo musculoskeletal environment itself. Remarkably, PubMed shows approximately 200,000 published articles when searching the term "stem cell" (Atala, 2012); that said, some think that maturation of new stem-cell therapies will likely take decades (Daley, 2012). Others are more optimistic, thinking development of efficacious approaches targeting cartilage damage and tendon repair, for example, to be only 5 to 10 years from clinical application (Schmitt et al., 2012).

12.6 Summary

The overwhelming majority of basic science innovations with perceived clinical relevance fail to meet expectations (Contopoulos-Ioannidis et al., 2003). For that to change, we must effectively target clinically relevant endpoints driven by end-user need (Functional Tissue Engineering Conference Group, 2008). More specifically, Spindler et al. (2010) suggest that the goal of "translational models should be to explore proven predictors of clinically relevant outcomes (i.e., 'bedside-to-bench') in sharp contrast to the traditional 'bench-to-bedside' approach." With the research field facing increasing performance scrutiny (Weber, 2013), facilitated preclinical progression and translation is critical. The International Conference of Translational Medicine (ICTM) fosters "bed-to-bench efforts" based on clinical observation (Chen et al., 2012).

Because there is no single or "ideal protocol" set of requirements for preclinical studies, successful, clinically focused hypotheses and animal-model design must reflect end-use therapy-specific factors, recognizing that multiple animal models are likely required to satisfactorily address efficacy, safety and translation. Industry assesses risk/benefit ratios that consider a spectrum of preclinical studies, clinical trials, and manufacturing implementation requiring regulatory approval pathways years in duration, with incumbent financial burden. In vivo data, in addition to basic characterization, elevates the perceived value of a technology and substantially allays proof-of-concept expectations and risk/benefit considerations. Ideally, this flow of research is bidirectional, fluidly moving either direction between basic science and clinical implementation, each informing the other, but ultimately a clinical need must be met to claim success.

Our purpose in this chapter was not to exhaustively review available animal-research models. There are a number of excellent and comprehensive such reviews (see, for example, An et al., 1999; Mooney et al., 2005). Rather, our goal is to emphasize, by way of example, that preclinical design and methods must be guided by, and therefore reflect, intended clinical use and outcome. Every step in that direction is of value. That is to say, expedited clinical translation can be achieved through judicious choice of model, reflecting a "modus operandi" of "bedside-to-bench" informed decision making, focusing ultimately on the desired clinical outcome. Design to succeed.

References

Ahern BJ, Parvizi J, Boston R, Schaer TP (2009) Preclinical animal models in single site cartilage defect testing: A systematic review. *Osteoarthritis Cartilage* 17:705.

Aigner T, Rose J, Martin J, et al. (2004) Aging theories of primary osteoarthritis: From epidemiology to molecular biology. *Rejuvenation Res.* 7:134–145.

Alden TD, Pittman DD, Beres EJ, et al. (1999) Percutaneous spinal fusion using bone morphogenetic protein-2 gene therapy. *J Neurosurg Spine* 90(1):109–114.

Alini M, Eisenstein SM, Ito K, et al. (2008) Are animal models useful for studying human disc disorders/degeneration? *Eur Spine J.* 17:2–19.

Allen MR, Kubek DJ, Burr DB, Ruggiero SL, Chu TG (2011) Compromised osseous healing of dental extraction sites in zoledronic acid-treated dogs. *Osteoporos Int.* 22(2):693–702.

Alman BA, Kelley SP, Nam D (2011) Heal thyself: Using endogenous regeneration to repair bone. *Tissue Eng Part B Rev.* 17(6):431–436.

Amini AR, Laurencin CT, Nukavarapu SP (2012) Bone tissue engineering: Recent advances and challenges. *Crit Rev Biomed Eng.* 40(5):363–408.

Amorosa LF, Lee CH, Aydemir AB, et al. (2013) Physiologic load-bearing characteristics of autografts, allografts, and polymer-based scaffolds in a critical sized segmental defect of long bone: An experimental study. *International J Nanomedicine* 8:1637–1643.

An YH, Friedman RJ (1999) *Animal Models in Orthopaedic Research*. Boca Raton, FL: CRC Press.

Antoci V Jr, Adams CS, Hickok NJ, Shapiro IM, Parvizi J (2007) Vancomycin bound to Ti rods reduces periprosthetic infection: Preliminary study. *Clin Orthop Relat Res* 461:88–95.

Atala A (2012) A new era in stem cells translational medicine. *Stem Cells Translational Med* 1:1–2.

Auer JA, Goodship A, Arnoczky S, et al. (2007) Refining animal models in fracture research: Seeking consensus in optimizing both animal welfare and scientific validity for appropriate biomedical use. *BMC Musculoskeletal Disorders* 8:72.

Bab I, Gazit D, Massarawa A, Sela J (1985) Removal of tibial marrow induces increased formation of bone and cartilage in rat mandibular condyle. *Calcif Tissue Int* 37:551–555.

Bab IA, Einhorn TA (1994) Polypeptide factors regulating osteogenesis and bone marrow repair. *J Cell Biochem* 55:358–365.

Badr CE, Tannous BA (2011) Bioluminescence imaging: Progress and applications. *Trends Biotechnol* 29:624–633.

Barboza EP, Caula AL, Caula FD, et al. (2004) Effect of recombinant human bone morphogenetic protein-2 in an absorbable collagen sponge with space-providing biomaterials on the augmentation of chronic alveolar ridge defects. *J Periodontol* 75:702.

Barkhordarian A, Pellionisz P, Dousti M, et al. (2013) Assessment of risk of bias in translational science. *J Translational Med.* 11:184.

Baroli B (2009) From natural bone grafts to tissue engineering therapeutics: Brainstorming on pharmaceutical formulative requirements and challenges. *J Pharm Sci.* 98(4):1317–1375.

Betz OB, Betz VM, Schröder C, et al. (2013) Repair of large segmental bone defects: BMP-2 gene activated muscle grafts vs. autologous bone grafting. *BMC Biotechnology* 13:65–73.

Bleich NK, Kallai I, Lieberman JR, Schwarz EM, Pelled G, Gazit D (2012) Gene therapy approaches to regenerating bone. *Adv Drug Deliv Rev.* 64(12):1320–1330.

Bobyn J, Rasch A, Little DG, Schindeler A (2013) Posterolateral inter-transverse lumbar fusion in a mouse model. *J Orthopaedic Surg Res* 8:2. http://www.josr-online -com/content/8/1/2

Boden SD. (2002) Overview of the biology of lumbar spine fusion and principles for selecting a bone graft substitute. *Spine* 27:S26–S31.

Boskey AL, Coleman R (2010) Aging and bone. *J Dent Res* 89(12):1333–1348.

Boulton AJ, Kirsner RS, Vileikyte L (2004) Clinical practice: Neuropathic diabetic foot ulcers. *N Engl J Med* 351: 48–55.

Brick KE, Chen X, Lohr J, Schmidt AH, Kidder LS, Lew WD (2009) rhBMP-2 modulation of gene expression in infected segmental bone defects. *Clin Orthop Relat Res.* 467:3096–3103.

Briel M, Müller KF, Meerpohl JJ, et al. (2013) Publication bias in animal research: A systematic review protocol. *Systematic Reviews* 2:23.

Brown KV, Walker JA, Cortez DS, Murray CK, Wenke JC (2010) Earlier debridement and antibiotic administration decrease infection. *J Surg Orthop Adv.* 19:18–22.

Buxton TB, Travis MT, O'shea KJ, et al. (2005) Low-dose infectivity of *Staphylococcus aureus* (SMH strain) in traumatized rat tibiae provides a model for studying early events in contaminated bone injuries. *Comp Med* 55:123–128.

Cahill, KS, Chi, JH, Day A, Claus EB (2009) Prevalence, complications, and hospital charges associated with use of bone-morphogenetic proteins in spinal fusion procedures. *JAMA* 302:58.

Cai W, Zheng L, Weber FE, et al. (2013) Heterotopic bone formation around vessels: Pilot study of a new animal model. *BioResearch Open Access* 2(4):266–272.

Chen HC, Santamaria E, Chen HH, Cheng MH, Chang CJ, Tang YB (1999) Microvascular vastus lateralis muscle flap for chronic empyema associated with a large cavity. *Ann Thorac Surg.* 67(3):866–869.

Chen X, Andersson R, Cho WCS, et al. (2012) The international effort: Building the bridge for Translational Medicine: Report of the 1st International Conference of Translational Medicine (ICTM). *Clinical Translational Med* 1:15.

Chu CR, Szczodry M, Bruno S (2010) Animal models for cartilage regeneration and repair. *Tissue Engineering: Part B* 16(1):105–115.

Clar C, Cummins E, McIntyre LN, et al. (2005) Clinical and cost effectiveness of autologous chondrocyte implantation for cartilage defects in knee joints: Systematic review and economic evaluation. *Health Technol Assess* 9:iii–iv, ix–x, 1.

Contopoulos-Ioannidis DG, Ntzani E, Ioannidis JP (2003) Translation of highly promising basic science research into clinical applications. *Am J Med* 114:477–484.

Costerton JW, Stewart PS, Greenberg EP (1999) Bacterial biofilms: A common cause of persistent infections. *Science* 284:1318–1322.

Cottrell J, O'Connor JP (2010) Effect of non-steroidal anti-inflammatory drugs on bone healing. *Pharmaceuticals* 3:1668–1693.

Cowie CC, Rust KF, Byrd-Holt DD, et al. (2010) Prevalence of diabetes and high risk for diabetes using A1C criteria in the U.S. population in 1988-2006. *Diabetes Care* 33(3):562–568.

Dai T, Kharkwal GB, Tanaka M, Huang Y, Bil de Arce VJ, Hamblin MR (2011) Animal models of external traumatic wound infections. *Virulence* 2(4):296–315.

Daley GQ (2012) The promise and perils of stem cell therapeutics. *Cell Stem Cell* 10(6):740–749.

Dede O, Akel I, Demirkiran G, Yalcin N, Marcucio R, Acaroglu E. (2011) Is decreased bone mineral density associated with development of scoliosis? A bipedal osteopenic rat model. *Scoliosis* 6(1):24.

Del Pozo JL, Patel R (2009) Clinical practice. Infection associated with prosthetic joints. *N Engl J Med* 361:787–794.

Derwin KA, Baker AR, Iannotti JP, et al. (2010) Preclinical models for translating regenerative medicine therapies for rotator cuff repair. *Tissue Eng Part B Rev* 16:21–30.

Dickerson DA, Misk TN, Van Sickle DC, Breur GJ, Nauman EA (2013) In vitro and in vivo evaluation of orthopedic interface repair using a tissue scaffold with a continuous hard tissue-soft tissue transition. *J Orthopaedic Surg Res* 8:18.

Dimitriou R, Mataliotakis GI, Calori GM, Giannoudis PV (2012) The role of barrier membranes for guided bone regeneration and restoration of large bone defects: Current experimental and clinical evidence. *BMC Medicine* 10:81.

Dmitriev AE, Lehman RA Jr, Symes AJ (2011) Bone morphogenetic protein-2 and spinal arthrodesis: The basic science perspective on protein interaction with the nervous system. *Spine J.* 11:500–505.

Donlan RM, Costerton JW (2002) Biofilms: Survival mechanisms of clinically relevant microorganisms. *Clin Microbiol Rev.* 15:167–193.

Egermann M, Goldhahn J, Schneider E (2005) Animal models for fracture treatment in osteoporosis. *Osteoporos Int* 16(suppl 2):S129–S138.

Elefteriou F, Yang X. (2011) Genetic mouse models for bone studies—Strengths and limitations. *Bone* 49(6):1242–1254.

Esther C, Novosel A, Kleinhans A, et al. (2011) Vascularization is the key challenge in tissue engineering. *Adv Drug Deliv Rev.* 63:300–311.

Evans CH (2011a) Barriers to the clinical translation of orthopedic tissue engineering. *Tissue Engineering Part B* 17(6):437–441.

Evans CH (2011b) Gene therapy for the regeneration of bone. *Injury* 42:599–604.

Evans CH, Palmer GD, Pascher A, et al. (2007) Facilitated endogenous repair: Making tissue engineering simple, practical, and economical. *Tissue Eng* 13:1987.

Fink DW Jr. (2009) FDA regulation of stem cell based products. *Science* 324:1662–1663.

Frey-Vasconcells J, Whittlesey KJ, Baum E, Feigal EG (2012) Translation of stem cell research: Points to consider in designing preclinical animal studies. *Stem Cells Translational Med* 1:353–358.

Functional Tissue Engineering Conference Group (2008) Evaluation criteria for musculoskeletal and craniofacial tissue engineering constructs: A conference report. *Tissue Engineering: Part A* 14(12):2089–2104.

Funk JF, Krummrey G, Perka C, Raschke MJ, Bail HJ (2009) Distraction osteogenesis enhances remodeling of remote bones of the skeleton. *Clin Orthop Relat Res* 467:3199–3205.

Gao X, et al. (2007) CHD7 gene polymorphisms are associated with susceptibility to idiopathic scoliosis. *Am J Hum Genet* 80(5):957–965.

Garcia P, Holstein JH, Histing T, et al. (2008) A new technique for internal fixation of femoral fractures in mice: Impact of stability on fracture healing. *J Biomech* 41:1689–1696.

Garrison KR, Donell S, Ryder J, et al. (2007) Clinical effectiveness and cost-effectiveness of bone morphogenetic proteins in the non-healing of fractures and spinal fusion: A systematic review. *Health Technol Assess.* 11:1–150.

Geris L, Reed AAC, Vander Sloten J, Simpson AHRW, Van Oosterwyck H (2010) Occurrence and treatment of bone atrophic non-unions investigated by an integrative approach. *PLoS Comput Biol* 6(9):e1000915.

Giraldo CE, López C, Álvarez ME, Samudio IJ, Prades M, Carmona JU (2013) Effects of the breed, sex and age on cellular content and growth factor release from equine pure-platelet rich plasma and pure-platelet rich gel. *BMC Veterinary Research* 9:29.

Giuliani A, Manescu A, Langer M, et al. (2013) Three years after transplants in human mandibles, histological and in-line holotomography revealed that stem cells regenerated a compact rather than a spongy bone: Biological and clinical implications. *Stem Cells Translational Med* 2:316–324.

Gokhale A, Rwigema J, Epperly M, et al. (2010) Small molecule GS-nitroxide ameliorates ionizing irradiation-induced delay in bone wound healing in a novel murine model. *In Vivo* 24(4):377–385.

Goldring MB, Goldring SR (2010) Articular cartilage and subchondral bone in the pathogenesis of osteoarthritis. *Ann N Y Acad Sci.* 1192:230–237.

Greek R, Menache A (2013) Systematic reviews of animal models: Methodology versus epistemology. *Int. J. Med. Sci.* 10:206–221.

Gregory MH, Capito N, Kuroki K, Stoker AM, Cook JL, Sherman SL (2012) A review of translational animal models for knee osteoarthritis. *Arthritis* Vol 2012, Article ID 764621.

Gulotta LV, Kovacevic D, Ehteshami JR, Dagher E, Packer JD, Rodeo SA (2009) Application of bone marrow derived mesenchymal stem cells in a rotator cuff repair model. *Am J Sports Med* 37(11):2126–2133.

Gulotta LV, Kovacevic D, Montgomery S, Ehteshami JR, Packer JD, Rodeo SA (2010) Stem cells genetically modified with the developmental gene MT1-MMP improve regeneration of the supraspinatus tendon-to-bone insertion site. *Am J Sports Med* 38(7):1429–1437.

Gulotta LV, Kovacevic D, Packer JD, Deng XH, Rodeo SA. (2011) Bone marrow-derived mesenchymal stem cells transduced with scleraxis improve rotator cuff healing in a rat model. *Am J Sports Med* 39(6):1282–1289.

Gutierrez-Aranda I, Ramos-Mejia V, Bueno C, et al. (2010) Human induced pluripotent stem cells develop teratoma more efficiently and faster than human embryonic stem cells regardless the site of injection. *Stem Cells* 28:1568–1570.

Halme DG, Kessler DA (2006) FDA regulation of stem cell-based therapies. *N Engl J Med.* 355, 1730.

Harris MT, Butler DL, Boivin GP, Florer JB, Schantz EJ, Wenstrup RJ (2004) Mesenchymal stem cells used for rabbit tendon repair can form ectopic bone and express alkaline phosphatase activity in constructs. *J Orthopaedic Res.* 22(5):998–1003.

Harvey EJ, Giannoudis PV, Martineau PA, et al. (2011) Preclinical animal models in trauma research. *J Orthop Trauma* 25:488–493.

Hasharoni A, et al. (2005) Murine spinal fusion induced by engineered mesenchymal stem cells that conditionally express bone morphogenetic protein-2. *J Neurosurg Spine* 3(1):47–52.

Hasty P, Campisi J, Hoeijmakers J, et al. (2003) Aging and genome maintenance: Lessons from the mouse? *Science* 299:1355–1359.

Hellman, KB, Johnson, PC, Bertram, TA, Tawil, B (2011) Challenges in tissue engineering and regenerative medicine product commercialization: Building an industry. *Tissue Eng Part A* 17(1–2):1–3.

Henderson VC, Kimmelman J, Fergusson D, Grimshaw JM, Hackam DG (2013) Threats to validity in the design and conduct of preclinical efficacy studies: A systematic review of guidelines for in vivo animal experiments. *PLoS Med* 10(7): e1001489.

Hickok NJ, Shapiro IM (2012) Immobilized antibiotics to prevent orthopedic implant infections. *Adv Drug Deliv Rev* 64(12):1165–1176.

Hoff AO, Toth BB, Altundag K, et al. (2008) Frequency and risk factors associated with osteonecrosis of the jaw in cancer patients treated with intravenous bisphosphonates. *J Bone Miner Res* 23:826–836.

Hoff BA, Kozloff KM, Boes JL, et al. (2010) Parametric response mapping of CT images provides early detection of local bone loss in a rat model of osteoporosis. *Bone* 51(1):78–84.

Hollister SJ, Murphy WL (2011) Scaffold translation: Barriers between concept and clinic. *Tissue Engineering: Part B* 17(6):459–474.

Hooijmans CR, Ritskes-Hoitinga M (2013) Progress in using systematic reviews of animal studies to improve translational research. *PLoS Med* 10(7):e1001482.

Hootman, JM, Helmick, CG (2006) Projections of US prevalence of arthritis and associated activity limitations. *Arthritis Rheum* 54(1):226–229.

Horner EA, Kirkham J, Wood D, et al. (2010) Long bone defect models for tissue engineering applications: Criteria for choice. *Tissue Engineering: Part B* 16(2):263–271.

Hunziker, EB (2002) Articular cartilage repair: Basic science and clinical progress. A review of the current status and prospects. *Osteoarthritis Cartilage* 10(6):432–463.

Hussein K, Zakhary I, Hailat D, Elrefai R, Sharawy M, Elsalanty M (2013) Delayed versus immediate reconstruction of mandibular segmental defects using recombinant human bone morphogenetic protein 2/absorbable collagen sponge. *J Oral Maxillofac Surg* 71(6):1107–1118.

Ishihara A, Shields KM, Litsky AS, et al. (2008) Osteogenic gene regulation and relative acceleration of healing by adenoviral-mediated transfer of human BMP-2 or -6 in equine osteotomy and ostectomy models. *J Orthop Res.* 26:764–771.

Jiang F, Zhang J, Wang X, Shen X (2013) Important steps to improve translation from medical research to health policy. *J Translational Med.* 11:33.

Johnson EN, Burns TC, Hayda RA, Hospenthal DR, Murray CK (2007) Infectious complications of open type III tibial fractures among combat casualties. *Clin Infect Dis* 45:409–415.

Johnson PC, Bertram TA, Tawil B, Hellman KB (2011) Hurdles in tissue engineering/regenerative medicine product commercialization: A survey of North American academia and industry. *Tissue Eng Part A* 17(1–2):5–15.

Jurgens WJFM, Kroeze RJ, Zandieh-Doulabi B, et al. (2013) One-step surgical procedure for the treatment of osteochondral defects with adipose-derived stem cells in a caprine knee defect: A pilot study. *BioResearch Open Access* 2(4):315–325.

Karageorgiou V, Kaplan D (2005) Porosity of 3D biomaterial scaffolds and osteogenesis. *Biomaterials* 26(27):5474–5491.

Kelley M, Edwards K, Starks H, et al. (2012) Values in translation: How asking the right questions can move translational science toward greater health impact. *Clin Trans Sci* 5:445–451.

Khan WS, Rayan F, Dhinsa BS, Marsh D (2012) An osteoconductive, osteoinductive, and osteogenic tissue-engineered product for trauma and orthopaedic surgery: How far are we? *Stem Cells International* Vol 2012, Article ID 236231.

Khosla S, Burr D, Cauley J, et al. (2007) Bisphosphonate-associated osteonecrosis of the jaw: Report of a task force of the American Society for Bone and Mineral Research. *J Bone Miner Res* 22:1479–1491.

Kilkenny C, Browne WJ, Cuthill IC, Emerson M, Altman DG (2010) Improving bioscience research reporting: The ARRIVE guidelines for reporting animal research. *J Pharmacol Pharmacother* 1:94–99.

Kim DH, Vaccaro AR (2006) Osteoporotic compression fractures of the spine; current options and considerations for treatment. *Spine J* 6:479–487.

Kinsella CR, Cray JJ, Smith DM, et al. (2012) Novel model of calvarial defect in an infected unfavorable wound: Reconstruction with rhBMP-2. Part II. *J Craniofac Surg* 23(2):410–414.

Klein K, Zamparo E, Kronen PW, et al. (2013) Bone augmentation for cancellous bone development of a new animal model. *BMC Musculoskeletal Disorders* 14:200.

Kleinbeck K, Anderson E, Ogle M, Burmania J, Kao WJ. (2012) The new (challenging) role of academia in biomaterial translational research and medical device development. *Biointerphases* 7(0):12.

Knight A (2008) Systematic reviews of animal experiments demonstrate poor contributions toward human healthcare. *Rev Recent Clin Trials* 3(2):89–96.

Kokubu T, Hak DJ, Hazelwood SJ, Reddi AH (2003) Development of an atrophic nonunion model and comparison to a closed healing fracture in rat femur. *J Orthop Res* 21:503–510.

Kratzel C, Bergmann C, Duda G, Greiner S, Schmidmaier G, Wildemann B (2008) Characterization of a rat osteotomy model with impaired healing. *BMC Musculoskeletal Disorders* 9:135.

Kuhn NZ, Tuan RS (2010) Regulation of stemness and stem cell niche of mesenchymal stem cells: Implications in tumorigenesis and metastasis. *J Cell Physiol* 222:268–277.

Kumagai K, Vasanji A, Drazba JA, Butler RS, Muschler GF (2008) Circulating cells with osteogenic potential are physiologically mobilized into the fracture healing site in the parabiotic mice model. *J Orthop Res* 26:165–175.

Kwan TS, Lajeunesse D, Pelletier JP, Martel-Pelletier J (2010) Targeting subchondral bone for treating osteoarthritis: What is the evidence? *Best Pract Res Clin Rheumatol.* 24:51–70.

Lazard ZW, Heggeness MH, Hipp JA, et al. (2011) Cell-based gene therapy for repair of critical size defects in the rat fibula. *J Cell Biochem* 112(6):1563–1571.

Le NN, Rose MB, Levinson H, Klitzman B (2011) Implant healing in experimental animal models of diabetes. *J Diabetes Sci Tech* 5(3):605–618.

Lindsey BA, Clovis NB, Smith ES, Salihu S, Hubbard DF (2010) An animal model for open femur fracture and osteomyelitis: Part I. *J Orthop Res* 28:38–42.

Liu F, Yu S, Wang Z, Sun X (2012) Biomimetic construction of large engineered bone using hemoperfusion and cyto-capture in traumatic bone defect. *BioResearch Open Access* 1(5):247–251.

Longo UG, Forriol F, Campi S, Maffulli N, Denaro V (2011) Animal models for translational research on shoulder pathologies: From bench to bedside. *Sports Med Arthrosc Rev* 19:184–193.

Longo UG, Loppini M, Fumo C, et al. (2012) Osteoarthritis: New insights in animal models. *Open Orthopaedics J* 6(3):M11, 558–563.

Lories RJ, Luyten FP (2011) The bone-cartilage unit in osteoarthritis. *Nat Rev Rheumatol.* 7(1):43–49.

Lovati AB, Drago L, Monti L, et al. (2013) Diabetic mouse model of orthopaedic implant-related *Staphylococcus aureus* infection. *PLoS ONE* 8(6):e67628.

Machida M, Murai I, Miyashita Y, Dubousset J, Yamada T, Kimura J (1999) Pathogenesis of idiopathic scoliosis. Experimental study in rats. *Spine* 24:1985–1989.

Manolagas SC, Parfitt AM (2010) What old means to bone. *Trends Endocrinol Metab* 21(6):369–374.

Markel DC, Guthrie ST, Wu B, Song Z, Wooley PH (2012) Characterization of the inflammatory response to four commercial bone graft substitutes using a murine biocompatibility model. *J Inflammation Res.* 5:13–18.

Mastrangelo AN, Magarian EM, Palmer MP, Vavken P, Murray MM (2010) The effect of skeletal maturity on the regenerative function of intrinsic ACL cells. *J Orthop Res.* 28(5):644–651.

Masuda K, Lotz, JC (2010) New challenges for intervertebral disc treatment using regenerative medicine. *Tissue Engineering, Part B* 16(1):147–158.

Matthys R, Perren SM (2009) Internal fixator for use in the mouse. *Injury* 40(suppl 4):S103–S109.

McGartland Rubio D, Schoenbaum EE, Lee LS, et al. (2010) Defining translational research: Implications for training. *Acad Med.* 85(3):470–475.

Meslin EM, Blasimme A, Cambon-Thomsen A (2013) Mapping the translational science policy 'valley of death.' *Clinical Translational Med* 2:14.

Mody RM, Zapor M, Hartzell JD, et al. (2009) Infectious complications of damage control orthopedics in war trauma. *J Trauma* 67:758–61.

Mooney MP and Siegel MI (2005) Animal models for bone tissue engineering of critical-sized defects (CSDs), bone pathologies and orthopedic disease states. In: Hollinger, J.O., Einhorn, T.A., Doll, B.A., Sfeir C. (Eds.). *Fundamentals of Bone Tissue Engineering*, pp. 217–244. Boca Raton, FL: CRC Press.

Moriarty TF, Schlegel U, Perren S, Richards RG (2010) Infection in fracture fixation: Can we influence infection rates through implant design? *J Mater Sci Mater Med* 21:1031–1035.

Muller M, Schilling T, Minne HW, Ziegler R (1991) A systemic acceleratory phenomenon (SAP) accompanies the regional acceleratory phenomenon (RAP) during healing of a bone defect in the rat. *J Bone Miner Res* 6:401–410.

Muller M, Schilling T, Minne HW, Ziegler R (1992) Does immobilization influence the systemic acceleratory phenomenon that accompanies local bone repair? *J Bone Miner Res* 7:S425–S427.

Munk B, Larsen CF (2004) Bone grafting the scaphoid nonunion: A systematic review of 147 publications including 5246 cases of scaphoid nonunion. *Acta Orthop Scand.* 75:618–629.

Muschler G, Raut V, Patterson T, Wenke J, Hollinger J (2010) The design and use of animal models for translational research in bone tissue engineering and regenerative medicine. *Tissue Eengineering. Part B* 16:123–145.

Nair M, Kretlow J, Mikos A, Kasper F (2011) Infection and tissue engineering in segmental bone defects—A mini review. *Curr Opin Biotechnol.* 22(5):721–725.

Neubauer T, Bayer GS, Wagner M (2006) Open fractures and infection. *Acta Chir Orthop Traumatol Cech* 73:301–12.

Niikura T, Hak DJ, Reddi AH (2006) Global gene profiling reveals a down regulation of BMP gene expression in experimental atrophic non-unions compared to standard healing fractures. *J Orthop Res* 24:1463–1471.

Nishioka M, Shiiya T, Ueno K, Suda H (1998) Tooth replantation in germ-free and conventional rats. *Endod Dent Traumatol* 14:163–73.

Niska JA, Meganck JA, Pribaz JR, et al. (2012) Monitoring bacterial burden, inflammation and bone damage longitudinally using optical and µCT imaging in an orthopaedic implant infection in mice. *PLoS ONE* 7(10):e47397.

Noth U, Rackwitz L, Steinert AF et al. (2010) Cell delivery therapeutics for musculoskeletal regeneration. *Adv Drug Deliv Rev* 62:765–783.

O'Keefe RJ, Mao J (2011) Bone tissue engineering and regeneration: From discovery to the clinic—An overview. *Tissue Engineering: Part B* 17(6):389–392.

Orth P, Madry H (2013a) A low morbidity surgical approach to the sheep femoral trochlea. *BMC Musculoskeletal Disorders* 14:5.

Orth P, Zurakowski D, Alini M, Cucchiarini M, Madry H (2013b) Reduction of sample size requirements by bilateral versus unilateral research designs in animal models for cartilage tissue engineering. *Tissue Engineering Part C* 19(11):885–891.

Osterhoff G, Loffler S, Steinke H, Feja C, Josten C, Hepp P (2011) Comparative anatomical measurements of osseous structures in the ovine and human knee. *Knee* 18:98–103.

Pan J, Wang B, Li W, et al. (2012) Elevated cross-talk between subchondral bone and cartilage in osteoarthritic joints. *Bone* 51(2):212–217.

Parenteau N, Hardin-Young J, Shannon W, Cantini P, Russell A (2012) Meeting the need for regenerative therapies I: Target-based incidence and its relationship to U.S. spending, productivity, and innovation. *Tissue Engineering: Part B* 18(2):139–154.

Park SH, Silva M, Bahk WJ, et al. (2002) Effect of repeated irrigation and debridement on fracture healing in an animal model. *J Orthop Res* 20:1197.

Patel M, Rojavin Y, Jamali AA, Wasielewski SJ, Salgado CJ (2009) Animal models for the study of osteomyelitis. *Seminars Plastic Surg* 23(2):148–15.

Pelled G, Ben-Arav A, Hock C, et al. (2010) Direct gene therapy for bone regeneration: Gene delivery, animal models, and outcome measures. *Tissue Engineering: Part B* 16(1):13–20.

Penteado FT, Faloppa F, Giusti G, Moraes VY, Belloti JC, Gomes dos Santos JB (2011) High-energy extracorporeal shockwave therapy in a patellar tendon animal model: A vascularization focused study. *Clinics* 66(9):1611–1614.

Pignolo RJ, Kassem M (2011) Circulating osteogenic cells: Implications for injury, repair, and regeneration. *J Bone Mineral Res.* 26(8):1685–1693.

Poole R, Blake S, Buschmann M, et al. (2010) Recommendations for the use of preclinical models in the study and treatment of osteoarthritis. *Osteoarthritis Cartilage* 18(Suppl 3):S10–16.

Porada CD, Almeida-Porada G (2010) Mesenchymal stem cells as therapeutics and vehicles for gene and drug delivery. *Advanced Drug Delivery Reviews* 62(12):1156–1166.

Preininger B, Bruckner J, Perka C, et al. (2012) An experimental setup to evaluate innovative therapy options for the enhancement of bone healing using BMP as a benchmark—A pilot study. *eCells Materials* 23:262–272.

Preininger B, Duda G, Gerigk H, et al. (2013) CD133: Enhancement of bone healing by local transplantation of peripheral blood cells in a biologically delayed rat osteotomy model. *PLoS ONE* 8(2):e52650.

Pribaz JR, Bernthal NM, Billi F, et al. (2012) Mouse model of chronic post-arthroplasty infection: Noninvasive in vivo bioluminescence imaging to monitor bacterial burden for long-term study. *J Orthop Res* 30:335–340.

Qin J, He X, Wang D et al. (2012) Artificial cervical vertebra and intervertebral complex replacement through the anterior approach in animal model: A biomechanical and in vivo evaluation of a successful goat model. *PLoS ONE* 7(12):e52910.

Recker RR, Kimmel DB, Dempster D, Weinstein RS, Wronski T, Burr, DB (2011) Issues in modern bone histomorphometry. *Bone* 49(5):955–964.

Reinwald S, Burr D (2008) Review of nonprimate, large animal models for osteoporosis research. *J Bone Miner Res* 23:1353–1368.

Ren G, Chen X, Dong F, Li W, Ren X, Zhang Y, Shia Y (2012) Concise review: Mesenchymal stem cells and translational medicine: Emerging issues. *Stem Cells Translational Med* 1:51–58.

Rouwkema J, Rivron NC, van Blitterswijk CA. (2008) Vascularization in tissue engineering. *Trends Biotechnology* 26(8):434–441.

Rundle, C.H., Wang, H., Yu, H. et al. (2006) Microarray analysis of gene expression during the inflammation and endochondral bone formation stages of rat femur fracture repair. *Bone* 38(4):521–529.

Rustad KC, Sorkin M, Levi B, Longaker MT, Gurtner GC (2010) Strategies for organ level tissue engineering. *Organogenesis* 6(3):151–157.

Sandercock P, Roberts I (2002) Systematic reviews of animal experiments. *Lancet* 360:586.

Schindeler A, Liu R, Little DG (2009) The contribution of different cell lineages to bone repair: Exploring a role for muscle stem cells. *Differentiation* 77(1):12–18.

Schmitt A, van Griensven M, Imhoff AB, Buchmann S (2012) Application of stem cells in orthopedics. *Stem Cells International*. Article ID 394962.

Scott M, Levi B, Askarinam A, et al. (2012) Brief review of models of ectopic bone formation. *Stem Cells Develop* 21(5):655–667.

Shelton TJ, Beck JP, Bloebaum RD, Bachus KN (2011) Percutaneous osseointegrated prostheses for amputees: Limb compensation in a 12-month ovine model. *J Biomech*. 44(15):2601–2606.

Shenaq DS, Rastegar F, Petkovic D, et al. (2010) Mesenchymal progenitor cells and their orthopedic applications: Forging a path towards clinical trials. *Stem Cells International*. Article ID 519028.

Simmons DJ (1985) Fracture healing perspectives. *Clin Orthop Relat Res* 200:100–113.

Smith CL, Jarrett M, Bierer SB (2013) Integrating clinical medicine into biomedical graduate education to promote translational research: Strategies from two new PhD programs. *Acad Med* 88(1):137–143.

Søe NH, Jensen NV, Nürnberg BM, et al. (2013) A novel knee prosthesis model of implant-related osteomyelitis in rats. *Acta Orthopaedica* 84(1):92–97.

Song G, Habibovic P, Bao C, et al. (2013) The homing of bone marrow MSCs to non-osseous sites for ectopic bone formation induced by osteoinductive calcium phosphate. *Biomaterials* 34(9):2167–2176.

Sonnabend DH, Young AA (2009) Comparative anatomy of the rotator cuff. *J Bone Joint Surg Br* 91:1632–1637.

Sonnabend DH, Howlett CR, Young AA (2010) Histological evaluation of repair of the rotator cuff in a primate model. *J Bone Joint Surg Br* 92:586–594.

Sood A, Cunningham C, Lin S. (2013) The BB Wistar rat as a diabetic model for fracture healing infections. *ISRN Endocrinology* Vol 2013, Article ID 349604.

Sorger JI, Hornicek FJ, Zavatta M, et al. (2001) Allograft fractures revisited. *Clin Orthop Relat Res*. (382):66–74.

Spindler KP, Dunn WR (2010) The rationale for identifying clinical predictors modifiable by tissue engineering for translational models. *Tissue Engineering: Part B* Vol 16(1):117–21.

Steinert AF, Rackwitz L, Gilbert F, Noth U, Tuan RS (2012) Concise review: The clinical application of mesenchymal stem cells for musculoskeletal regeneration: Current status and perspectives. *Stem Cells Translational Med* 1:237–247.

Stinner DJ, Keeney JA, Hsu JR, et al. (2010) Outcomes of internal fixation in a combat environment. *J Surg Orthop Adv*. 19:49–53.

Swain L, Cornet D, Manwaring M, Collins B, Singh VK, Beniker DH, Carnes DL Jr. (2013) Negative pressure therapy stimulates healing of critical-size calvarial defects in rabbits. *BoneKEy Reports* 2, Article #299.

The PLOS Medicine Editors (2013) Translating translational research into global health gains. *PLoS Med* 10(7):e1001493.

Topolinski T, Mazurkiewicz A, Jung S, Cichanski A, Nowicki K (2012) Microarchitecture parameters describe bone structure and its strength better than BMD. *Scientific World J* Vol 2012, Article ID 502781.

Trochim W, Kane C, Graham M, Pincus H (2011) Evaluating translational research: A process marker model. *Clin Transl Sci.* 4(3):153–162.

van den Berg WB. (2009) Lessons from animal models of arthritis over the past decade. *Arthritis Research Therapy* 11:250.

van Gaalen SM, Kruyt MC, Geuze RE, de Bruijn JD, Alblas J, Dhert WJA. (2010) Use of fluorochrome labels in in vivo bone tissue engineering research. *Tissue Eng Part B Rev.* 16:209–217.

Vignola-Gagné E, Rantanen E, Lehner D, Hüsing B. (2013) Translational research policies: Disruptions and continuities in biomedical innovation systems in Austria, Finland and Germany. *J Community Genet* 4:189–201.

Vo N, Seo HY, Robinson A, et al. 2010. Accelerated aging of intervertebral discs in a mouse model of progeria. *J Orthop Res.* 28:1600–1607.

Vo N, Niedernhofer LJ, Nasto LA, et al. (2013) An overview of underlying causes and animal models for the study of age-related degenerative disorders of the spine and synovial joints. *J Orthop Res* 31:831–837.

Von Herrath M, Nepom GT (2009) Animal models of human type 1 diabetes. *Nat Immunol.* 10(2):129–132.

Wang X, Thibodeau B, Trope M, Lin L, Huang G (2010) Histologic characterization of regenerated tissues in canal space after the revitalization/revascularization procedure of immature dog teeth with apical periodontitis. *J Endod* 36:56–63.

Weber GM (2013) Identifying translational science within the triangle of biomedicine. *J Translational Med* 11:126.

Wilson, JM (2009) Medicine. A history lesson for stem cells. *Science* 324(5928):727–728.

Wong, D.A., Kumar, A., Jatana, S., Ghiselli, G., and Wong, K (2008) Neurologic impairment from ectopic bone in the lumbar canal: A potential complication of off-label PLIF/TLIF use of bone morphogenetic protein-2 (BMP-2). *Spine J* 8(6):1011–1018.

Woolfson, DN, Mahmoud, ZN (2010) More than just bare scaffolds: Towards multicomponent and decorated fibrous biomaterials *Chem Soc Rev* 39:3464.

Xie L, Lin ASP, Kundu K, Levenston ME, Murthy N, Goldberg RE (2012) Quantitative imaging of cartilage and bone morphology, reactive oxygen species, and vascularization in a rodent model of osteoarthritis. *Arthritis Rheum* 64(6):1899–1908.

Xue X, Zheng Q, Wu H, Zou L, Li P (2013) Different responses to mechanical injury in neonatal and adult ovine articular cartilage. *BioMedical Engineering OnLine* 12:53.

Yamaguchi K, Ditsios K, Middleton WD, Hildebolt CF, Galatz LM, Teefey SA (2006) The demographic and morphological features of rotator cuff disease. A comparison of asymptomatic and symptomatic shoulders. *J Bone Joint Surg Am* 88(8):1699–1704.

Yang HL, Zhu XS, Chen L, et al. (2012) Bone healing response to a synthetic calcium sulfate/b-tricalcium phosphate graft material in a sheep vertebral body defect model. *J Biomed Mater Res Part B* 100B:1911–1921.

Zerhouni EA (2005) Translational and clinical science—Time for a new vision. *N Engl J Med* 353(15):1621–1623.

Zimmerli W, Trampuz A, Ochsner PE (2004) Prosthetic-joint infections. *N Engl J Med* 351:1645–1654.

13

Regulatory Premarketing Processes

Patsy J. Trisler

CONTENTS

13.1 Introduction and Scope

The Food and Drug Administration (FDA) is the gatekeeper for the clinical evaluation and ultimate marketing of all products classified as medical devices. Bone graft substitute (also referred to as bone void filler) products, regardless of the medical indication, specified intended use, and composition of the product, are medical devices. As described below, some may be considered Combination Products, but if the primary intended purpose (primary mode of action [PMOA]) is to serve as a graft filler for osteoconductive purposes, under the current regulatory approach, the product will be considered to have a device PMOA and it will be regulated primarily as a device.

The FDA Centers that could be involved in regulation of these products are noted here and described further below. The primary FDA Center with regulatory authority over bone grafts is the Center for Devices and Radiological Health (CDRH). Within CDRH, three different Divisions manage submissions, depending on the intended use. The Center for Biologics Evaluation and Research (CBER) and the Center for Drug Evaluation and Research (CDER) will become more and more involved in the bone graft substitute product area as development continues with use of cells, tissues, blood products, proteins, and growth factors, as well as traditional drugs, such as antibiotics, when included as components or constituents of the final product.

Most new products which are composed of a traditional device (a synthetic or natural substance that serves as an osteoconductive scaffold) and a biologic or drug will be considered Combination Products by the FDA; many will continue to be regulated primarily by CDRH, depending on the determination of PMOA. Unless a very similar combination has been previously "regulated," it is advisable and may be necessary to obtain a reading or determination from the FDA's Office of Combination Products (OCP), in response to submission of a Request for Designation (RFD).

13.2 Regulatory Definitions

The following definitions and references are pertinent to the information presented in this chapter. Regulated products are either categorized as a medical device, biological, or drugs. Definitions for each category are as follows:

13.2.1 Medical Device

(Section 201(h) of the FD&C Act) The term "device" means an instrument, apparatus, implement, machine, contrivance, implant, in vitro reagent, or other similar or related article, including any component, part, or accessory, which is (1) recognized in the official National Formulary, or the United States Pharmacopeia, or any supplement to them; (2) intended for use in the diagnosis of disease or other conditions, or in the cure, mitigation, treatment, or prevention of disease, in man or other animals; or (3) intended to affect the structure or any function of the body of man or other animals, and which does not achieve its primary intended purposes through chemical action within or on the body of man or other animals and which is not dependent upon being metabolized for the achievement of its primary intended purposes. Medical devices are regulated primarily under the requirements in 21 CFR Sections 800-1050 primarily by the CDRH.

13.2.2 Biological

The definition of a biological is not as precise as a medical device. The FDA's regulatory authority for biologics is found in the Public Health Service (PHS) Act as well as the FD&C Act under the "Drugs" definition. The FDA has divided biologics into those that will be regulated by CBER and those regulated by CDER. Those categories regulated by CBER include human tissue and cellular products used in transplantation, gene therapy products, vaccines, allergenic extracts (for allergy shots and tests), antitoxins/antivenins/ venoms, and blood/blood components/plasma-derived products (including recombinant and transgenic versions). The categories regulated by CDER include those products mostly produced by biotechnology methods, including monoclonal antibodies designed as targeted therapies in cancer and other diseases, cytokines (proteins involved in immune response), immunomodulators (non-vaccine and non-allergenic agents that affect immune response), growth factors (proteins that affect the growth of a cell), and enzymes that speed up biochemical reactions.

13.2.3 Drug

Under Section 201(g) of the FD&C Act, the term "drug" means: (1) articles recognized in the official United States Pharmacopoeia, official Homoeopathic

Pharmacopoeia of the United States, or official National Formulary, or any supplement to any of them; (2) articles intended for use in the diagnosis, cure, mitigation, treatment, or prevention of disease in man or other animals; (3) articles (other than food) intended to affect the structure or any function of the body of man or other animals; and/or (4) articles intended for use as a component of any article specified in clause (1), (2), or (3) of this sub-section.

13.3 Medical Device Classification System

General Controls (Table 13.1), described in the FD&C Act, are basic provisions that provide the FDA with the means to regulate devices so as to ensure that these devices are safe and effective. Manufacturers of all products that are considered medical devices must comply with these General

TABLE 13.1

FD&C Act Sections for General Controls Categories

Section	General Control	Section	General Control
501	Adulterated devices	518	Notifications and other remedies • Notification • Repair • Replacement • Refund • Reimbursement • Mandatory recall
502	Misbranded devices	519	Records and reports on devices • Adverse event report • Device tracking • Unique device identification system • Reports of removals and corrections
510	Registration of producers of devices • Establishment registration and device listing • Premarket Notification (510k) • Reprocessed single-use devices	520	General provisions respecting control of devices intended for human use • Custom device • Restricted device • Good manufacturing practice requirements • Exemptions for devices for investigational use • Transitional provisions for devices considered as new drugs • Humanitarian device exemption
516	Banned devices		

Controls. Special Controls are usually device-specific and are listed in Table 13.2. Depending on the product types and risk, these products are then classified into one of the following three classes and the regulatory requirements: (1) Class I (low to moderate risk) General Controls, whereby devices are exempt from premarketing review; (2) Class II (moderate to high risk) General and Special Controls, whereby devices require the FDA's review and clearance of a 510(k) before marketing the device; and (3) Class III (high risk) General Controls, whereby devices require the FDA's review and approval of a Premarket Approval (PMA) Application.

13.4 Medical Device Regulatory Submissions

Note that reference to www.fda.gov/MedicalDevices/default.htm will take you to the CDRH home page where a search for guidance documents and other resource materials related to the following submission types is readily accessible. Except as noted, most of these submissions would be made to CDRH, but as relevant CBER might be the recipient FDA Center.

13.4.1 Investigational Device Exemption (IDE)

21 CFR 812: An application requesting the FDA's approval to conduct a clinical trial of a significant risk (SR) medical device. Bone graft products are considered SR primarily because they are implanted materials.

13.4.2 510(k) Premarket Notification

21 CFR 807: An application (notification) requesting clearance to market a device that is presented as being substantially equivalent (SE) to another device (a predicated device) legally on the market. The substantial equivalence is based on having the same intended use and similar technological characteristics as the predicate device(s). The 510(k) pathway is primarily for Class II devices and most bone graft products receiving permission to market via the 510(k) pathway.

TABLE 13.2

Special Controls

Performance standards
Postmarket surveillance
Patient registries
Special labeling requirements
Premarket data requirements
Guidelines

13.4.3 De Novo

Evaluation of Automatic Class III Determination (added as an option in FDAMA, 1997 and modified in FDASIA, 2012): An application for classification of (and permission to market) a novel device that is low to moderate risk and which has no predicate. Examples are bone graft substitutes that do qualify for De Novo are under the current interpretation of "low to moderate risk" devices.

13.4.4 Humanitarian Device Exemption (HDE)

An application to market a device determined to be a Humanitarian Use Device (HUD). An HUD is a medical device intended to benefit patients in treatment or diagnosis of a condition or disease that affects fewer than 4,000 persons in the US per year.

13.4.5 Premarket Approval (PMA) Application

21 CFR 814: An application for a Class III medical device. The standard for approval of a PMA is higher than for clearance of a 510(k): *reasonable assurance of safety and effectiveness.* For most PMA products, this must be demonstrated with data from a multi center human clinical trial and substantial supporting safety and device characterization data, as well as manufacturing information. Most PMA applications are reviewed by the FDA's Orthopedic and Restorative Devices advisory panel in an open public hearing. Combinations of bone graft substitutes with biologics or drugs that are designated to have a device PMOA will likely require PMA approval for marketing.

13.4.6 Request For Designation (RFD)

21 CFR 3: An application submitted to the FDA's Office of Combination Products (OCP) for designation of the FDA Center that will have primary premarket review responsibility for a new Combination Product (based on the determined PMOA) or for any product requiring a jurisdictional designation.

13.4.7 Pre-Submission (Pre-Sub)

An application requesting the FDA's feedback prior to the submission of an IDE, 510(k), HDE, or PMA application. This is the primary mechanism for obtaining Pre-IDE feedback (as this program replaces the previous Pre-IDE program); however, there are other mechanisms for obtaining feedback to questions pertaining to other regulatory submissions. It also is being used as the mechanism to receive feedback and direction for products that may qualify for De Novo. As of this writing, the guidance document made available for comments purposes in July, 2012, has not yet been finalized, but from experience, it is being used by the FDA.

13.5 Guidances and FDA-Referenced Standards

Following are the FDA Class II Special Controls Guidance Documents, which contain advice to guide the development of Dental and Orthopedics bone graft substitute 510(k) applications. There is no published guidance document for the neurological (cranial bone graft) application, although it is being developed by the FDA review branch. Review of the FDA guidance documents, as well as posted summaries of recently cleared 510(k)s will provide good information on the appropriate standards, such as ISO, ASTM, etc., to reference for various testing parameters.

13.5.1 Dental

Class II Special Controls Guidance Document: Dental Bone Grafting Material Devices (April 28, 2005).

13.5.2 Orthopedics

Class II Special Controls Guidance Document: Resorbable Calcium Salt Bone Void Filler Device (June 2, 2003).

13.6 Regulatory Premarketing Discussion

13.6.1 Lead Regulatory Review Center

The focus in this chapter is on the CDRH and the medical device regulatory premarketing pathways, since the vast majority of bone graft products fall within the realm of the CDRH. Included are products that contain a biologic or drug component, as long as the PMOA is the osteoconductive function of a scaffold, e.g., bone conduction that is intended for regeneration or filling a bony void caused by trauma or disease or for other reconstructive purposes.

13.6.2 Prevailing Law and Regulations

The original Food and Drug law was passed by Congress in 1906. This was superseded by the Federal Food, Drug and Cosmetic Act (FD&C Act) enacted in 1938. It has been amended many times. For the medical device world, the first significant amendment was in 1976 when the Medical Device Amendments were enacted. The purpose was to assure the safety and effectiveness of medical devices. Since then many significant "device" amendments have been passed and enacted, including the authorization in 2002 to collect User Fees for premarketing submissions. As of this date, the last significant one is the Medical Device User Fee Amendment of 2012 (referred to as MDUFA III), which has resulted in implementation of a revised Premarket Notification [510(k)] review process with a goal to achieve a more "predictable" process as well as accomplishment of the complete 510(k) review within 90 calendar days.

13.7 Medical Device Pathways and Processes

When the Device Amendments were passed in 1976, 1700 categories of existing generic types of devices were identified and classified into one of three regulatory classes, based on known or perceived risk and the level of control necessary to assure the safety and effectiveness of the device for its intended use. They were each assigned into a regulatory classification (21 CFR xxx.xxxx) with a numbering system developed according to therapeutic/diagnostic field, such as Orthopedics, Dental, Neurological. Within those classifications, unique product codes (a three-letter designation) were assigned for each generic type of device (the pertinent codes for bone filler/ graft products are noted in Table 13.3).

There are two primary paths to the market for medical devices: the 510(k) Premarket Notification [510(k)] and the Premarket Approval (PMA) Application pathways. In addition, the other two pathways are the De Novo and the Humanitarian Device Exemption (HDE) pathways, which were briefly described previously when discussing regulatory definitions in Section 13.2.

At the present time, De Novo is not an option for bone graft substitutes; however the HDE process is, for products intended to treat a condition with a prevalence of 4000 or less in the US population per year. The PMA, as noted, is likely to be the regulatory premarketing pathway for combinations of bone graft materials plus added biologicals or drugs.

The 510(k) has been the pathway to the market for hundreds of existing bone graft substitute products (Table 13.4). As noted, a 510(k) is an application/notification which must demonstrate substantial equivalence (SE) to a predicate device. The SE standard means the "new" product can be shown to be "as safe and effective" as the identified predicate device. In some product areas, this may be done with a side-by-side demonstration of SE parameters that are non-test-based.

TABLE 13.3

Bone Void Filler Regulatory Classification Information

Therapeutic area/ class/submission type	Regulation and name (21 CFR §...)	Regulatory description and reference to Special Controls Guidance document	Product code and associated name (if unique or specifically defined)
Dental Class II—510(k)	§872.3930 Bone grafting material	*A material such as hydroxyapatite, tricalcium phosphate, polylactic and polyglycolic acids, or collagen,* that is intended to fill, augment, or reconstruct periodontal or bony defects of the oral and maxillofacial region. Class II Special Controls Guidance Document: Dental Bone Grafting Material Devices (2005)	LYC LPK NUN (human source) NPL (animal source) NPK (including PTFE) NPM (animal source)
Dental Class III—PMA	§872.3930	(same definition) Products in these product codes are considered "Combinations."	NQA (biologic material including growth factors) NPZ (same)
Orthopedic (Extremities, Posterolaeral Spine & Pelvis) Class II— 510(k)	§888.3045	*A resorbable calcium salt bone void filler* device is a resorbable implant intended to fill bony voids or gaps of the extremities, spine, and pelvis that are caused by trauma or surgery and are not intrinsic to the stability of the bony structure. Class II Special Controls Guidance Document: Resorbable Calcium Salt Bone Void Filler Device (20__)	MQV MBP (w/o human growth factor) OIS (drillable, non-screw augmentation)
Orthopedic Class III—PMA	Unclassified	*Filler, recombinant human bone morphogenetic protein, collagen scaffold, osteoinduction*	MPW
Orthopedic Class III—PMA	Unclassified	*Filler, recombinant human bone morphogenetic protein, collagen scaffold with metal prosthesis, osteoinduction*	NEK

(Continued)

TABLE 13.3 *(Continued)*

Bone Void Filler Regulatory Classification Information

Therapeutic area/ class/submission type	Regulation and name (21 CFR §...)	Regulatory description and reference to Special Controls Guidance document	Product code and associated name (if unique or specifically defined)
Orthopedic Class III—PMA	§888.3015	*Bone heterograft is a device intended to be implanted that is made from mature (adult) bovine bones and used to replace human bone following surgery in the cervical region of the spinal column.*	NVC
Orthopedic (Spine)— HDE	Unclassified	*Filler, recombinant human bone morphogenetic protein, collagen scaffold, osteoinduction, revision spine surgery. Replacement for autograft bone in patients where autograft is unavailable or not feasible to harvest. Not feasible to harvest is intended to mean presence of a condition where normal bone metabolism would be expected to prevent healing, e.g., smokers and diabetics. Revision spine surgery to treat pseudarthrosis.*	OJZ
Orthopedic (Long bone)— HDE	Unclassified	*Filler, recombinant human bone morphogenetic protein, collagen scaffold, osteoinduction, long bone nonunion. Bone graft substitute when autograft is unavailable or unfeasible to harvest for treatment of recalcitrant long bone non unions where normal bone metabolism and healing is not present, e.g., smokers and diabetics.*	OKD

(Continued)

TABLE 13.3 (*Continued*)

Bone Void Filler Regulatory Classification Information

Therapeutic area/ class/submission type	Regulation and name (21 CFR §...)	Regulatory description and reference to Special Controls Guidance document	Product code and associated name (if unique or specifically defined)
Orthopedic (hindfoot & ankle fusion) (For export only)	Unclassified	*Filler, bone void,* **recombinant platelet-derived growth factor.** *For use as an alternative to autograft in hindfoot and ankle fusion procedures that require supplemental graft material, including tibiotalar, tibiocalcaneal, talonavicular and calcaneocuboid fusions.*	OYR
Neurology Class II—PMA	§882.5300	*Poly methyl methacrylate for cranioplasty (skull repair) is a self-curing acrylic that a surgeon uses to repair a skull defect in a patient. At the time of surgery, the surgeon initiates polymerization of the material and forms it into a plate or other appropriate shape to repair the defect.*	GXP

*Note: Not included is the bone cement (PMMA) category.

TABLE 13.4

Number of Cleared/Approved Regulatory Submissions by Product Code (as of January 2014)

Ortho (extremities, pelvis and/or Spine)	Dental (oral and maxillo-facial)	Neuro (cranial)
MQV = 320 510(k)s	LYC = 220 510(k)s	GXP = 41 510(k)s
MBP = 63 510(k)s	LPK = 2 510(k)s	
MPW = 1 PMA	NUN = 18 510(k)s	
NEK = 1 PMA		
NVC = 0 PMA	NPL = 27 510(k)s	
OIS = 1 510(k)	NPK = 23 510(k)s	
OJZ = 1 HDE	NPM = 16 510(k)s	
OKD = 1 HDE	NQA = 1 PMA	
OYR = 1 (for export only)	NPZ = 3 PMAs	

However, for most bone graft products, the FDA requires "characterization" testing that describes the device's chemical composition and physical properties, demonstrates safety of the manufactured product (including biocompatibility), and provides performance testing by laboratory (bench) evaluations as well as in vivo testing in an acceptable animal model. These test requirements are outlined by the FDA in the referenced guidance documents.

13.8 Classification of Bone Graft Substitutes

Most bone graft substitute/bone void filler devices are Class II and require clearance of a 510(k) prior to marketing. Bone graft substitutes for dental and orthopedics (extremities, spine and pelvis) indications also are subject to Special Controls guidance documents (described in Sections 13.10.1 and 13.10.2).

Bone grafting products that include an active drug, a growth factor, or biological or human cellular/tissue (non-DBM) component will likely be considered combination products and regulated as Class III devices, requiring PMA approval prior to marketing. Regulation as a medical device will prevail assuming they retain the osteoconductive "device" PMOA.

Table 13.3 lists the bone void filler/graft product (intended use) area, regulations, and relevant product codes for reference. Following this in Table 13.4 is a listing of those product codes and the number of regulatory applications that have been cleared or approved by the FDA since the first 510(k) clearances of the Wright Medical Technology Plaster of Paris pellets and bone void filler products in 1996 and 1997 respectively; the predicate technology was a pre-amendments product, Ethicon's Plaster of Paris Pellets. At that time, the FDA placed "calcium sulfate dehydrate" in the classification regulation, 21 CFR 888.3045, and established the MQV product code for "Filler, Bone Void, Calcium Compound." This was the beginning of the current regulatory pathway for bone graft substitutes.

These referenced product codes may be used in the FDA premarketing submission database search engines for 510(k) summaries for potential predicate devices, as well as to obtain the *Summary of Safety and Effectiveness* documents for PMA products and *Summary of Safety and Probable Benefit* documents for HDE products.

13.9 Clinical Studies

Bone graft substitute products are considered *significant risk* (SR) medical devices, primarily because they are implanted materials. As such, clinical studies for SR devices must be conducted under an IDE application approved by FDA, as well as by an Institutional Review Board (IRB)/Ethics Committee. Bone graft substitutes that require a PMA or HDE noted in Table 13.4 will require clinical trial data to support the premarketing application. Those include products that have an osteoconductive or osteoinductive scaffold that acts as the carrier for recombinant human bone morphogenetic proteins, or other proteins, growth factors, or drugs.

13.10 Advisories According to Therapeutic Areas

This subsection includes specific advice related to product development and 510(k) content requirements. Reference to above tables will lead to the device categories regulated by the Divisions and Branches noted in Section 13.9.

These advisories are based on recent FDA feedback during the review and processing of several 510(k)s. Since specific reviewers were not consulted for their consent, no names are provided. Rather, the comments here are presented by review Division and intended use of the bone graft substitutes. Further, no 510(k) sponsors were consulted for their permission; therefore, neither device composition nor any other identifiable specifics are detailed.

13.10.1 Division of Orthopedic Devices

13.10.1.1 Intended Uses/Indications for Use

This Division contains the Restorative and Repair Devices Branch, which regulates bone void filler applications for the extremities, pelvis, and posterolateral spine indications. The FDA requires animal performance data specific to the extremities and the posterolateral fusion (PLF), e.g., two performance studies need to be submitted in order to obtain the Indications for Use (IFU), which have been "refined" and limited by the FDA in the last several years. The current general IFU statement, which includes both indications, is as follows: *Device X is a bone void filler device intended for use in bony voids or gaps that are not intrinsic to the stability of the bony structure. These defects may be surgically created osseous defects or osseous defects created from traumatic injury to the bone. Device X is indicated to be packed gently into bony voids or gaps of the skeletal system (e.g., extremities, pelvis and posterolateral spine fusion procedures). The device provides a bone void filler that is resorbed and replaced with host bone during the healing process.*

Note that the statement may vary in a reference application as it relates to the physical form of the product, e.g. granular, moldable, or injectable. However, when the device has been tested as an extender with autograft, the following may be added to the IFU statement: *Device X also can be used with autograft as a bone graft extender in the posterolateral spine (and/or in the extremities – as tested).*

Additional claims that may be obtained, with supporting animal study data, are femoral osteotomy and tibial osteotomy. If autogenous bone marrow aspirate (BMA) is requested as an ingredient that may be mixed with the bone graft substitute as an autograft extender, an animal study which demonstrates safety and performance for each of the indications requested must be provided in the 510(k).

13.10.1.2 General Comments Related to Test Data Required for 510(k)s: Orthopedics Indications

The first step is to reference and follow the Calcium Salts guidance document. The second step is to review the most recent 510(k) summaries from the FDA's database of cleared 510(k)s for products of similar composition for discussions of the testing performed. Nothing new may be learned; however, it is important to check for tidbits of information not previously considered.

13.10.1.3 Specific Comments Based on Recent Experience

The reason this section is important is that the bar for 510(k) clearance for all bone graft substitute products has been raised substantially by the FDA during recent years. Many of the 510(k)s submitted more than 3 years ago would be subject to considerably greater scrutiny during their reviews if submitted today and might not receive clearance without additional testing. This additional scrutiny includes:

- *Labeling*: The FDA now requires that the product components (material composition) be specified on the package labels.
- *Sterilization and Shelf-Life Testing*: A few years ago the FDA accepted a promise of sterilization validation prior to clearance of the 510(k). This is no longer acceptable; sterilization validation must be completed and information presented in the 510(k). Likewise, a commitment regarding shelf-life testing was acceptable for the 510(k). Now the FDA expects a first reasonable time point to have been reached for the shelf life and data discussed in the submission. Real-time testing is required, but it may be extended with accelerated testing if appropriate for the material composition.
- *Biocompatibility and Other Safety Testing/Information*: Testing according to ISO 10993 must be completed on the final, sterile, packaged device and presented in the 510(k). If the product contains human donor bone, including demineralized bone matrix (DBM), validation of the viral inactivation potency of the manufacturing and sterilization processes needs to be included in the 510(k). Alternatively, if the product contains animal-sourced material, additional documentation will be required in the 510(k)

regarding the source and testing to assure the transmissible disease potential is thoroughly controlled. Reference is made to the FDA's January 23, 2014 Draft Guidance (issued for comment purposes only) "Medical Devices Containing Materials Derived from Animal Sources (Except for In Vitro Diagnostic Devices)." When final, this document will replace the November, 1998 guidance by the same name.

- *Device Characterization*: The FDA's suggestions in the Calcium Salts guidance document should be closely followed as a guide for the testing to be performed to fully characterize the device. Note that the porosity data must be submitted on the final finished device, not just on the separate materials/components in the device.

- *Performance Testing (In Vivo)—General Comments*: This topic is subject to very intense scrutiny and review by the FDA. Staff biologists who are experts in animal study design and conduct participate in reviews across Divisions. Endpoints should include osteoconduction, graft resorption, and osteoinduction. In general the FDA requires specific and detailed documentation that demonstrates over time the resorption of the graft material (including a baseline especially for resorption), osteoconduction, e.g., regeneration of bone or fusion (as relevant), as well as osteoinduction (if appropriate for the graft composition and the "osteoinductive potential" claim). There should be at least three time points from which data and measurements will be generated. Those data must be include the following:

  - Labeled radiographs must be provided. The FDA acknowledges that radiographs alone are not definitive; however, they are used by the FDA along with other data to make a final determination of new bone formation and graft resorption. Analysis of radiographs must be performed using an acceptable radiograph scale. The amount of defect healing may be scored with a 3- or 4-point scale ranging from "none" to "extensive." The grading should be performed by independent reviewers.

  - MicroCTs for all time points, analyzed and presented with accompanying descriptions, are recommended. Validation of the accuracy of the microCT results is required.

  - Histology images in color and labeled, accompanied by histopathologic descriptions of the defect area, test and control articles, new bone formation, surrounding bone, bone marrow, fibrous tissue, and all cell types present should be presented for all animals at all time points. Histomorphometry must be performed to determine/measure the amount of implant, new bone, and soft tissue during the course of the study.

- Osteoinductive parameters: If the product contains a component that is considered osteoinductive, additional testing, such as the athymic rat muscle pouch model, must be provided to prove it has osteoinductive potential. However, "labeling" conclusions regarding the osteoinductive potential are limited to a statement similar to "Osteoinduction assay results observed in surrogate assessments should not be interpreted to predict clinical performance in human subjects."

- Bioactivity parameter: Similarly, if the product composition includes a bioactive glass material and a claim related to the bioactivity is requested, in vitro bioactivity testing is necessary. The study may be described in the 510(k) summary, similar to the osteoinductive potential study, and a similar disclaimer needs to be made which says "the results have not been correlated to clinical performance."

13.10.1.4 Specific Comments on Posterolateral Spine Study

The acceptable and preferred model is the Boden posterolateral fusion (PLF) using adult rabbits. If the test plan includes any variation to the validated Boden model, it is imperative that the FDA be consulted prior to conducting the study. A vertebral defect model is not acceptable to support the PLF indication. Controls used for the study should include autograph and a predicate device and evaluation time points should include at a minimum 4, 8, and 12 weeks. Healing, graft migration, osteolysis, fracture, and any other adverse events should be assessed using radiographs. Healing in this study refers to fusion, which is bilateral bridging bone between transverse processes (TPs). Fusion mass needs to be graded using a scale, which the FDA recommends to include (1) bilateral bridging bone between TP, (2) unilateral bridging bone, (3) no bone on either side, or (4) indeterminate; this scoring needs to be performed by "blinded" radiographic reviewers. The FDA has noted that plain x-rays are sufficient, but suggestions have been made to consider microCT, which provides additional detail and information.

Mechanical evaluation for the study should include (1) manual palpation (a subjective, nondestructive evaluation of stiffness of the fused motion segments) to assess fusion, and (2) biomechanical assessment to assess the fusion stiffness using flexion/extension, lateral bending and torsion testing. Providing a table which presents a final (average) fusion rate as determined from the rates obtained from radiographic, manual palpation, and biomechanical evaluations is helpful to the FDA. In addition to mechanical assessments, the FDA also requires complete histological evaluations of all the sections obtained rather than a sampling of the sections so as to provide a more comprehensive evaluation of bone formation, implant resorption, and the nature of the tissue response at the fusion masses. Histomorphometry is also strongly recommended by the FDA, which provides quantitative information such as the amount of new bone formation, implant resorption, and possible areas of fibrotic tissue and bone marrow for all treatment groups at all time points of the study.

13.10.1.5 Specific Comments on Extremities Study

An acceptable model is the femoral critical-size defect in adult rabbits. If another model that has not been validated as critically sized is chosen, an empty defect arm needs to be added to the controls. Controls used should include a predicate device (indicated for use in the extremities) and/or autograft bone. The use of bone wax should also be included in the study design because it is not cleared for use with bone graft substitutes, and the FDA has concerns about its effect on bone growth. Time points for evaluation should include at least 4, 8, and 12 weeks and last for sufficient duration so that the resorption of the device can be adequately assessed. Additionally the FDA has recommended the used of four to five animals per time point per treatment group. At each time point, radiographs should be used to assess healing, graft migration, osteolysis, fracture, and any other adverse events. The complete graft site needs to be x-rayed and healing needs to be graded by "blinded" radiographic reviewers using a scale similar to "none," "some," "moderate," and "extensive" or "complete." The histomorphometric analysis should be representative of an average of multiple slices obtained at different levels throughout the sample, including an assessment for the presence of inflammatory cells.

13.10.2 Division of Anesthesiology, General Hospital, Respiratory, Infection Control and Dental Devices

This "catchall" division contains the Dental Devices Branch, which regulates bone void filler applications for the intraoral and maxillo-facial indications. The generally acceptable IFU, at the time of writing this chapter, is: *Device X is a bone filling material indicated for dental intraosseous, oral and maxillofacial defects, including periodontal/infrabony defects; alveolar ridge augmentation; dental extraction sites; sinus lifts; cystic defects.*

13.10.2.1 General Comments for 510(k)s for the Dental Indications

As suggested for the other bone grafting applications, the first step is to reference and follow the guidance document, in this case the Dental Bone Grafting guidance. The second step is to review the most recent 510(k) summaries from the FDA's database of cleared 510(k)s for products of similar composition for discussions of the testing performed.

13.10.2.2 Specific Comments Based on Recent Experience

Similar to the comments in Section 13.10.2, this section is important because of the FDA's increased scrutiny of the performance and characterization testing provided to support new product clearances in the Dental Devices Branch. Products with components derived from human cadaveric tissue must include evidence of testing according to all the serological tests listed in 21 CFR 1271.85, despite a reduction of the testing requirements according to the American Association of Tissue Banks (AATB). If a product offering includes different forms of the same basic product composition, the FDA will require characterization and performance testing specific to each form.

As described earlier in this chapter, when a model chosen is not exactly the model the FDA recommends, the submitter needs to be prepared to justify fully, with reference to literature and data, that the model chosen is appropriate and that the controls were appropriate and the results fully document the endpoints required by the FDA. A very recent submission included an issue related to the "critical size" definition and resulted in multiple challenges from the FDA, but in the end the applicant was able to satisfy the FDA's questions. Additionally, histology and histomorphometry need to be performed as noted earlier regarding how fully assessing bone regeneration and device resorption, including immediate and adjacent tissue response, pertains to the dental products review.

13.10.3 Division of Neurological and Physical Medicine Devices

This Division contains the Neurodiagnostic and Neurosurgical Devices Branch, which regulates bone void filler applications for the cranial repair indications. The general acceptable IFU statement is: *Device X is indicated for repairing or filling cranial defects and craniotomy cuts with a surface area no larger than 25 cm² Device X also is indicated for the restoration and augmentation of bony contours of the cranial skeleton (including fronto-orbital areas), such as burr holes and other cranial defects.* It is important to note that the material composition of bone graft substitutes cleared in the GXP product code is not limited to methyl methacrylate (bone cement) despite the regulatory definition. DBM and synthetic resorbable materials fall within this product code as well as PMMA.

13.10.3.1 General Comments Related to Test Data Required for 510(k)s for the Cranial Indication

Unfortunately, unlike the orthopedics/spine and dental indications, the FDA has not made available a guidance document for this product area. Therefore, the steps to follow are not as defined in preparing for a 510(k) as they are for the previously discussed applications. As starting steps, it is advisable to review the recommendations in both the above-referenced guidance documents as well as review the posted summaries of recently cleared 510(k)s in the GXP product code. It also may be useful to contact the CDRH review branch for informal advice or submit a Pre-Submission as described above in Section 13.4. The animal model generally recommended by the FDA to evaluate performance is the rabbit or canine critical-size calvarial defect using skeletally mature animals.

13.10.3.2 Specific Comments Based on Informal Guidance from FDA and Recent Submission-Specific Experience

Similar to the comments in Sections 13.10.1 and 13.10.2, this section is important because of the FDA's increased scrutiny of the performance and characterization testing provided to support new product clearances in the neurological devices review branch—in particular, if the composition contains "non-standard" materials, the FDA is overly cautious because of possible contact with brain and neural tissues. The controls for the study design should include empty defect and predicate device controls. Because the FDA is concerned about animal welfare, it has been stated that the sample size or the number of animals used per treatment group does not need to be based on a statistical size determination. Additionally, the number of animals for empty, the defect group, may be reduced. It is also important to review ISO 10993-11 for guidance on group size determination as well as testing site. Under ISO 10993, the FDA has required that biocompatibility testing be performed at the intended implant site, rather than the standard test sites. The length of the study is to be based on the known chemistry of the device in combination with prior performance data, in particular resorption of the device. However, if no prior data exist, FDA suggests that a study endpoint of 1 year will be acceptable if at least 85% of the device is resorbed, and there are no clinical signs of toxicity or histopathological signs of active inflammation at the implant site and adjacent tissues.

The FDA has also suggested that the same animals may be used for both the biocompatibility/toxicological and performance evaluations if it is possible to bisect the calvarial implant sites for the separate evaluations. For implants other than bone graft substitute uses, the recommended limit is 0.5 EU/mL. However, for the devices used in the cranial application, the FDA has advised the bacterial endotoxin level must be shown to be below the recommended limit for intrathecal devices of 0.06 EU/mL or 2.5 EU/device. If the product contains nano-sized particles (<100nm), the FDA is concerned about possible release into the brain; therefore testing must be provided to demonstrate the particles are not released from the implanted materials in a clinically relevant, worst-case scenario. When that cannot be demonstrated, additional biocompatibility testing, such as biodistribution, may need to be provided.

At each time point, it is also important to evaluate the explant macroscopically during necropsy before removal from the animal to assure there are no significant differences between the two halves. In the evaluation, the investigator should also include toxicity parameters such as general health, signs of neurobehavioral dysfunction, clinical chemistry, blood chemistry, and histopathology of tissue response at implant site and adjacent tissues. Evaluation on toxicity parameters needs to be performed on all animals at 52 weeks. The study performance characteristics should also include the standard osteointegration and resorption of the device over the course of healing, as well as demonstration of bone regeneration and biomechanical testing of the newly formed bone.

13.11 Concluding Advice

For manufacturers who are developing new bone graft substitute products and/or planning regulatory submissions to the FDA, the FDA CDRH website should always be consulted for (1) newly released guidance documents pertinent to the product type, product use, and submission-specific needs such as preclinical, clinical, or premarketing; and (2) general advisories at the following website: http://www.fda.gov/MedicalDevices /DeviceRegulationandGuidance/default.htm.

Index